D1409458

GRETCHEN DAHL REEVES, Ph.D.
MEDICAL COLLEGE OF OHIO
SAH-DEPT. OF O. T.
TOLEDO, OHIO 43614-5608
(419) 383-5498 FAX: (419) 383-5880

Mosby's Resource Guide

to
Children
with
Disabilities
and
Chronic Illness

WALLACE ■ BIEHL ■ MACQUEEN ■ BLACKMAN

with foreword by
C. Everett Koop

Mosby's Resource Guide

to
Children
with
Disabilities
and
Chronic Illness

Helen M. Wallace, MD, MPH,
Professor of Maternal and Child Health,
Graduate School of Public Health,
San Diego State University,
San Diego, California

John C. MacQueen, MD,
Professor of Pediatrics Emeritus,
College of Medicine;
Director,
National Maternal and Child
Health Resource Center,
College of Law,
University of Iowa,
Iowa City, Iowa

Robert F. Biehl, MD, MPH,
Director,
Division of Specialized Care for Children;
Clinical Professor of Pediatrics,
University of Chicago,
Chicago, Illinois

James A. Blackman, MD, MPH,
Professor of Pediatrics,
Director of Research,
Kluge Children's Rehabilitation Center,
University of Virginia,
Charlottesville, Virginia

with foreword by C. Everett Koop

with 42 illustrations

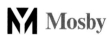 Mosby

St. Louis   Baltimore   Boston   Carlsbad   Chicago   Naples   New York   Philadelphia   Portland
London   Madrid   Mexico City   Singapore   Sydney   Tokyo   Toronto   Wiesbaden

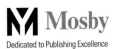
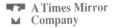

Publisher: Don Ladig
Executive Editor: Martha Sasser
Developmental Editor: Kellie F. White
Project Manager: Mark Spann
Production Editor: Holly Roseman
Designer: Judi Lang
Manufacturing Manager: Tony McAllister

Printed in the United States of America
Composition by Mosby Electronic Production
Printing/binding by R.R. Donnelley & Sons Company

Mosby–Year Book, Inc.
11830 Westline Industrial Drive
St. Louis, Missouri 63146

Library of Congress Cataloging-in-Publication Data

Mosby's resource guide to children with disabilities and chronic illness /
    [edited by] Helen M. Wallace ... [et al.].
        p.   cm.
        Includes bibliographical references and index.
        ISBN 0-8151-9051-4
        1. Chronically ill children—Services for. 2. Exceptional children—
    Services for. 3. Exceptional children—Rehabilitation. 4. Chronically ill
    children—Rehabilitation.   I. Wallace, Helen M.
        [DNLM: 1. Disabled—rehabilitation. 2. Child, Exceptional. 3. Chron-
    ic Disease—in infancy & childhood. 4. Chronic Disease—rehabilitation.
    5. Community Health Services—United States. WS 368 M894 1996]
    RJ380.M66   1996
    362/1'9892—dc20
    DNLM/DLC
    for Library of Congress   96-10609
                                                                        CIP

97 98 99 00 01 / 9 8 7 6 5 4 3 2 1

Contributor List

Myron J. Adams, Jr., MD,
Associate Director for Program
  Development,
Division for Birth Defects and Develop-
  mental Disabilities,
National Center for Environmental
  Health,
Centers for Disease Control and
  Prevention,
Atlanta, Georgia

Gary L. Albrecht, PhD,
Professor, Health Policy and
  Administration,
School of Public Health,
University of Illinois,
Chicago, Illinois

Marion Taylor Baer, PhD, RD
Associate Professor of Clinical Pediatrics,
Department of Pediatrics;
Associate Director,
University Affiliated Program,
Children's Hospital,
University of Southern California
  Medical School,
Los Angeles, California

L. Kay Bartholomew, EdD, MPH,
University of Texas Houston Health
  Science Center,
School of Public Health,
Center for Health Promotion Research
  and Development,
Houston, Texas

Forrest C. Bennett, MD,
Professor of Pediatrics,
Center on Human Development
  and Disability
University of Washington School
  of Medicine,
Seattle, Washington

Arnold Birenbaum, PhD,
Associate Director,
Rose F. Kennedy Center,
University Affiliated Program;
Professor of Pediatrics,
Albert Einstein College of Medicine,
New York, New York

Suzanne M. Bronheim, PhD,
Associate Professor of Pediatrics,
Georgetown University Child
  Development Center,
Georgetown University Medical Center,
Washington, D.C.

John C. Carey, MD
Professor of Pediatrics;
Chief,
Division of Medical Genetics,
University of Utah,
School of Medicine,
Salt Lake City, Utah

Elizabeth A. Cassidy, MA,
Jefferson County School System,
Denver, Colorado

Jennifer M. Cernoch, PhD,
Director,
Texas Respite Resource Network,
Texas Planning Council for
  Developmental Disabilities,
Santa Rosa Children's Hospital,
San Antonio, Texas

Herbert J. Cohen, MD,
Director,
Children's Evaluation and Rehabilitation
    Center,
Rose F. Kennedy Center,
University Affiliated Program;
Professor of Pediatrics and
    Rehabilitation Medicine,
Albert Einstein College of Medicine,
New York, New York

Brenda G. Considine,
Education Policy Advisor and Consultant
    on Disability Issues,
Former Director of Government
    Relations,
The Arc of New Jersey,
North Brunswick, New Jersey

William C. Cooley, MD
Director,
Dartmouth Center for Genetics and
    Child Development,
Dartmouth Medical School,
Lebanon, New Hampshire

Lisa T. Craft, MD,
Assistant Professor of Pediatrics,
Vanderbilt Child Development Center,
Nashville, Tennessee

Allen C. Crocker, MD,
Program Director,
Institute for Community Inclusion,
Children's Hospital;
Associate Professor of Maternal and
    Child Health,
Harvard School of Public Health;
Associate Professor of Pediatrics,
Harvard Medical School,
Boston, Massachusetts

Danita I. Czyzewski, PhD,
Assistant Professor of Psychiatry and
    Behavioral Sciences and Pediatrics,
Baylor College of Medicine,
Texas Children's Hospital,
Houston, Texas

Susan G. Epstein, MSW,
Co-Director,
New England SERVE,
Boston, Massachusetts

John E. Evans, MS,
Executive Director,
Centers for Minority Health Initiatives
    and Cultural Competency,
Texas Department of Health,
Austin, Texas

Anita M. Farel, DPH,
Clinical Associate Professor,
Department of Maternal and
    Child Health,
School of Public Health,
University of North Carolina,
Chapel Hill, North Carolina

Douglas Fisher, MPH, PhD,
Consortium on Inclusive
    Schooling Practices,
Interwork Institute,
San Diego State University,
San Diego, California

Josephine Gittler, JD,
Professor of Law,
College of Law;
Co-Director,
National Maternal and Child Health
    Resource Center;
Director,
Institute on Conflict Management, Health
    Care and Disability
University of Iowa,
Iowa City, Iowa

Glenn E. Hedman, MEng,
Coordinator,
Assistive Technology Unit,
Institute of Disability and Human
    Development,
College of Associated Health Professions,
University of Illinois,
Chicago, Illinois

Lola J. Hobbs, MA, MSW,
Title 4-E Faculty,
School of Social Work,
San Diego State University,
San Diego, California

Joseph Hollowell, Jr., MD, MPH,
Disabilities Prevention Program,
National Center for Environmental
    Health,
Centers for Disease Control
    and Prevention,
Atlanta, Georgia

John E. Hutchins,
Senior Program Associate,
Family Impact Seminar,
Washington, D.C.

Vince L. Hutchins, MD, MPH,
Distinguished Research Professor,
National Center for Education in
    Maternal and Child Health,
Graduate Public Policy Program,
Georgetown University,
Arlington, Virginia

Henry T. Ireys, PhD,
Assistant Professor,
Department of Maternal and
    Child Health,
School of Hygiene and Public Health,
Johns Hopkins University,
Baltimore, Maryland

Beverley H. Johnson,
President and Chief Executive Officer,
Institute for Family-Centered Care,
Bethesda, Maryland

Scott Katz, RN, MPH,
School of Hygiene and Public Health,
Johns Hopkins University,
Baltimore, Maryland

Joanna Kaufman, RN, MS,
Vice President for Care Management,
Health Services for Children with Special
    Needs, Inc.,
Washington, D.C.

Tina Ciesiel Kitchin, MD, FAAP,
Medical Director,
Office of Developmental Disability
    Services,
State of Oregon,
Salem, Oregon

Marilyn J. Krajicek, EdD, RN, FAAN,
Associate Professor,
School of Nursing,
University of Colorado Health Sciences
    Center,
Denver, Colorado

Richard D. Krugman, MD,
Director,
Henry Kempe National Center for the
    Prevention and Treatment of Child
    Abuse and Neglect;
Professor and Dean of Pediatrics,
University of Colorado School
    of Medicine,
Denver, Colorado

Arthur F. Kohrman, MD,
President,
LaRabida Children's Hospital and
    Research Center,
Chicago, Illinois

Lynette A. Lancial, RDH, MS, MA,
Program Associate,
College of Medicine,
University of Iowa,
Iowa City, Iowa

Pamela Luft, MEd, MS,
Kent State University,
Educational Foundations and
    Special Services,
Kent, Ohio

Eleanor W. Lynch, PhD,
Professor of Special Education,
College of Education,
San Diego State University,
San Diego, California

Carolyn Maddy-Bernstein, MS, EdD,
Director of the Office of Student Services,
National Center for Research in
    Vocational Education,
University of California, Berkeley,
University of Illinois Site,
Champaign, Illinois

Colleen Monahan, DC, MPH,
Assistant Director for Research and
    Development,
Division of Specialized Care for Children,
University of Illinois at Chicago,
Chicago, Illinois

Thomas R. Montgomery, MD,
Director,
Developmental Disabilities,
Eastern Virginia Medical School,
Children's Hospital of the
    King's Daughters,
Norfolk, Virginia

John T. Neisworth, PhD,
Professor of Special Education and
    Early Intervention,
Department of Educational and School
    Psychology and Special Education,
Pennsylvania State University,
University Park, Pennsylvania

Elizabeth E. Newhouse, MTS,
Assistant Director,
Texas Respite Resource Network,
Texas Planning Council for
    Developmental Disabilities,
Santa Rosa Children's Hospital,
San Antonio, Texas

Robert E. Nickel, MD,
Clinical Director,
Regional Service Center,
Child Development and Rehabilitation
    Center;
Associate Professor of Pediatrics,
Oregon Health Sciences University,
Eugene, Oregon

Guy S. Parcel, PhD,
Director,
Center for Health Promotion Research
    and Development;
Professor of Behavioral Sciences
    and Pediatrics,
University of Texas Health
    Science Center
University of Texas School of
    Public Health,
Houston, Texas

James M. Perrin, MD,
Director,
Ambulatory Care Programs and
    General Pediatrics,
Pediatric Services,
Massachusetts General Hospital,
Wang Ambulatory Care Center;
Associate Professor of Pediatrics,
Harvard Medical School,
Boston, Massachusetts

Margo I. Peter, MEd,
Former Co-Director
Medical Home Project,
Hawaii Medical Association,
Honolulu, Hawaii

Susan Reichert, MD,
Director,
EPIC Center for Child Maltreatment,
Children's Hospital Oakland,
Oakland, California

Beverly Schenkman Roberts,
Program Director,
Mainstreaming Medical Care Project,
The Arc of New Jersey,
North Brunswick, New Jersey

Richard N. Roberts, PhD,
Director,
Early Intervention Research Institute;
Director of Research and Evaluation,
Center for Persons with Disabilities;
Professor,
Psychology Department,
Utah State University,
Logan, Utah

Cordelia Robinson, PhD, RN
Director,
Colorado University Affiliated Program,
University of Colorado Health Sciences
    Center,
Denver, Colorado

Elizabeth S. Ruppert, MD,
Emeritus Professor of Pediatrics,
Medical College of Ohio,
Toledo, Ohio

Frank R. Rusch, PhD,
Director,
Transition Research Institute;
Professor of Special Education,
University of Illinois at
    Champaign-Urbana,
Champaign, Illinois

Lawrence W. Schneider, BSE, MSE, PhD,
Research Scientist and Head,
Transportation Research Institute,
Biosciences Division,
University of Michigan,
Ann Arbor, Michigan

Lisa A. Schneider, PhD,
Director of Children's Services,
ARC Allegheny,
Pittsburgh, Pennsylvania

Calvin C.J. Sia, MD,
Clinical Professor of Pediatrics,
University of Hawaii School of Medicine,
Honolulu, Hawaii

Jane Squires, PhD,
Assistant Professor of Special Education,
University of Oregon,
Eugene, Oregon

Ann B. Taylor, EdD,
Co-Director,
New England SERVE,
Boston, Massachusetts

Josie Thomas,
Director for Family Issues,
Institute for Family-Centered Care;
State Coordinator,
Family Voices,
Bethesda, Maryland

Mark L. Wolraich, MD,
Professor of Pediatrics,
Vanderbilt Child Development Center,
Nashville, Tennessee

Barbara J. Woodward, MPH, OT/R
Children's Hospital of New Mexico,
Albuquerque, New Mexico

Dedication

To special children and their families
To the care providers who support them

Foreword

C. EVERETT KOOP

For nearly 50 years I have had a deep commitment to children with special health care needs and their families. During my tenure as Surgeon General of the United States, one of my major goals was to improve the lives of children with special health care needs and their families. At a time when our nation's health care system is in crisis and reforms in the system are being proposed, adopted, and implemented, it is important not to lose our focus on these children and their families.

As physicians at one of the country's leading children's hospitals, my colleagues and I were privileged to be in the forefront of providing new and improved types of surgical and medical care for children with special health care needs. Despite the many advances in medical science and technology that have benefited these children, I came to recognize that significant changes must be made in the ways in which services for them were organized, financed, and provided.

As Surgeon General I launched several initiatives designed to bring about such changes. These initiatives were launched with the invaluable assistance of the Bureau of Maternal and Child Health and Resources Development under the leadership of its director, Vince Hutchins, MD, and the Bureau's Division of Services for Children With Special Health Care Needs under the leadership of its director, Merle McPherson, MD.

One of the most significant of these initiatives was the convening of the Surgeon General's workshop on *Children with Handicaps and Their Families* in 1982. This workshop was designed to promote an understanding of the needs of children with special health care needs and their families and to develop strategies to meet them. This was followed by a series of activities culminating in the issuance of the *Surgeon General's Report on Children with Special Health Care Needs* in 1987. In this report I issued a call to action to join in a campaign to take the action steps necessary to meet the needs of children with special health care needs and their families. Two Surgeon General's conferences were held in 1987 and 1988 that brought together health professionals and other providers of services, family members of children with special health care needs, elected officials, and other public policy makers for the purpose of enlisting them in this campaign.

As a result of these initiatives the provision of family-centered, community-based, coordinated care for children with special health care needs and their families was enunciated as a national goal. In recent years much has been done to achieve this goal but the task is far from finished.

This book explains and expands upon the concepts underlying the goal of family-centered, community-based, coordinated care, and it discusses how this goal can and should be made a reality in this era of sweeping changes that could undermine health care financing and delivery. It brings together as authors a wide variety of individuals from different professional backgrounds who have been leaders in improving services for children with special health care needs and their families, and I am confident it will make a significant contribution to the body of knowledge concerning these children and their families.

Preface

The needs of children and youth with disabilities and chronic illness, frequently referred to as children with special health care needs, have become increasingly complex, the number of children requiring services progressively larger, and the world of those serving the children and their families exceedingly complicated. Professionals seeking to serve children with special needs commonly learn their craft and practice among others of their own kind, and there is a growing risk of professional isolation as disciplines become more specialized and services more sophisticated. We wrote this book in recognition of this risk, and we hope to provide the reader with an overview of the many different needs of children with disabilities and their families, the broad array of services created to meet those needs, and the people who devote their professional lives to the task.

We, the editors, have a strong bias toward interdisciplinary service delivery. This book is intended to facilitate that process and encourage collaboration through greater mutual understanding. For that reason we address the book to our peers in all the disciplines important to children with special needs, to our students, and to the many advocates seeking to understand and make better this complex service system.

We recognized early in the formative process that a book attempting to address so large a subject would need to sacrifice detail for breadth of coverage. Authors were asked to address their topics so that someone new to the material would obtain a comprehensive overview of the subject. Those already familiar with a specific issue or field of study will find little that is controversial in these pages, though the readings and references offered with each chapter do provide an open door to a more indepth understanding.

We have organized this work into six parts.

Part One introduces the population in need and the growing and evolving effect of chronic illness and disability on children, their families, and the communities in which they live. This part then describes the development of public programs for these children and mechanisms for financing their health care.

Part Two addresses the future directions of services and programs for children with disabilities and chronic illness and their families.

In Part Three the reader learns about issues of particular importance to children with special needs and their families as they seek to live normal and productive lives in their own communities. Although most of the issues described are held in common with all members of society (i.e., privacy and confidentiality, cultural sensitivity, legal rights and responsibilities, access to needed services, etc.) they carry special significance for children and youth with chronic conditions.

The more important services needed by children with special needs and their families are addressed in Part Four. The intent of these chapters is to describe the services, their scope, and their objectives in a manner that will increase the understanding of readers not regularly engaged in their supervision or delivery. This effort is taken a step further by the discipline descriptions contained in Part Six. Here the reader will learn about the preparation and skills of the other members of the interdisciplinary team and gain a better understanding of what each can bring to the collaborative process.

Part Five describes common chronic conditions using a standardized format that permits easy comparison. The descriptions are not intended to be comprehensive. Rather they have been included for students and readers who may be less familiar with the conditions or the needs they create.

We invite our readers to begin their journey wherever they will. Every effort has been made to offer chapters and parts that can stand alone as well as contribute to greater understanding of other chapters and the book as a whole. A student may find value in starting at the beginning and taking each offering in turn. A new member of an interdisciplinary team might find it more useful to focus on the parts that describe other team members and the services that they provide. An advocate or policy maker might spend time most profitably in the sections that describe the populations in need, the efforts made by society to address their needs, and the issues that must be considered in future measures.

Wherever begun, we hope the journey will be judged to be valuable and instructive.

The Editors

Acknowledgments

The completion of this book would not have been possible without the valuable input and assistance from Josephine Gittler, JD and Susan Overstreet.

Contents

PART ONE

BACKGROUND AND CHALLENGES

The care of children with disabilities and chronic illnesses, often referred to as children with special health care needs, poses challenges not only for families and communities but also for society as a whole. Part I of this text contains five chapters aimed at providing the reader with the factual background necessary for an understanding of the nature and scope of these challenges.

Chapter 1 deals with the epidemiology and demography of childhood disability and illness. It furnishes answers to basic questions regarding the prevalence of disabilities and chronic illnesses among children, the distribution of such disabilities and chronic illnesses in terms of age, gender, race, and socioeconomic status, and finally the changing patterns in prevalence and distribution of such disabilities and chronic conditions.

The focus of Chapters 2 and 3 is children with disabilities and chronic illnesses in relation to their families and their communities. Chapter 2 explores the multiple and ongoing needs of these children and the role of families and communities in meeting these needs. Chapter 3 describes the specific effect of disability and chronic illness on children, families, and communities.

The focus of Chapters 4 and 5 is the health service needs of children with disabilities and chronic illnesses who, as a group, require specialized health services and use a disproportionately large share of child health services. Chapter 4 describes the critical role the public sector has played in expanding and improving health services for these children. Chapter 5 examines the financing of needed health services for these children, including the cost and the sources of payment for such services.

CHAPTER 1

The Demography of Disability and Chronic Illness Among Children

HENRY T. IREYS
SCOTT KATZ

GENERAL PREVALENCE ESTIMATES

Estimates of the prevalence of children with disabilities and chronic illnesses vary from 2% to 32% of the nation's children, depending on the definition of the terms *disability* and *chronic illness* and on the source of data. Larger estimates typically include children with conditions that place few or no limitations on the child's functioning. Smaller estimates include children with conditions that place comparatively severe limitations on the child's functioning.

For example, analyses of data from the National Health Interview Survey (NHIS) suggest that 31% of children in the United States 18 years of age or younger had one or more chronic health conditions in 1988, excluding chronic mental health problems and learning disabilities.[27] The chronic conditions most frequently reported were respiratory allergies and repeated ear infections. Nine percent of children had moderately severe conditions, defined as conditions that result in some bothersome consequence or some activity limitation; 2% of children had conditions that cause frequent bother and lead to numerous limitations in daily activities.[27]

Recent estimates indicate that 32% of teenagers in the U.S. have one or more chronic conditions.[24] The most frequently reported conditions among that age group include allergies, asthma, and frequent headaches, which generally lead to minimal or no functional impairment. Adolescents with more than one condition report substantially more school absences and days of

3

restricted activity. Using a more restrictive definition of the population, Newacheck[22] reported that 6% of individuals from 10 to 18 years of age had a chronic condition that resulted in some degree of disability or limitation in usual daily activities.

Analyses of data from a 1981 NHIS suggest that 9% of children in the United States have at least 1 of 19 selected serious, ongoing physical health conditions, such as arthritis, hearing problems, or sickle-cell anemia.[11] In a 1981 community-based sample of families in Ontario, Canada, 20% of children were found to have either or both an activity-limiting condition or a chronic illness.[6]

The range of estimates reflected in these and other studies underscores the lack of a broadly accepted definition of this population and the inherent difficulty in sampling rare populations.[38] Although analyses of the 1981 and 1988 NHIS data have yielded important prevalence estimates, the data have serious limitations. For example, the surveys included a limited list of specific chronic conditions, and therefore data are unavailable on children with chronic conditions that are not included on the list. Moreover, measuring the functional severity and the effect of a condition was quite limited, making it difficult to assess the actual consequences of a child's chronic conditions.

Recently, a more generic or noncategorical approach to defining this population has been advocated.[31,37] With this new approach the population is defined by the consequences a chronic condition has on a child's growth, development, and age-appropriate activity. The 1994 to 1995 NHIS has a special supplement that includes a childhood disability section. Partly because items in this section derive from a noncategorical definition of the population,[37] analysis of this survey data will yield comparatively accurate estimates of the prevalence of children with serious, ongoing physical health conditions, as well as comprehensive information on their health and functional status, service use, and social and family functioning. These analyses should provide important new national data for policy analysis and program planning. However, state-based or country-based information will be limited because of constraints in the NHIS sampling frame.

CONDITION-SPECIFIC PREVALENCE ESTIMATES

In adults there is a limited number of major chronic diseases and disabilities (e.g., stroke-related conditions, cardiovascular disorders, arthritis, cancer, hearing and vision limitations, orthopedic conditions), each of which occurs with high frequency. In children the pattern is reversed: There are more than 200 chronic conditions and disabilities that affect youth.[14] With the exception of asthma and other chronic respiratory or allergic conditions, most of these conditions are rare, and prevalence estimates based on national or community-based samples are often unavailable. However, prevalence estimates have been made for some of the more common chronic conditions based on populations served through major tertiary care centers, state surveys, and condition-specific registries.[4,10,13]

Prevalence rates have also been estimated for specific subgroups of disabled or chronically ill children defined by their reliance on particular medical technologies or services, such as ventilators or extensive home-based medical care. These children have varying diagnoses that lead to a common need for specific medical services. Estimates of these populations are important for policy purposes because these children frequently use costly medical services. In 1987, for example, a statewide census of technology-dependent children was completed in Massachusetts to determine the prevalence of this population. Approximately 1250 children were identified for a minimum prevalence rate of .08% of all children.[29,30] A review of research studies on children dependent on medical technology estimated that there was a maximum of 100,000 of these children in the U.S. in 1988.[28]

DEMOGRAPHIC DISTRIBUTION OF CONDITIONS

Age. The functional consequences of many chronic illnesses interact with age to produce complex patterns of disability and service use across developmental stages. For example, infants born with a very low birthweight may need intensive medical treatments throughout their first year of life. As acute medical issues resolve, many of these children will require developmental interventions during their preschool years. To use another example, children with diabetes may maintain good control of insulin levels throughout middle school but may experience more difficulty in early adolescence as hormonal changes occur in conjunction with normal adolescent acting out. These youth and their families will then need special support or counseling services to assist in negotiating new social challenges.[2]

Improved survival patterns of children with many formerly fatal diseases raise complex new issues for the transition to adulthood. Dramatic increases in the survival of children with cystic fibrosis, sickle-cell anemia, and other disorders have led to questions about how these youth find employment, form intimate relationships, and make the transition to adult medical service systems.[18]

Another issue associated with the transition to adulthood is that young adults with disabilities and chronic illnesses are at high risk for limited access to medical care and supportive services.[25] This problem usually results from age-based eligibility criteria for pediatric services, disruptions in insurance coverage, or both. Several anecdotal accounts[20,36] indicate a dearth of carefully planned transition services. However, few studies have systematically addressed the process whereby older adolescents with chronic illnesses and disabilities leave pediatric health services and move into adult-oriented service systems.[3] This transition is critical because disruptions in access to appropriate services may have particularly severe consequences for the continuity and quality of health care for this population of young persons and thereby lead to otherwise preventable secondary health and mental health conditions.[21]

Gender. Gender-linked disorders are common among disabled or chronically ill children. For example, hemophilia rarely occurs in females, but survival rates for females with cystic fibrosis are lower than they are for males.[40] Additional information on gender differences in prevalence rates for other chronic conditions may be found in a sourcebook of rates published for the southeastern states.[13]

Poverty. Poverty is associated with increased risk of disability and with increased hospitalization for problems related to chronic health conditions.[22,41] Diminished access to service as a result of inadequate insurance coverage is considered to be a key factor in the relationship between low socioeconomic status and disability.[12]

Race. The effects of race are difficult to separate from the effects of poverty. However, for certain conditions race is a primary determinant of occurrence. For example, sickle cell anemia occurs primarily in African-American children; cystic fibrosis occurs primarily in children of European descent. From a national perspective white children are more likely to have at least one chronic condition than African-American or Hispanic children.[26] However, the latter two groups, more than white children, experience more limitation in their usual activities and more days of restricted activity as a result of a chronic condition. Thus, absolute prevalence differences among races appear to result from higher prevalence of comparatively mild conditions (e.g., respiratory conditions, skin allergies) among white children. Minority children may experience more severe consequences of their conditions,[26,39] although these differences may result in part from heightened exposure to social and economic impoverishment and associated deficits in access to health services.

Although recent publications have added considerably to knowledge about the associations between prevalence and racial and income factors, much remains unknown about the relationships between the health status of children with special needs and their ethnic or cultural background, especially when economic status is taken into account.

TRENDS IN PREVALENCE AND DISTRIBUTION

Changes in the prevalence of children with a disability or chronic condition are determined by changes in the size of overall birth cohorts, incidence rates (the number of new cases in a given year per population unit), survival rates, and classification or diagnostic practices (e.g., adopting a noncategorical approach, more sensitive screening approaches, or new definitions of disease states). Since 1975 birth cohorts have been increasing but are expected to remain relatively stable for the next decade. There is little evidence that incidence rates will change substantially for most of the major chronic illnesses with the possible exception of HIV infection, which will increase.[9] Survival rates of children with chronic illnesses have increased substantially during the last 20 years,[7,10] but further increases will probably contribute marginally to increased prevalence. Better reporting, more sensitive screening procedures, and changes in survey techniques have been seen as contributing to increased prevalence estimates,[23] but future effects of these factors are difficult to estimate.

Although a major increase in the overall prevalence of chronic illnesses is unlikely in the next decade, several critical service-delivery trends are emerging. First, continued advances in biomedical research are likely to increase the number of children living with severe medical conditions requiring major emotional, family, and financial investment.[34] Second, more children with complex medical needs will be cared for in the home as a result of health policies emphasizing rapid hospital discharge and greater use of home care services.[30] This trend, in turn, will increase the need for more specialized health and educational services at the community level. Third, in some American communities children with disabilities and chronic illnesses have become increasingly involved in mainstream activities—largely as a result of continued advocacy efforts on the part of families. During the next decade at least, children with special health needs will play more active roles in community life as state governments implement policies to promote more comprehensive, community-based, family-centered service systems.[17] In turn, families will play increasingly collaborative roles in policy development, program implementation, and the training of health care professionals.[19]

Interest in the prevention of secondary health and mental health conditions is likely to increase, especially as managed care programs provide coverage to increasing numbers of children with disabilities and chronic illnesses. Many of these children are at high risk for secondary health problems, such as decubitus ulcers, obesity, contractures, respiratory insufficiency, and depression, and family members of these children are at risk for a wide range of mental health problems.[83] Despite this increased risk, however, preventive interventions have been largely neglected.[15]

Trends in the demography of this population of disabled and ill children also underscore the need for informed and innovative community responses to them and their families. Improved systems of services, prevention of secondary health problems, and continued integration of these children into mainstream society and adequate financing of high-quality care will require sustained collaboration among concerned families, professionals, and communities. Public health personnel and community-based health professionals have important roles to play in shaping how communities and new managed care organizations respond to this population of children and families.[16]

POPULATION SUBGROUPS FACING
CRITICAL PROBLEMS AND CHALLENGES

At any one point in time 10% to 20% of children with disabilities or chronic illnesses have no insurance coverage.[5,22] From a demographic perspective, this subpopulation represents a group that is at very high risk for inadequate care. Other children who do have insurance are often enrolled in policies that may cover certain medical services (e.g., hospitalization) but not other, equally needed services, such as transportation, home health care, or counseling services. Identification of underinsured or uninsured children with chronic health conditions represents an important public health objective.

Like most children in America, most children with disabilities and chronic illnesses have private health insurance through one or both of their parents' employers.[5] However, because private insurance fails to cover many costs that are not strictly medical, out-of-pocket expenses can be extremely high for some families.[1] Moreover, restrictions in private insurance plans (e.g., expenditure caps, preexisting condition exclusions, and policies designed to limit reimbursement to certain providers) may discourage the use of needed treatment or preventive services or may impede transfers to better positions with new employers whose health-insurance coverage may not be as complete.

Poor children with chronic illnesses or disabilities may be eligible for publicly financed health care programs, such as Medicaid and other state programs.[32] Services available through Medicaid, however, vary from state to state and numerous obstacles (e.g., long waiting times, administrative paperwork, lack of providers, and eligibility restrictions) interfere with access to program coverage. As a result, many poor children with disabilities are not enrolled in Medicaid. Liberalization of criteria for eligibility to the Supplemental Security Income (SSI) program in the early 1990s improved access to Medicaid for some children with disabilities; in about 35 states SSI eligibility automatically links the child to Medicaid benefits.[35]

While states implement health system reforms, new problems are emerging in the organization and financing of care for children with disabilities and chronic illnesses. Many families, pediatricians, and other health care professionals are concerned, for example, that managed care programs in both the public and private sectors will decrease access to needed subspecialty and supportive services and undermine recent efforts to develop community-based systems of care for these children and their families.[16] Increased monitoring of medical costs and greater recognition of limited public resources will raise difficult questions about supporting care for children who require long-term health and education services. Moreover, statewide implementation of Medicaid managed care programs and anticipated reductions in state Medicaid expenditures may affect this population of children disproportionately. Little baseline data are available to assess the influence of these changes on the health status and quality of life for these children and families.

Children with disabilities and chronic illnesses are often seen as a separate population of children for whom a separate set of public health and education programs has been established. In fact, however, many of these children are integrated into programs for children in general. Head Start, for example, now requires that 10% of enrolled children have disabilities. Many local school districts are integrating into general classrooms some children who were formerly placed in special education. As a result, additional expectations may be placed on teachers who are inadequately trained to respond effectively to the accompanying challenges. In some communities the movement toward integration of children with disabilities into regular school classrooms may contribute to an increase in social rejection of these children. Here again public health personnel and health professionals can play key roles in the ongoing debate pertaining to the integration of children with disabilities and chronic illnesses.

Many children with disabilities and chronic illnesses are eligible for numerous services and programs. However, costly duplication of administrative procedures and heightened stress for families result when each program has its own set of eligibility guidelines and forms. In recognition of poor coordination among service programs, there have been numerous calls for an organizational infrastructure that will establish and sustain a coherent community-based system of care.[17] For example, federal law now explicitly mandates the development of working relationships between state programs for children with special health care needs and SSI programs. From a health service planning perspective it is important to identify and provide coordination services to assist the subgroup of this population of disabled and chronically ill children who are involved in numerous programs.

EMERGING POPULATIONS

If history is any guide, new populations of children with serious, ongoing health conditions are likely to emerge. Children infected with HIV, infants born at a low birthweight with severe complications, and infants or toddlers diagnosed with fetal alcohol syndrome represent newly identified groups of children with serious, ongoing health conditions. From a national perspective these events are rare and therefore these populations will only marginally increase total prevalence rates.[10] However, new services will be required as new needs are identified.

For example, increased numbers of children with serious, ongoing physical health conditions are living into adulthood. In addition, children who may have had certain chronic conditions (such as leukemia) but who have been technically cured may nonetheless face increased risk for secondary problems or reoccurrences in early adulthood.[8] Existing health-, education-, and employment-related services are generally ill-equipped to respond to many of the needs of young adults who have been living with chronic health conditions since childhood.[36]

Over the last 20 years major advances in prenatal and perinatal screening and diagnosis have led to earlier identification of many chronic illnesses and disabilities. For example, with alpha-fetoprotein (AFP) testing it is now possible to identify whether a fetus is likely to be born with spina bifida; amniocentesis enables detection of fetuses with sickle cell anemia, cystic fibrosis, Tay-Sachs disease, and other genetic disorders. With continued progress it is likely that more conditions will be identified before the onset of symptomatology, leading to a new cohort of children (e.g., HIV-infected children) who are asymptomatic but incipient patients. In turn, these children will require more preventive and early intervention services.

CONCLUSION

Although the total size of the population of children with disabilities and chronic illnesses will probably remain stable for the foreseeable future, the needs of these children and their families will continue to evolve. The families of children dependent on costly medical treatments will require ongoing assistance in paying for and coordinating services. Regardless of the changes that ensue from proposed health care reforms, this population will still require a broad array of complex health, mental health, and social services. Continued migration of these children into community institutions and primary health care settings will force the need for new accommodations and will potentially raise divisive issues of resource allocation. Because it is comparatively small and requires a disproportionate amount of resources, this population risks being disenfranchised from core health and community-based services. Continued advocacy will be needed to assure that program planners and policy makers take into account the needs of children with disabilities and chronic illnesses and the families of such children.

REFERENCES

1. Birenbaum A, Guyot D, and Cohen H: Health care financing for severe developmental disabilities, number 14. In Begab M, editor: *Monographs of the American Association on Mental Retardation*, Washington DC, 1990, The Association.
2. Blum RW, editor: *Chronic illness and disability in childhood and adolescence*, Orlando, Fla, 1984, Grune & Stratton, Inc.
3. Blum R et al: Transition from child-centered to adult health-care systems for adolescents with chronic conditions, *Journal of Adolescent Health* 14:570-576, 1993.
4. Boyle CA, Decoufle P, and Yeargin-Allsopp M: Prevalence and health impact of developmental disabilities in U.S. children. *Pediatrics* 93:399-403, 1994.
5. Butler J et al: Health care expenditures for children with chronic illnesses. In Hobbs N and Perrin JM, editors: *Issues in the care of children with chronic illness: a sourcebook on problems, services, and policies*, San Francisco, 1985, Jossey-Bass.
6. Cadman D et al: Chronic illness, disability, and mental and social well-being: findings of the Ontario Child Health Study, *Pediatrics* 79:805-813, 1987.
7. FitzSimmons S: The changing epidemiology of cystic fibrosis, *Journal of Pediatrics* 122:1-9, 1993.
8. Fritz G and Williams J: After treatment ends: psychosocial sequelae in pediatric cancer survivors, *American Journal of Orthopsychiatry* 58:552-561, 1988.
9. Gortmaker S: Demography of chronic childhood diseases. In Hobbs N and Perrin JM, editors: *Issues in the care of children with chronic illness: a sourcebook on problems, services, and policies*, San Francisco, 1985, Jossey-Bass.
10. Gortmaker SL and Sappenfield W: Chronic childhood disorders: prevalence and impact, *Pediatric Clinics of North America* 31:3-18, 1984.
11. Gortmaker SL et al: Chronic conditions, socioeconomic risks, and behavioral problems in children and adolescents, *Pediatrics* 85:267-276, 1990.
12. Halfon N and Newacheck P: Childhood asthma and poverty: differential impacts and utilization of health services, *Pediatrics* 91:56-61, 1993.
13. Health and Education Collaboration for Children with Handicaps (HECCH): *The incidence and prevalence of conditions in children: a sourcebook of rates and state-specific estimates for DHHS Region IV*, ed 2, Chapel Hill, NC, 1990, University of North Carolina.
14. Hobbs N, Perrin J, and Ireys HT: Health and social services. In *Chronically ill children and their families*, San Francisco, 1985, Jossey-Bass.
15. Institute of Medicine: *Disability in America: toward a national agenda for prevention*. Washington DC, 1991, National Academy Press.
16. Ireys H, Grason H, and Guyer B: Assuring quality of care for children with special health care needs in managed care organizations: roles for pediatricians, *Pediatrics*, 1995 (in press).
17. Ireys HT, and Nelson R: New federal policy for children with special health care needs: implications for pediatricians, *Pediatrics* 90:321-327, 1992.
18. Ireys HT et al: Schooling employment and idleness in young adults with chronic conditions, *Journal of Adolescent Health*, 1995 (in press).
19. Johnson B, Jeppson E, and Redburn E: *Caring for children and families: guidelines for hospitals*, Bethesda, Md, 1992, Association for the Care of Children's Health.

20. Knowles M and Fernald G: Diabetes and cystic fibrosis: new questions emerging from increased longevity, *Journal of Pediatrics* 112:415-416, 1988.
21. Kokkonen J et al: Social outcome of handicapped children as adults, *Developmental Medicine and Child Neurology* 33:1095-1100, 1991.
22. Newacheck PW: Adolescents with special health needs: prevalence, severity, and access to health services, *Pediatrics* 84:872-881, 1989.
23. Newacheck PW, Budetti PP, and Halfon N: Trends in activity-limiting chronic conditions among children, *American Journal of Public Health* 76:179-184, 1986.
24. Newacheck PW, McManus MA, and Fox HB: Prevalence and impact of chronic illness among adolescents, *American Journal of Diseases of Children* 145: 1367-1373, 1991.
25. Newacheck P, McManus M, and Gepart J: Health insurance coverage of adolescents: a current profile and assessment of trends, *Pediatrics* 90:589-596, 1992.
26. Newacheck PW, Stoddard JJ, and McManus M: Ethnocultural variations in the prevalence and impact of childhood chronic conditions, *Pediatrics* 91:1031-1039, 1993.
27. Newacheck PW and Taylor WR: Childhood chronic illness: prevalence, severity, and impact, *American Journal of Public Health* 82:364-371, 1992.
28. Office of Technology Assessment: *Technology-dependent children: hospital v. home care—a technical memorandum*, Washington DC, 1987, U.S. Government Printing Office.
29. Palfrey JS et al: Technology's children: report of a statewide census of children dependent on medical supports, *Pediatrics* 87:611-618, 1991.
30. Palfrey JS et al: Prevalence of medical technology assistance among children in Massachusetts in 1987 and 1990, *Public Health Reports* 109:226-233, 1994.
31. Perrin E et al: Issues involved in the definition and classification of chronic health conditions, *Pediatrics* 91:787-793, 1993.
32. Perrin J, and Ireys HT: Organization of services for chronically ill children. *Pediatric Clinics of North America* 31:235-258, 1984.
33. Perrin J, and MacLean W: Children with chronic illness: the prevention of dysfunction, *Pediatric Clinics of North America* 35:1325-1337, 1988.
34. Perrin J, Shayne M, and Bloom S: *Home and Community care for chronically ill children*, New York, 1993, Oxford University Press.
35. Perrin J, and Stein R: Reinterpreting disability: changes in Supplemental Security Income for children, *Pediatrics* 88:1047-1051, 1991.
36. Schidlow D, and Fiel S: Life beyond pediatrics: transition of chronically ill adolescents from pediatric to adult health care systems, *Medical Clinics of North America* 74:1113-1120, 1990.
37. Stein R et al: A framework for identifying children who have chronic conditions: the case for a new definition, *American Journal of Diseases of Children* 122:342-347, 1993.
38. Sudman S, Sirken M, and Cowan C: Sampling rare and elusive populations, *Science* 240:991-996, 1988.
39. Weitzman M, Gortmaker S, and Sobol A: Racial, social, and environmental risks for childhood asthma, *American Journal of Diseases of Children* 144:1189-1194, 1990.
40. Wielinski C, Budd J, and Warwick W: Measures of prognosis and survival for cystic fibrosis, *American Review of Respiratory Disease* 141:A813-819, 1990.
41. Wissow L et al: Poverty, race, and hospitalization for childhood asthma, *American Journal of Public Health* 78:777-782, 1988.

CHAPTER 2

Families and Communities

GARY L. ALBRECHT

The civility of a nation is judged by how it treats its children, its persons with disabilities, and its poor and elderly citizens. However, intense financial pressures on all levels of government place these populations at particular risk. Some health care reformers, while well intentioned, generally argue that health services must be rationed and that many citizens will pay more for less health care. The intent of this reform is to introduce equity in medical care for the disenfranchised, those that have no or little health insurance or other resources, at a cost the nation can afford.

Children and youth with disabilities often belong to poor and/or dysfunctional families and live in disadvantaged communities so their opportunities for a high quality of life are limited, and their accumulated risks are considerable.[32] To be effective, health care reform must include these children and not leave them isolated and neglected. This is a real danger because, as Frenkel[13] points out, reformers are calling for a complete reassessment of entitlement programs like Medicare and Medicaid so that costs can be contained. The questions persist: Who will benefit, and who will suffer from these reforms? Will the nation take care of its children and youth with disabilities?

This chapter emphasizes the critical role that families and communities play in habilitating children and youth with disabilities. The family traditionally is the primary social unit and support group for dependent members of society; the community provides the environment and an additional source of support for those in need. The functional independence and quality of life of disabled children and youth, then, are in large part dependent on family and community resources. Therefore, a key priority of health and social service reform should be strengthening family and community resources designed to fulfill the needs of children and youth with disabilities. This can be accomplished through special-education programs in the schools, construction of a barrier-free environment, crime reduction, community-education programs to reduce bias and stigma, the availability of day care centers to relieve family responsibilities, and job training programs.[17] Community-based self-help groups are also effective in meeting the needs of persons with disabilities.

Under the new reforms government probably will guarantee basic services to children and youth with disabilities.[3] These will be most effectively delivered through family and community-based programs where they can be custom delivered at a lower price. Certainly delivering services at home is less costly than in institutions.

THE IMPORTANCE OF THE FAMILY IN HABILITATION

The family is the cornerstone of American society. When all else fails, we generally can depend on our families to offer support and a safe haven if needed. Although structure and activities of the family have been adjusted over the years to fit an industrialized and information-oriented society, families continue to provide a basic foundation and context for individual behavior.[29] Families set values, draw boundaries, provide role models, and teach members how to behave.[10] Regardless of age, children and youth tend to turn to their family for advice and support. In many ways the future of children depends on the strength and resources of their families.

When disability strikes children, medical and rehabilitation services can mend bodies and restore function but it is the family that provides a home, context, and the environment in which children can grow at their own pace. Substantial evidence indicates that the rehabilitation success of children and adolescents depends in large part on family support.[1] Families that are neither too controlling nor too laissez-faire appear to offer the type of support that best enhances rehabilitation progress. Therefore, a primary task of the health care worker in rehabilitation is to support family structures and strengths so that a child with a disability is returned to a secure environment where he or she can function as independently as possible.

In the last 30 years myriad social changes have redefined how we think of families. In 1970 only about 11% of adults lived with each other before their first marriage but by the early 1980s that number had increased to 44%. People are marrying later, cohabiting more often and even bearing children before marriage. The Census Bureau takes these dynamics into account with its definition of a family or family household, which requires the presence of at least two persons, the householder (the person in whose name the housing unit is owned or rented), and one or more additional family members related to the householder by birth, adoption, or marriage.[34]

The structure and living arrangements of children and young adults has also changed dramatically over the last 20 years. Since 1970 the number of children and youth under age 18 living with only one parent has doubled. In 1990 more than 25% of all children lived with only one parent compared to less than 12% in 1970. This trend reflects the soaring divorce rate of the period. The majority of African-American children (54.8%) lived with only one parent in 1990, and slightly more than 50% of them were born to unmarried mothers, a 50% increase since 1980. These structural changes have staggering consequences for families with disabled children and youth. These families are less likely today to have the stability, social support, and economic resources of families of previous generations. For these reasons today's families are more vulnerable to stress and often break down under the pressures of moving a child back and forth between informal and formal systems of care.[14]

Regardless of imperfect structure and limited resources, the family remains the principal source of survival and nurturance for the child with disabilities. A parent's legal responsibility for a child lasts until the child reaches age 18. However, because many of the disabling conditions of children and youth are hereditary or developmental in nature, such as Down syndrome, fetal alcohol syndrome, and mental retardation, they are likely to have lifelong effects requiring continual attention.[28] In such cases the disabled person often becomes a ward of the state and is handled in an institution if the parents are no longer willing or able to care for him or her. However, the family generally continues to assume responsibility for children with disabilities throughout the life course[26] and for most families these burdens of care and support fall upon mothers and grandmothers.[12,18] These are the individuals and family units that need strengthening, encouragement, resources, and support.

HABILITATION

The goal of treating children and youth with disabilities is to enable them to live at their highest level of function and with a high quality of life. Habilitation is a method of achieving these goals. Habilitation refers to a continuous process of assessing persons with disabilities, measuring their needs, identifying barriers, and developing a treatment plan based on this assessment.[33] This customized care approach concentrates on reducing barriers and teaching the skills necessary for independent functioning. Early intervention with disabled children, youth, and their families to identify concrete treatment goals and construct adaptive strategies enhances the family's ability to cope and maximizes the child's chances of achieving a high level of functioning.[30]

Current trends in family structure and social conditions threaten the realization of these goals and objectives. A family's ability to cope with a child who has a serious disability is dependent on the integrity of the family unit and its resources. In a study of cancer survivors and their families, Bloom et al[6] suggest that a person's social network and perceived family cohesiveness increases psychological well being. In a longitudinal study of long-term survivors of endstage renal disease in England, Gerhardt[15] discovered that patients who did well had families that were economically stable, provided security, and had an emotionally supportive environment. Pescosolido[27] argues that appropriate service utilization and compliance with prescribed treatment regimens is contingent on a stable and functional social network that provides support across the life course. This is particularly important in the case of children in which the disability could well persist for life.

Breakdowns in the structure and dynamics of the contemporary American family put children and youth with disabilities at risks rarely experienced even two generations ago. Many infants are born out of wedlock, large numbers of children live in one-parent households, minority families with limited resources are more likely to be broken, and connections to the extended family are weakened by geographical and social distances. One in four American families moves every year. Children do not have contact with grandparents, cousins, aunts, and uncles as they did some years ago. This level of social disintegration and the weakening of social networks makes families less able to deal with setbacks and stress.

Poverty exacerbates these burdens. Disability exerts continuous financial and social stress on families so that even those with means may see their resources eroded until they reach a subsistence or poverty level. Some parents have even lost or quit their jobs because they needed a flexible work schedule to care for their children. Unemployment translates into reduced income and health benefits, and as this occurs the child and family find that they cannot obtain the level of care that they once enjoyed. St. Peter et al[31] in a national sample of 17,710 children found that poor children do not have access to the same level and type of care as children with more financial means. This is catastrophic for a child with disabilities because the nature of his or her problem is complex and demands continuous, integrated, and comprehensive care that is not generally available to those without their own resources.

For these reasons the present structure of care for children and youth with disabilities appears discriminatory.[9] Wealthier families receive markedly better care for their disabled children than do those families with limited means.[7] Poor families often have to seek care for their children at general or community hospitals or even through emergency rooms. This type of care is not integrated and has no continuity. In addition, medical staff at these locations are acute care oriented and they do not have the perspective or training required to provide optimal rehabilitation services. Parents rarely have the expertise to be a case manager for their own children's care. As a consequence, disabled children who could be helped by early intervention and continuity of care suffer by having their conditions worsen before being detected. Many preventable conditions and sequelae then swamp the beleaguered health care system because early, preventive actions were not taken.

These problems in achieving equity and appropriateness of care are exacerbated by the long-term nature of the child's condition. Families who have children with disabilities continue to be at risk for years or even across the entire life course. Children with disabilities that used to result in early mortality now live longer. With improved treatment and drugs, children with AIDS, for example, will soon live for years with serious disabilities before dying.[20] Others have conditions that affect the child and family for decades. Children with craniofacial anomalies experience behavioral and psychological problems in addition to any required medical interventions.[5] In cases like mental retardation and cerebral palsy the question remains: Who will care for these children with disabilities when their parents die? Will they all become wards of the state? If so, the economic cost to the nation and the emotional costs to individuals and their families will be enormous.

EFFECT OF LIMITED RESOURCES AND STRESS ON COPING

Well-designed adaptive strategies for families with disabled children focus on strengthening and supporting the family unit so that it can function to care for the child.[21] Family support strategies need to take the age, gender, social and cultural characteristics of the family, and the nature of the disability into account. Needs and resources differ across the life course. Avison et al[4] found that mothers bear the brunt of the care giving and experience a disproportionate amount of stress in doing so. Furthermore, parents of children with Down syndrome and infantile autism experience more stress-related problems than parents of children with cancer. Social support and the provision of health care services alleviate this stress and are related to improved family functioning. In a review of 66 studies Andersen and Telleen[3] note that mothers function much better with the problems of their disabled children when they are provided with resources and consistent social support. Interventions, then, to be effective must be designed for the family and the disability condition.

Social and cultural characteristics affect how families cope with children with disabilities and therefore should be reflected in intervention strategies. For example, African-American families are more likely than other families to have a single-parent household and have fewer resources. These single mothers often are young and can benefit from parenting skills classes and from help in navigating the disability system. As another example, families in smaller towns are more likely to have integrated social support networks than those in large metropolises. Where such networks are missing, self help and special interest groups can be formed around the disability type to help people help themselves.[19] Different periods in the course of the disability are more burdensome for one family member than another. In families with cerebral palsy children, for example, infancy and toddlerhood are often most demanding for mothers whereas fathers find the school-age and adolescence periods most stressful.[16] Counseling and social support mechanisms can be designed to take these differences into account.

THE COMMUNITY CONTEXT OF DISABILITY

Recognition that families have striking problems in caring for children with disabilities and that institutional help from the government is impersonal and restricted turns attention to the development and utilization of community resources. Churches, schools, community centers, and neighborhood health clinics are institutions that can be enlisted and strengthened to support families and deliver services. These institutions represent stability and community values. Although population mobility can affect community services, those neighborhoods with strong local institutions provide an infrastructure and a set of social networks that are accessible even to the newcomer. This mix of institutions ensures both public and private programs in the community.

Problems arise, however, in the level of support across communities. Government programs, including entitlements, often provide different amounts and types of resources to families with disabled children depending on state and local conditions. Rural and inner-city communities have felt the loss of community hospitals and clinics. As a consequence, residents of rural areas are experiencing reduced standards of care and inner-city residents are forced to travel outside their communities to large public hospital emergency rooms. In these instances strong tax bases and loud political voices usually translate into more and better programs. The resource problem is further compounded by intense competition for public funds as most recently expressed in the government budget battles between competing interest groups over defense, health care, and education spending. The social class of a community will also dictate the level of contributions to charitable local institutions. Inner-city communities, however, can often make up for lack of money by building resilient social networks and contributing labor and time to local causes.

To build community resources, families with disabled children and youth must organize and become vocal or they will not be heard. This means demanding clear communication, continuity of care, and physician referrals to appropriate specialists.[11] On a community level this activism includes building public and private community resources by insisting that services be delivered in the neighborhood and be accessible to all. Because money is limited, innovative programs can be developed by building on local resources.

Brewer et al[8] cite growing evidence to show that coordinated care for children with disabilities can be effectively delivered through a family-centered, community-based model. Such an approach is possible by forging relationships with physicians in the community, by building teams of parents who are knowledgeable and supportive of families with disabled children, by developing health care teams in community health centers who are familiar with the local neighborhood's culture and resources, and by utilizing case-management techniques to attack continuity-of-care issues.[22] Community acceptance of people with disabilities can be improved by implementing low-cost public-education programs through the local media and in schools and the workplace.

In addition, Olds and Kitzman[25] report that home visitations by trained health care workers have been used to improve mothers' health-related behaviors during pregnancy, the birthweight and health of newborns, children's developmental status, and parents interactions with children. Related studies suggest that home visitation by nurses can reduce the incidence of child abuse and neglect, childhood behavioral problems, and hospital visits.[24] O'Grady et al[23] even suggest that early identification and treatment of children with disabilities in the community will prevent more severe health problems in the future and will not necessarily increase health services utilization. This body of evidence taken as a whole suggests that the community is the desirable and effective location to address the needs of families with disabled children. The programs that improve the accessibility and quality of care are those that centrally involve the community, parents, and children in the solution. This reorganization of health care for children with disabilities would shift the locus of treatment from remote tertiary care facilities to the local community and would change the focus from the individual patient to the family and social networks.

CONCLUSION

This chapter calls for a reorientation in addressing the needs of children and youth with disabilities and the needs of their families. Merely providing medical care to children ignores the social dynamics of the problem. Children with disabilities share the fate of their families and communities; they are inextricably intertwined. A constructive approach to addressing the problems of children with disabilities is to strengthen families and enable them to develop and use available resources to deal with their problems. Likewise, families are embedded in communities. Bringing services to the community and delivering them in the home places help in the context where it is needed. Education is needed to improve the knowledge and skills of these families and to reduce bias and stigma toward disability in the community. Prevention efforts to avoid disability-producing behavior and to help in early identification and treatment of disabling conditions also are critical components in controlling disability in the family and community.

REFERENCES

1. Albrecht G and Higgins P: Rehabilitation success: the interrelationships of multiple criteria, *J Health and Soc Behavior* 18:36-45, 1977.
2. Albrecht GL: *The disability business: rehabilitation in America*, Newbury Park, Calif, 1992, Sage.
3. Andersen PA and Telleen SL: The relationship between social support and maternal behaviors and attitudes: a meta-analytic review, *J Com Ment Health*, 1991, (in press).
4. Avison WR, Noh S, and Speechley KN: Parents as caregivers: caring for children with health problems. In Albrecht GL and Levy JA, editors: *Advances in medical sociology*, vol 2, Chronic illness and disability as life course events, Greenwich, Conn, 1991, JAI Press.
5. Benson BA et al: Social support among families of children with craniofacial anomalies, *Health Psych* 10:252, 1991.
6. Bloom JR et al: Social supports and the social well-being of cancer survivors. In Albrecht GL and Levy JA, editors: *Advances in medical sociology*, vol 2, Chronic illness and disability as life course events, Greenwich, Conn, 1991, JAI Press.
7. Breslau N and Mortimer EA: Seeing the same doctor: determinants of satisfaction with specialty care for disabled children, *Med Care* 19:741, 1981.
8. Brewer EJ et al: Family centered, community-based, coordinated care for children with special health needs, *Pediatrics* 83:1055, 1989.
9. Butler JA, Rosenbaum S, and Palfrey JS: Ensuring access to health care for children with disabilities, *NEJM* 317:162, 1987.
10. Coleman J: *Foundations of social theory*, Cambridge, Mass, 1990, The Belknap Press of Harvard University Press.
11. Emanuel EJ and Emanuel LL: Four models of the physician-patient relationship, *JAMA* 267:2221, 1992.
12. Erickson ME and Upshur CC: Caretaking burden and social support: comparison of mothers with infants with and without disabilities, *Am J Mental Retardation* 94:250-256, 1989.
13. Frenkel M: What should Mr. Clinton do to reform America's health care system? *J Med Practice Management* 4:147, 1993.

14. Garmezy N: Resiliency and vulnerability to adverse developmental outcomes associated with poverty. In Thompson T and Hupp S, editors: *Saving children at risk: poverty and disabilities*, Newbury Park, Calif, 1992, Sage.

15. Gerhardt U: Family rehabilitation and long-term survival in end-stage renal failure. In Albrecht GL and Levy JA, editors: *Advances in medical sociology*, vol 2, Chronic illness and disability as life course events, Greenwich, Conn, 1991, JAI Press.

16. Hirose, T and Ueda R: Long-term follow-up study of cerebral palsy children and coping behaviour of parents, *J of Ad Nursing 15*:762, 1990.

17. Kozol J: Savage inequalities: children in America's schools, New York, 1991, Crown.

18. LaPlante MP: *Data on disability from the national health interview survey, 1983-1985*, Washington DC, 1988, U.S. National Institute on Disability and Rehabilitation Research.

19. Maines DR: The storied nature of health and diabetic self-help groups: In Albrecht GL and Levy JA, editors: *Advances in medical sociology*, vol 2, Chronic illness and disability as life course events, Greenwich, Conn, 1991, JAI Press.

20. Mangos JA et al: Pediatric AIDS: treatment and outcome of patients, *Texas Med 86*:40, 1990.

21. Moen P and Wethington E: The concept of family adaptive strategies, *Annu Rev Soc 18*:233, 1992.

22. Moxley DP: *The practice of case management*, Newbury Park, Calif, 1989, Sage.

23. O'Grady RS, Baruffi G, and Strofino DM: The use of preventive health services by disabled children, *Am J Prev Med 1*:31, 1985.

24. Olds DL et al: Preventing child abuse and neglect: a randomized trial of nurse home visitation, *Pediatrics 78*:65, 1986.

25. Olds DL, and Kitzman H: Can home visitation improve the health of women and children at environmental risk? *Pediatrics 86*:108, 1990.

26. *Parham v JR*, 442 US 584, 1978.

27. Pescosolido BA: Illness careers and network ties: a conceptual model of utilization and compliance. In Albrecht GL and Levy JA, editors: *Advances In medical sociology*, vol 2, Chronic illness and disability as life course events, Greenwich, Conn, 1991, JAI Press.

28. Pope AM and Tarlov, editors: Disability in America: toward a national agenda for prevention. Washington DC, 1991, National Academy Press.

29. Seccombe W: *A millennium of family change*, London, 1992, Verso.

30. Simeonson RJ et al: Scaling and attainment of goals in family-focused early intervention, *Com Mental Health J 27*:77, 1991.

31. St. Peter RF, Newacheck PW, and Halfon N: Access to care for poor children, *JAMA 267*:2760, 1992.

32. Thompson T: For the sake of our children. In Thompson T and Hupp S, editors: *Saving our children at risk: poverty and disabilities*, Newbury Park, Calif, 1992, Sage.

33. Wielkiewicz RM and Calvert CR: *Training and habilitating developmentally disabled people*, Newbury Park, Calif, 1989, Sage.

34. Wright JW: *The universal almanac*, Kansas City, 1992, Andrews and McMeel.

CHAPTER **3**

The Impact of Disabling Conditions

ALLEN C. CROCKER

Disabling conditions have effects that extend well beyond the individual, affecting family, caregiver, and community in ways not always immediately obvious. The following discussion identifies some of the more notable consequences to consider when seeking to understand and serve this population.

IMPACT ON THE CHILD
Creating Differentness

The presence of one or more disabilities in the personal world of a child defines a degree of exceptionality. The meaning of the disability to the individual, and its intrusiveness regarding daily function are potentially quite variable. However, the varying effects of disabilities are similar at least in that they create "differentness."

One aspect of differentness that may be significant to individuals with disabilities relates to *performance or achievement*. Attainment of certain skills may be below age expectation, based on normed scales, or may be qualitatively unusual. However, good adaptive skills can compensate for some cognitive limitation, and situations do vary regarding the achievements needed.

An additional differentness in the life of a child with disability is that of the *services required*. All of us draw on inside and outside services in this social world. For persons with significant exceptionality the urgency is greater. Alliances for safety, for transportation, for technologic solutions, and for learning, are beneficial.

Another dissimilarity of importance in the life of a person with disability is that of *participation* because this relates to life events and sequences. The traditional isolation experienced by persons with disabilities has now received energetic attention, resulting in less restrictive and more normalized and inclusive program planning. This has become a major human rights and legislative concern.

A final component of possible differentness relates to participation but goes further, dealing with attainment of *connectedness*, which refers to substantial interrelationships and interactions with other persons. Here rests the responsibility for all human beings to maintain the life-sharing and fellowship that keeps us a "family."[4]

Expression of Developmental Disability

The characteristics of developmental disabilities and their effects were delineated in the basic definition that appeared in Public Law 95-602 in 1978. There it spoke of mental and/or physical impairments manifest in childhood and continuing indefinitely. The functional implications most commonly involve self-care, language, learning, mobility, self-direction, independent living, and economic sufficiency. The developmental disabilities constitute an important source of childhood infirmity; in sum they involve about 3% of the population. They arise from hereditary, prenatal, perinatal, and acquired childhood origins, and involve processes in which there is particular impingement on the central nervous system. The affected young people may show mental retardation, cerebral palsy, seizure disorders, or various multiple phenomena. In a population of children with mental retardation, for example, about one third will have physical disability and motor function problems, 10% may have seizures, and a similar number will have sensory disabilities. A group of youngsters with cerebral palsy will include an appreciable number with mental retardation, as will those with epilepsy.[8] Impairment in communication skills is also widespread, illustrating the sensitivity of language function to alterations in nervous system or physical integrity.

Health Care Needs

There are health concerns closely linked to many of the syndromes that carry disabilities. A care model has been formulated that is referred to as "alike/unalike," acknowledging that much of health management of children with disabilities is comparable to that for typical children but there is also the need for vigilance in special areas of vulnerability. The child with Down syndrome, for example, requires a watchful regard for cardiac, otologic, orthopedic, endocrine, gastrointestinal, ocular, and other systems. The youngster with myelodysplasia is often troubled with hydrocephalus, paraplegia, scoliosis, complications of neurogenic bladder and bowel disability, skin trauma, seizures, and so on. For children with cerebral palsy attention may be needed for weakness, spasticity, contractures, dislocations, strabismus, seizures, hearing impairment, and/or nutritional problems.

Behavioral Effects

Behavioral effects are also components of certain disability states. Some can be viewed as part of the adaptational challenge in a setting of personal idiosyncrasy. In other situations there are characteristic features of social interaction to some degree associated with the disorder, such as those in persons with fragile X syndrome, Williams syndrome, autism, and Down syndrome. Most concerning are the troubled behavioral responses that may complicate severe developmental disorders, with pica, self-injury, or aggression. Skilled program guidance is needed in such situations for best personal progress.

IMPACT ON FAMILIES

Membership within the family of a young person with a disability or chronic illness secures the parent or parents and others in the home as partners in special support and treatment. The home becomes the site of the sought-after "family-based, community-centered" care, as promoted by the federal Maternal and Child Health Bureau, which carries out the provisions of Title V of the Social Security Act. Depending on the degree of specialness involved, modifications in the home and in the parental activities may or may not be substantial.

Family as Caregiver

It is only recently that we have come to honor the family as caregiver. To this effort families bring usual or natural parental resources but also acquire additional special knowledge and skills. Characteristic requirements include the following:

- *Physical maintenance*—The practical logistics of diets, adaptive equipment, home modifications, and access to specialized health care. To be geographically close to necessary providers parents may have to limit their career opportunities. To pay for the care as well as other physical needs of children, parents may choose to stay with a job that offers responsive health insurance.
- *Emotional and psychological support*—Including assistance in emerging self-concept, personality definition, and in developing autonomy and needed interactive skills.
- *Access to education and planning*—Pursuit of the best embodiment of this important educational entitlement for the child, where much must be learned by all.

- *Social and recreational opportunities*—May have to be encouraged because of limited natural availability.
- *Transition to adulthood*—Including acquisition of the new knowledge necessary regarding the employment, service, and community-living worlds.

This empirical expansion of family expertise is well described by Featherstone[5] in *A Difference in the Family* and by Callanan[2] in *Since Owen*.

Supports Needed

Interviews with families of children with disabilities about the pressures felt and the supports desired have revealed certain strategic requirements as most prominent[14]:

- parent education on rights and entitlements
- financial counseling
- information on community resources
- recreational opportunities
- parent support groups
- parent training for child's health needs
- transportation
- respite care
- legal services

It should be noted that these are the nonreimbursable reinforcements commonly referred to now as *family support services* by public and private agencies. They are the useful tools of daily management for a family of a child with disabilities.

Family Growth

However, there are other kinds of responses engendered by the impact a child with special needs has on a family. These are the pieces that become what has been referred to as "the awesome adventure"—the elements of child and family growing together. There is so much to become familiar with, both from a conceptual point of view and pragmatically. The search for information and understanding is a powerful drive and it must be as personal and accurate as possible. A family learns to reach out, to share, to trust, to become allied, to contend, to strive, and to struggle on behalf of the child with particular needs.

Cognitive Coping

Part of the excitement of the strengthening consumer position established in the last two decades has been the potential for putting a child with exceptionality in a more creative context, which renders the effect on the family more manageable. This philosophy of valuing the child with special needs is found in parent support groups, peer counseling, numerous consumer-based publications (including the magazine *Exceptional Parent*), and the examples of many families. Particular purposeful behavior in this constructive vein is referred to as *cognitive coping* by the Beach Center on Families and Disability at the University of Kansas in Lawrence. An elaboration of cognitive coping strategies would include the following:

- Making favorable comparisons of one's situation to others.
- Finding positive benefits from an event or choosing to selectively ignore negative aspects. For example, family members may concentrate on the positive contribution of the person with a disability in being the catalyst for assertiveness, sensitivity, and family unity.
- Attributing a meaningful and self-enhancing cause of the event. For example, a family may decide that a person with a disability has a special purpose in life.
- Having a sense of control or influence over the event. For example, a family may perceive that they can shape educational or employment opportunities for their family member, thus reducing their feelings of helplessness or despair.
- Finding humor. For example, families may find something humorous about inappropriate behavior in public and thus transform the situation from one of embarrassment to one of light-heartedness.[13]

Sisters and Brothers

A vigorous portion of life within the family involves the contributions and perceptions of the sisters and brothers of the principally affected child. A compassionate acknowledgement of the elements of potential impact for these fellow travelers in the home scene would consider the following:

- Alteration in the normalcy of family rhythm, conformity, and image (an adapted home, loss of some flexibility, need to attend to other than their own gratification);
- Competition for parental resources and attention (priorities for parents' energy and time, demands for family funds);
- Misconceptions that the normal child may carry (puzzlement about causation, possible genetic issues, what will happen to the involved child);
- Need for the normal child to act as a surrogate parent (share in care, child coverage, conflict in social activities, possible lifelong responsibility); and
- Obligation to meet enhanced parental expectations (need to "make up" for frustrations, prove parental normalcy).[3]

Early studies in this field expected and found some short- and long-term psychologic distress among sisters and brothers of children with disabilities.

More searching work in recent years has, on the other hand, provided documentation of predominantly positive adjustment for these family members.[1,3,10] Outreach to them in program involvement, support groups, newsletters, and especially in respected participation in decision-making has built a critically valuable cohort of advocates. Grossman,[6] Featherstone,[5] and others have especially noted insights gained by sisters and brothers relating to human differences and various patterns of achievement.

EFFECT ON THE COMMUNITY

It is difficult to know how to most fairly approach the question of the effect of disability or chronic illness on society. The involved phenomena are deeply rooted, an almost anticipatable element of human variation and part of our definition as a culture. Further, it must be acknowledged that some of this basic diversity among people is a source of important richness. In our heterogeneous society we are continually exchanging special understanding and values. We all have a complex interdependence with one another. We need each other and gain from each other. Thus there must be caution about reckoning the impact of disability.

Community economics provide systems for the possible assignment of costs (i.e., extensions beyond average circumstances), but one must be careful that such insinuations about cost are fair, relevant, and accurate. Four circumstances or approaches are noted here for reflection.

Securing Access

The concept of full community access for individuals with disabilities has had historic barriers, both physical and conceptual. With the signing of the Americans with Disabilities Act in July 1990, commitment was begun in earnest to bring adjustments in line regarding employment practices, public accommodations, transportation, government offices, and telecommunication services. These actions will assist in the rectification of many of the prejudicial conditions that exist for persons with disabilities, both child and adult.

Costs and Productivity

Care costs and productivity lost because of disability are complex to track and, when aggregated, are overwhelming. One such analysis[9] of all U.S. persons regardless of age, suggests that in 1980 disability was attributed with a net consumption (difference in medical care utilization and costs before and after the disabling condition occurred) of $91 billion plus $68 billion for primary market time (reduced productivity) and $18 billion additional for secondary market time (household members).

Special Education

Special education is a community-based service directly relating to children's special needs. The required costs for special personnel and other resources come from the local school district (city, town), with some assistance from the state and dedicated federal funds. The majority of children for whom special-education planning is carried out have mild degrees of assistance needed (e.g., learning disabilities and language problems). Some others, with complex developmental disability, may require more extensive supports. Tuition can rise to 30 or more times that expended for average students. Taken in the sum, the numbers of all types of children in special education is about 10% to 11% of the total, while their costs represent about 20% of the school department budget.

Personal Costs

A final model sometimes used in measurement is that of summed personal costs, most commonly generated in discussions regarding prevention. The study of Sadovnick and Baird[11] looked at the presumed costs of caring for a person with Down syndrome on a lifetime basis as viewed in 1981 in Vancouver. This study concentrated on expenses ultimately accruing to the provincial government. The authors identified particular costs of $26,600 for medical care, $55,500 for education, and $113,900 for residence assistance in adult life. The total thus becomes $196,000, a figure that needs enormous qualification (historically, culturally, and otherwise) and yet is still being quoted at this time. In a similar study, although grossly overdeveloped, Lauria et al[7] sought to account for the base costs in the life of an individual with fragile X syndrome. This reaches $237,000 for the family in the first 18 years for each person and $1.61 million for public systems costs during an additional 54 years.

CONCLUSION

This discussion principally considers the impact of disabling conditions on the involved person and on the world around her or him. Also appropriate for reflection would be the converse of this, the effect of surrounding matters on the disability itself. Inclusive environments commonly lead to improved function. Constructive planning can minimize troubling secondary events or complications and add to the joy of life. Gifts of empowerment, the chance for self-development, sharing, and an atmosphere that promotes wellness are important as impacts on rather than of disability.

REFERENCES

1. Boyce GC and Barnett WS: Siblings of persons with mental retardation. In Stoneman Z and Berman PW, editors: *The effects of mental retardation, disability, and illness on siblings relationships*, Baltimore, 1993, Paul H. Brookes.
2. Callanan CR: *Since Owen*, Baltimore, 1990, Johns Hopkins University.
3. Crocker AC: Sisters and brothers. In Mulick JA and Pueschel SM, editors: *Parent-professional partnerships in developmental disability services*, 1983, Ware Press.
4. Crocker AC and Nelson RP: Mental retardation. In Levine MD, Carey WB, and Crocker AC, editors: *Developmental-behavioral pediatrics*, ed 2, Philadelphia, 1992, WB Saunders.
5. Featherstone H: *A Difference in the family: life with a disabled child*, New York, 1980, Basic Books.
6. Grossman FK: *Brothers and sisters of retarded children*, Syracuse, NY, 1972, Syracuse University Press.
7. Lauria DP et al: The economic impact of the Fragile X syndrome on the state of Colorado, In Hagerman RJ and McKenzie P, editors: *International Fragile X Conference Proceedings*, Dillon, Colo, 1992, Spectra Publishing Co.
8. Murphy A and Crocker AC: Impact of handicapping conditions on the child and family. In Wallace et al, editors: *Handicapped children and youth*, New York, 1987, Human Sciences Press.
9. Pope AM and Tarlov AR: *Disability in America: toward a national agenda for prevention*, Washington DC, 1991, National Academy Press.
10. Powell TH and Gallagher PA: *Brothers & sisters—a special part of exceptional families*, ed 2, Baltimore, 1992, Paul H. Brookes.
11. Sadovnick AD and Baird PA: A cost-benefit analysis of prenatal detection of Down syndrome and neural tube defects in older mothers. *Am J Med Genet 10*:367, 1981.
12. Taylor AB, Epstein SG, and Crocker AC: Health care for children with special needs. In Schlesinger MJ and Eisenberg L, editors: *Children in a changing health system*, Baltimore, 1990, Johns Hopkins University.
13. Turnbull AP and Turnbull HR III: Participatory research on cognitive coping. In Turnbull AP et al, editors: *Cognitive coping, families, & disability*, Baltimore, 1993, Paul H. Brookes.
14. Walker DK et al: Perceived needs of families with children who have chronic health conditions, *Children's Health Care 18*:196, 1989.

CHAPTER **4**

Public Sector Health Services for Children with Special Health Care Needs

VINCE L. HUTCHINS
JOHN E. HUTCHINS

During the last several decades the public sector, consisting of legislatures, administrative agencies, and courts at the federal, state, and local levels, participated in and responded to an ongoing evolution in the care of children with special health care needs. This population of children encompasses those who have health problems requiring more than routine and basic care, including those with or at risk of disabilities, chronic illnesses, and health-related educational and behavioral problems.

This evolution, which might be more properly characterized as a revolution, is the product of a complex interplay of biomedical advances and political, social, and economic forces. A highlight of this evolution has been a series of federal government initiatives directed at the development of systems of health services and other services that are family-centered, community-based, and coordinated. This important concept and its implications for the delivery of health and other services to children with special health care needs is described in detail by other contributors to this book.*

---

*Dr. C. Everett Koop, the former United States Surgeon General has been a leader in the launching of federal initiatives to develop family-centered, community-based, coordinated care and he summarizes the history of these initiatives in his foreword to this book. Various aspects of family-centered, community-based, coordinated care are discussed in the following chapters: Families and Communities by Gary L. Albrecht; Future Development of Community-Based Service Systems by John MacQueen and Josephine Gittler; Family Roles: The Most Relevant Aspect of Family-Centered Care by Josie Thomas and Beverley H. Johnson; Systems of Care for Children and Adolescents with Chronic Illness by James A. Perrin; Children with Disabilities and Chronic Illness: Challenges and Solutions by Beverly Schenkman Roberts and Brenda G. Considine; and Inter-Organizational Collaboration by Margo I. Peter and Calvin C.J. Sia.

The purpose of this chapter is to present a brief overview of public sector health services for children with special health care needs. The presentation of such an overview poses definitional problems because the line between the public and private sectors is often blurred in the provision of health services. Although the provision of health services may be wholly within either the private or public sector, it often involves both. For example, the vast majority of children obtain medical services from private physicians in private offices, clinics, and hospitals, but these medical services are often publicly funded.

At the present time the federal and state governments play a critical and essential role in the delivery of health services to children with special health care needs. That role may take the form of providing services, funding services, organizing services, promoting services, or some combination of the foregoing. Brief descriptions of some of the major federal and federal-state programs that fill these roles appear in the following pages.

MATERNAL AND CHILD HEALTH SERVICES BLOCK GRANT

Title V of the Social Security Act, enacted in 1935, gave states the impetus and means to design and implement state public health programs serving children with special health care needs. These programs were called the State Crippled Children's Services Programs and the purpose of them was to expand and improve services for identifying crippled children and services for the diagnosis, treatment, and aftercare of crippled children and those suffering from conditions that lead to crippling. The 1935 Title V legislation also furnished support for State Maternal and Child Health Programs for the purpose of promoting the health of mothers and children.

In 1981 Title V was amended and the State Crippled Children's Services and Maternal and Child Health Programs were consolidated with other programs under the Maternal and Child Health Services Block Grant (MCH Block Grant).[15] Since 1989 the stated mission of the MCH Block Grant has been the improvement of the health of all mothers and children in accordance with the national health promotion and disease prevention objectives for the year 2000.[12] An important component of the MCH Block Grant remains the state programs that serve children with special health care needs.

Originally the State Crippled Children's Services Programs largely served children with orthopedic problems. Over the years these programs extended their coverage to children with a variety of other physical disabilities, sensory impairments, developmental disabilities, and chronic illnesses. In 1986 Congress recognized the expanding coverage of these programs and responded to criticism of the use of the term *crippled children* as stigmatizing by changing the name of these programs to State Programs for Children with Special Health Care Needs (CSHCN). However, the MCH Block

Grant legislation does not define the terminology *children with special health care needs*, and each state is allowed to determine its own eligibility requirements for its CSHCN Program.

The MCH Block Grant programs, including the State CSHCN Programs, are administered by the Maternal and Child Health Bureau, which is part of the Public Health Service in the United States Department of Health and Human Services. At the state level the programs are usually administered by the state health agencies, although a few are administered by other state entities. Because of the block grant nature of the State CSHCN Programs, these state agencies have flexibility to design and implement these programs to meet the specific needs of the population of children with special health care needs in their state. This flexibility has led to a wide variation in the State CSHCN Programs in terms of the children served, the services funded and provided, and other program functions and activities.

Although there is considerable variation in the State CSHCN Programs, a hallmark of these programs from their inception has been a medically directed, interdisciplinary, comprehensive approach to the care of children with special health care needs. They have emphasized the provision of a continuum of primary, secondary, and tertiary level diagnostic and treatment services. The programs also have emphasized the prevention as well as the diagnosis and treatment of disabilities and chronic conditions.

In addition to providing or funding diagnostic and treatment services, the programs may provide or fund a wide variety of habilitation and rehabilitation and support services. Other needs that may be met by the programs include medications, medical supplies, special adaptive equipment, assistive communication devices, prosthesis, and special formulas and nutritional supplements. The programs also perform other types of valuable functions directed at expanding and improving health services for children with special health care needs. They organize statewide service infrastructures, provide care coordination or case management services, and formulate standards for care.

The most recent Title V amendments require these programs "to provide and promote family-centered, community-based, coordinated care (including care coordination services as defined in the legislation) for children with special health care needs and to facilitate the development of community-based systems of services for such children and their families."* In the current era of limited resources, this mandate is creating tension in the states between the need to provide and fund direct services and the need to develop community-based service systems.

In 1989 Congress mandated that once the total MCH appropriation exceeded $600 million, 12.75% of the amount above $600 million had to be set aside to support discretionary grants referred to as Community Integrated Service Systems (CISS) projects. Eighty-five percent of the remaining funds are dispersed as MCH Block Grants to states. Since 1990 each state is required to use at least 30% of its annual MCH Block Grant allocation for services for children with special health care needs. Tables 4-1 and 4-2 set forth the MCH Block Grant appropriations and the allocation of these appropriations among different components of the Block Grant.

The first $422.05 million of Title V money is distributed to the states proportionally on the basis of the 1980 pre-Block Grant funding levels. The

Table 4-1. Federal Funding* for Selected Federal and Federal-State Programs Serving Children with Special Health Care Needs, 1984, 1990, 1993, 1994, and 1995 (in millions)

Program	Federal Fiscal Year				
	1984	1990	1993	1994	1995
Maternal and Child Health Services Block Grant	$399	$554	$665	$687	$684
Medical Assistance (Medicaid) Program†	20,061	41,103	75,774	82,034	88,438 (estimated)
Supplemental Security Income Program (SSI)†	17,797	24,423	33,709	36,966	40,491 (estimated)
Pediatric AIDS	—	15	21	22	26
Emergency Medical Services for Children	—	4	5	8	10
Community and Migrant Health Centers	373	457	616	663	757
Head Start	996	1,448	2,779	3,326	3,534

*The figures for the Medicaid and SSI programs, which are entitlement programs, represent annual outlays of federal funds. The figures for other programs represent annual appropriations of federal funds.
†The figures for the Medicaid and SSI Programs represent total expenditures for beneficiaries, including but not limited to children.
From Office of Management and Budget: *Historical tables: budget of the United States government, fiscal year 1996*, Washington DC, 1995, U.S. Government Printing Office. Health Resources and Services Administration, PHS, U.S. Department of Health and Human Services: *Appropriations Summary*, (undated), (unpublished). Maternal and Child Health Bureau, HRSA, PHS, U.S. Department of Health and Human Services: *Summary of Federal Appropriations for MCH Bureau Programs*, (undated), (unpublished).

*Social Security Act (Title V), Maternal and Child Health Services Block Grant, 42 U.S.C. §§701(a)(1)(D) (Supp V 1994).

amount above $422.05 million is distributed in proportion to the number of low-income children in each state in relation to the number of such children nationally. States must provide a three-dollar match for every four federal dollars allocated. In-kind matching is permitted, but federal funds from other sources may not be utilized. Historically, because of strong state support for MCH Block Grant programs for children with special health care needs, most states have overmatched.

Fifteen percent of the MCH Block Grant appropriation is reserved for Special Projects of Regional and National Significance (SPRANS). Many of these SPRANS have as their target population, in whole or in part, children with special health care needs and their families. Table 4-3 sets forth SPRANS funding for different SPRANS categories from 1982 to 1995.

Table 4-2. Maternal and Child Health Appropriation Levels by Type of Grant, 1982-1995 (in millions)

Federal Fiscal Year	Total	Block Grants to States	Children with Special Health Care Needs Allocation[||]	Discretionary Grants
1982	$373.8	$316.2		$57.6
1983	478.0	422.1*		55.9
1984	399.0	339.2		59.8
1985	478.0	406.3		71.7
1986	457.4[†]	388.8		68.6
1987	496.8[‡§]	421.1		75.7
1988	526.6[§]	444.3		82.3
1989	554.3[§]	465.3		89.0
1990	553.6	470.6	$141.2	83.0
1991	587.3	499.2	149.8	88.1
1992	649.7	547.1	164.1	102.6[¶]
1993	664.4	557.9	167.4	106.7[¶]
1994	687.0	574.5	172.4	112.5[¶]
1995	684.0	572.2	171.7	111.8[¶]

*Includes $105 million designated funds from the Jobs Bill Urgent Supplemental Legislation (PL 98-8).
†Reflects a $20.6 million reduction stemming from the Gramm-Rudman Act (PL 97-216).
‡Includes a Supplemental Appropriation for $18.8 million.
§Includes funds for projects to screen for sickle cell anemia and other hemoglobinopathies as well as new child health demonstration projects for primary care services and community network and case management services for children with special health care needs.
||Minimum 30% of allocation for children with special health care needs.
¶Includes $6.4 million for the first year, $8.2 million for the second year, $11.1 million for the third year, and $10.7 million for the fourth year of Community Integrated Service Systems Projects (CISS).
From Maternal and Child Health Bureau, HRSA, PHS, U.S. Department of Health and Human Services: *Summary of Federal Appropriations for MCH Bureau Programs*, (undated), (unpublished).

MEDICAL ASSISTANCE (MEDICAID) PROGRAM

Title XIX of the Social Security Act, enacted in 1965, established the Medical Assistance Program, known as Medicaid.* Since its enactment Medicaid has become the major source of health insurance for poor and near poor children.

Medicaid is a federal-state program. At the federal level Medicaid administration is the responsibility of the Health Care Financing Administration of the United States Department of Health and Human Services and at the state level Medicaid administration is usually the responsibility of the state human services or social services agencies. State agencies have authority to structure the program within overall federal requirements and guidelines.

Medicaid is jointly financed by the federal government and by state governments. In contrast to the MCH Block Grant, Medicaid is an entitlement

Table 4-3. SPRANS Grant Funding Levels by Category of SPRANS Grant, 1982 to 1995 (in millions)

Year	Total	Research	Training	Genetics	Hemophilia*	Other
1982	$57.55	$2.35	$27.92	$7.25	$2.60	$17.43
1983	55.95	3.70	26.66	7.33	2.60	15.66
1984	59.85	4.70	27.50	7.40	3.03	17.22
1985	71.70	6.00	29.50	8.00	3.60	24.60
1986	68.62	5.35	28.28	7.50	3.45	24.04
1987	75.62	6.20	28.40	8.81†	3.69	30.97
1988	82.28	7.20	29.43	10.89†	3.69	30.97
1989	88.98	7.20	30.33	13.87†	4.70	32.88
1990	83.04	7.60	30.86	7.00	4.70	32.88
1991	88.10	7.60	32.87	7.50	4.70	35.43
1992	96.19	7.75	33.67	9.10	5.20	40.47
1993	98.37	7.00	35.19	9.29	5.36	41.53
1994	101.39	6.72	37.09	9.29	5.30	42.99
1995	101.00	8.10	35.10	9.00	5.30	43.50

*Does not include transfer of funds from CDC for AIDS service programming in hemophilia, 1986 to 1995 ($2.5, $3.5, $6.3, $7.2, $7.5, $8.5 $7.6, $7.6, $7.6, and $6.0 million in successive years).
†Includes funds for projects to screen for sickle cell anemia and other hemoglobinopathies as well as new child health demonstration projects for primary care services and community network and case management services for children with special health care needs.
From Maternal and Child Health Bureau, HRSA, PHS, U.S. Department of Health and Human Services: *Summary of Federal Appropriations for MCH Bureau Programs,* (undated), (unpublished).

*Social Security Act (Title XIX), Grants to States for Medical Assistance Programs, 42 U.S.C. §§1396a-1396v (1988 & Supp V 1994).

program. This means that individuals who meet program eligibility requirements are "entitled" to receive authorized benefits and that funds sufficient to cover program expenditures must be appropriated by Congress and state legislatures. Table 4-1 indicates the level of federal funding for Medicaid services during the last decade.

Eligibility of children for Medicaid was originally linked to eligibility for the Aid to Families with Dependent Children Program (AFDC), a welfare program that provides cash payments for eligible children. Children eligible for the AFDC program were and are automatically eligible for Medicaid. During the period from 1986 to 1990 Congress amended the Title XIX legislation so as to sever, or at least reduce, the linkage between Medicaid eligibility and AFDC eligibility. All states are now required to furnish Medicaid coverage to children up to 6 years of age in families with incomes at or below 133% of the federal poverty level and to phase in by the year 2001 coverage of all children up to age 19 below 100% of the poverty level.

This congressionally mandated expansion of Medicaid eligibility has led to a dramatic increase in Medicaid coverage of children. A 1995 American Academy of Pediatrics report stated that the percentage of all children through age 21 covered by Medicaid increased from 16.9% in 1990 to 20.1% in 1992.[4] This dramatic increase was due to Medicaid eligibility expansion begun in the mid 1980s. Medicaid has become by far the largest payor for health services for the poor in this country.[4] Children comprise one half to three quarters of all Medicaid recipients and account for about one fifth of all expenditures,[5] but existing data does not reveal what proportion of these expenditures go to children with special health care needs.

State Medicaid programs must provide reimbursement for certain types of services; such mandatory services include inpatient and outpatient hospital services, physician services, laboratory tests, and other primary services. States can choose to fund additional services; such optional services include prescription drugs, physical, occupational, and speech therapy, case management, and hospice, dental, and respiratory care.

States that participate in Medicaid must conduct an Early and Periodic Screening, Diagnosis, and Treatment (EPSDT) program for children under age 21. Recent amendments to the Medicaid legislation give the EPSDT program, at least in theory, the potential to provide a comprehensive process through which children are screened for disabilities and chronic illnesses, diagnosed, and provided with all the services necessary to treat their diagnosed conditions—whether or not those services are covered by their state Medicaid plan. Surveys reveal that the progress made by EPSDT programs in realizing this potential has been slow. In 1989 only 39% of eligible children participated in EPSDT in the average state.[5]

States increasingly rely on managed care to deliver health services to Medicaid beneficiaries. According to the Kaiser Family Foundation, nearly 8 million beneficiaries (of the 35 million served by Medicaid) now receive Medicaid services through health maintenance organizations (HMOs) and other less structured primary care case management systems.[6] These beneficiaries are predominantly poor children and their families. There are concerns that managed care organizations will not meet the needs of children who need complex and high cost health services, and it has sometimes proved difficult for managed care organizations and state Medicaid agencies to arrive at acceptable capitation rates for such services. Therefore some state Medicaid agencies have thus far avoided enrolling in managed care plans children with special health care needs.

Collaboration between the Medicaid program and other public health programs serving children is important to assure the effective and efficient delivery of health services to children, including children with special health care needs. To foster such collaboration state Medicaid agencies and state Title V agencies, administering the State CSHCN Programs, have entered into interagency agreements.[1] For example, there are a number of interagency agreements dealing with Medicaid reimbursement for services furnished to Medicaid eligible children by Title V supported institutions and organizations.

SUPPLEMENTAL SECURITY INCOME

Title XVI of the Social Security Act, enacted in 1972, created the Supplemental Security Income (SSI) Program for the Aged, Blind, and Disabled.* SSI provides cash benefits to low-income blind and disabled children as well as adults who meet the Social Security Act's definition of disability and income eligibility requirements.

SSI is a federal program administered by the Social Security Administration (SSA) and, like Medicaid, is an entitlement program. Table 4-1 summarizes federal SSI funding during the last 10 years. There traditionally has been a close relationship between the SSI program and the State CSHCN Programs. In 1976 Congress established the SSI/Disabled Children's Program through amendment of the SSI legislation. This amendment required SSI recipients under age 16 to be referred to the State Crippled Children's Services Programs (State Programs for CSHCN) for counseling, for the establishment of individual service plans, and for referrals to other agencies for needed services and for monitoring of compliance with individual ser-

---

*Social Security Act (Title XVI), Supplemental Security Income for Aged, Blind and Disabled, 42 U.S.C. §§1382-1383(d) (1988 & Supp V 1994).

vice plans. In addition, the state programs were directed to provide medical, social, developmental, and rehabilitative services for children under age 7 and for children, age 7 and over, who had never attended school. This latter group of children were to receive the listed services in order to enhance their ability to benefit from education and training.

There is also a strong link between SSI program eligibility and Medicaid eligibility. In most states children determined to be eligible for SSI benefits are eligible for Medicaid benefits. In short the SSI program is of significance to children with special health care needs not only because it may furnish them with needed financial assistance but also because it may enable them to obtain needed health services.

Determining for the purpose of SSI eligibility whether a child is disabled has been a continuing problem and has generated controversy. In a 1990 decision, *Sullivan v. Zebley,*[11] the United States Supreme Court ruled that the process used by SSA for determining disability of children violated the Social Security Act because children were subject to a more restrictive standard than adults and did not receive the same kind of individual assessment that adults received. In response to Zebley SSA issued new regulations under which children applying for SSI receive individual functional assessments of how their claimed impairment limits their ability to act and behave in an age-appropriate manner.

In the wake of expanded SSI eligibility criteria and outreach efforts by SSA, there was a large and rapid increase in the population of children receiving benefits under the SSI program. From 1989 to 1994 the number of SSI recipients who were children grew from 300,000 to 900,000, and the proportion of children making up the SSI recipient pool grew from 6.5% to 14.2%.[9] The growth in child SSI recipients and the corresponding growth in the cost of the program, together with widely publicized claims that fraud has contributed to children on the SSI rolls, has given rise to efforts to amend the SSI legislation so as to limit the eligibility of children for the SSI program.

PEDIATRIC AIDS PROGRAM

In 1987 Congress appropriated funds under the authority of the Public Health Service Act for the Pediatric AIDS Health Care Demonstration Program, which is now referred to as the Pediatric/Family HIV Health Care Demonstration Program. This program subsequently was incorporated into the HIV Health Care Program authorized by legislation known as the Ryan White Act.* This program was directed toward a relatively new population of children with

---

*Public Health Service Act (Title XXVI), HIV Health Care Services Program, 42 U.S.C. §§300ff-21-300ff-30 (Supp VI 1995).

special health care needs—children infected with human immunodeficiency virus (HIV) that produces acquired immunodeficiency syndrome (AIDS).

In the 1990s, the second decade of the American HIV epidemic, HIV infection has become a leading cause of morbidity and mortality among children. The vast majority, nearly 90%, of reported pediatric AIDS cases are attributable to perinatal transmission of the virus from an infected woman to her fetus or newborn.[2] It is estimated that between the years 1988 and 1992 there were 1000 to 2000 HIV-infected infants born annually and by 1995 there were more than 5500 reported AIDS cases of children under age 13.[2]

The Pediatric AIDS Program is administered by the Federal Maternal and Child Health Bureau. Table 4-1 lists the federal appropriations for this program. The Pediatric AIDS Program represents the federal government's principal effort to respond to the challenge posed by pediatric AIDS. The projects funded under the program have demonstrated effective ways to prevent HIV infection among children and to deliver family-centered, community-based, coordinated care for infants, children, adolescents, and their families affected by HIV/AIDS.[7] These projects provide comprehensive health services to children infected with HIV, have successfully integrated research findings into their actual clinical care, and provide social support for affected families. They stress the identification of HIV-positive pregnant women through outreach, counseling, and testing, which in turn enables better follow-up care. The projects also stress the link of families whose members have HIV infection or are at risk of HIV infection with other sources of prevention, health, and social support services.

EMERGENCY MEDICAL SERVICES FOR CHILDREN

In 1984 Congress created the Emergency Medical Services for Children (EMSC) Program under the Public Health Service Act.* The purpose of the EMSC program was to reduce morbidity and mortality among children by expanding and improving emergency transportation and medical services for children. This program is of particular relevance to children with special health care needs inasmuch as the emergency medical services reduce disability and chronic conditions among children. The creation of this program was a response to the fact that emergency medical service systems around the country had largely ignored the special needs of children in need of emergency treatment for trauma or acute illnesses. Not all emergency medical personnel had adequate training necessary to care for children and the special pediatric equipment necessary for this care was not widely available.

*Public Health Service Act, Preventive Health and Health Services Block Grant, Emergency Medical Services for Children, 42 U.S.C. §300w-9 (Supp V 1993).

The EMSC Program is jointly administered by the Federal Maternal and Child Health Bureau and the National Highway Traffic Safety Administration. Table 4-1 details the history of federal appropriations for this program.

In the last decade the EMSC Program has assisted 36 states, the District of Columbia, and Puerto Rico in incorporating pediatric components into their emergency medical systems.[5] During this period the program has also furnished support to two resource centers for information dissemination and technical assistance and consultation activities.

OTHER PROGRAMS

There are a host of other federal and federal-state health programs that serve children with special health care needs. Many of these programs have as their focus preventive and primary care for poor and low-income individuals, medically underserved individuals, or both. An example is the previously mentioned State Maternal and Child Health Programs authorized under the Title V MCH Block Grant. Another example is the community health centers and the migrant health centers authorized by the Public Health Service Act.* The former centers provide primary health care to medically underserved areas. The latter centers provide primary health care to migrant and seasonal farm workers. These centers provide immunizations and other care to children, including children with special health care needs.

There also are programs that target various categories of disadvantaged children and have a health component as well as other types of service components. An example is the Head Start Program authorized under the Community Services Act.† Head Start is a comprehensive child development program for preschool children from economically disadvantaged families. All Head Start programs have a health component. In 1972 Congress mandated that at least 10% of Head Start enrollees be children with disabilities, and in 1993 nearly 100,000 children enrolled in Head Start were identified as having disabilities.[10]

The United States Department of Health and Human Services is responsible for the administration of the community health centers, the migrant health centers, and Head Start. Within the Department of Health and Human Services, the Primary Health Care Bureau, which is part of the Public Health Service, administers the community health centers and the migrant health centers, and the Head Start Bureau, which is part of the Administration for Children and Families administers Head Start. Table 4-1 sets forth the federal appropriations for these programs during the last decade.

---

*Public Health Service Act, Primary Health Care, Primary Health Centers, 42 U.S.C. §§254b-254c (1988 & Supp V 1994).

†Community Services Act, Head Start Programs, 42 U.S.C. §§9831-9848 (1988 & Supp V 1994).

CONCLUSION

For more than half a century federal and federal-state health programs have been at the forefront of the improvement and expansion of health services for children with special health care needs. These programs have become an integral part of the health care infrastructure and they fund and provide many of the health services these children receive.

The American health care system is currently in flux, and both public and private health care sectors are being fundamentally restructured. Changes are being proposed and are actually taking place in federal and federal-state health programs serving children with special health care needs. In this environment it is of critical importance that the federal leadership role in the care of children with special health care needs be preserved.

REFERENCES

1. Association of Maternal and Child Health Programs: *State MCH-Medicaid coordination: a review of Title V and Title XIX interagency agreements,* Washington DC, 1992, The Association.
2. Centers for Disease Control, U.S. Public Health Services: Recommendations for human immunodeficiency virus counseling and voluntary testing for pregnant women, *Morbidity and Mortality Weekly Report* 44(7):2-3, 1995.
3. Feely HB and Athey JL: *Emergency medical services for children: 10 year report,* Arlington, VA, 1995, National Center for Education in Maternal and Child Health.
4. Fleming G: *The health insurance status of children: 1990 to 1992,* Elk Grove Village, Ill., 1993, American Academy of Pediatrics.
5. Hill IT: The role of medicaid and other government programs in providing medical care for children and pregnant women, *The Future of Children* 2(2): 134-153, 1992.
6. Kaiser Commission on the Future of Medicaid: *Medicaid and Managed Care* Policy brief, Washington DC, 1995, Kaiser Family Foundation.
7. National Pediatric HIV Resource Center: *Pediatric/family HIV health care demonstration grant program,* Newark, NJ, 1992, The Center.
8. Public Health Service, U.S. Department of Health and Human Services: *Healthy children 2000: national health promotion and disease prevention objectives,* Washington DC, 1991, Government Printing Office.
9. Ross JL, U.S. General Accounting Office: *Supplemental Security Income: recent growth in the rolls raises fundamental program concerns.* Testimony before the Subcommittee on Human Resources, Committee on Ways and Means, U.S. House of Representatives, Washington DC, January 27, 1995.
10. Stubbs PE: Personal communication, April 1993 and August 1995.
11. *Sullivan v. Zebley,* 493 US 521, 1991.

CHAPTER **5**

Overview of Health Care Financing for Children with Severe Developmental Disabilities

HERBERT J. COHEN
ARNOLD BIRENBAUM

Assuring the delivery of adequate health care in the United States and finding the best mechanisms to pay for it are issues of major national concern. Contributing to the current high level of interest are the recognition of the rapidly rising cost of health care, the large number of individuals who are now uninsured, and questions about what the dollars now being spent on health care are actually buying and why the current organization of health care results in a very uneven distribution of services. Compounding the problem are the increasing difficulties that Americans have paying for insurance coverage, the negative effect of rising health insurance costs on industry profits, and the escalating national debt to which the costs of Medicaid and Medicare are significant contributors. Because of cost shifting to pay for uncompensated care received by uninsured patients, the premiums for insurance increase at a rate above inflation. Medicaid costs escalate as individuals with special needs are denied private insurance and spend down their cash reserves so they can join the Medicaid system. However, despite the major national investment in health care, the U.S. lags embarrassingly behind many other countries in providing universal health care and has a relatively poor showing, as compared with other industrial countries, in its longevity figures and particularly in infant mortality statistics. Moreover, changes in labor-force participation in the United States have made it more likely that part-time workers will not have access to employer-based health insurance.[2] Families of children with severe developmental disabilities are caught in these national trends, as are all families.

RISING COSTS

In 1993 the U.S. spent $888.4 billion (13.9%) of its gross domestic product (GDP) on health care.[7] This compares to 1992 figures of 10.3% in Canada, 6.9% in Japan, and 7.1% in England.[13] If the current rate of increase continues, the U.S. will be spending 20% of its GDP on health care by the year 2000. However, current indications are that the rate of increase appears to be slowing somewhat. Figs. 5-1 and 5-2 illustrate the rapid rise in health care costs nationally and to American families.

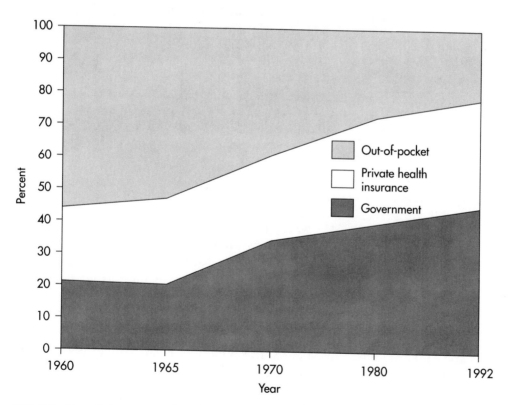

FIG. 5-1. Growth in personal health care expenditures by source of funds: selected CYs 1960 to 1992.

From Health Care Financing Administration: *Data from the Office of the Actuary and the Office of National Cost Estimators.*

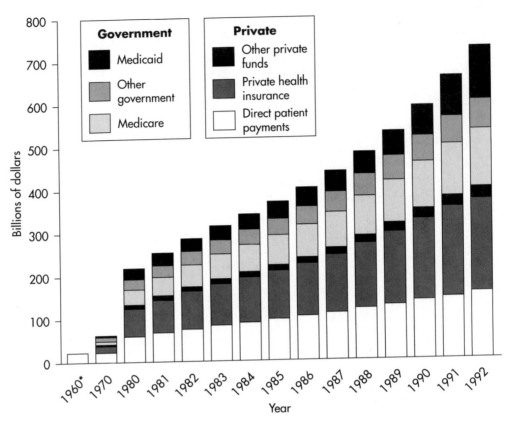

FIG. 5-2. Personal health care expenditures, by source of funds: CYs 1960 to 1992.

From Health Care Financing Administration: *Data from the Office of the Actuary and the Office of National Cost Estimators.*

Private health insurance costs have also been increasing rapidly, until recently at a rate of more than 20% per year. Costs for persons with severe disabilities can be more than $100,000 per year and can reach $1 million per year when a prolonged hospitalization and advanced life support systems are required. The cost of public programs are rising the fastest.[7] Medicaid and Medicare programs spent $272.1 billion for health care in 1993, which is 30.8% of all health care spending. According to the U.S. General Accounting Office the estimated total federal and state costs of Medicaid from 1991 to 1993 are as follows:

1991—$92.2 Billion

1992—127.2 Billion (34% increase)

1993—153+ Billion (20+ % increase)

THE UNINSURED

The U.S. Bureau of the Census estimated that 15.3% of all Americans were without health insurance.[14] Pearl[11] reported that a Census Bureau study of a 30-month period during 1990 to 1992 found that 25% of Americans were uninsured for at least one month and that among children 29% under age 18 were insured. Rowland et al[12] estimated that 51.3 million people— "one in five Americans"—were without health coverage for at least some period during 1993.

Similar patterns of deteriorating coverage exist for children and adolescents, presenting challenges to pediatricians and other health care providers.[9,10] The actual number of uninsured children has increased 30% in the last decade despite a 28.4% increase in the number of children, ages 0 to 6 years covered by Medicaid in the 1987 to 1990 period.[8] Past surveys have shown that among disabled children below the poverty level 63% are in public programs, 17.5% are in private plans, and 19.5% are uninsured.[4] The inadequacy or unavailability of prenatal care is striking, as well, in that 24.4% of U.S. women receive no prenatal care in the first trimester and 6.3% receive no prenatal care at all.

INADEQUACIES OF THE SYSTEM

A 1992 report from the Center for The Future of Children[5] of the David and Lucile Packard Foundation describes seven key weaknesses in the current system of care for children attending school. These could apply as well to all aspects of the health care system and especially to children with disabilities. The problems are fragmentation of care, excess specialization, complexity of the service delivery system, limited access, poor mechanisms for follow-up, and poor collaboration with other systems (e.g. health systems and schools). To this list could be added the following major problems: (1) there is a clear emphasis on reimbursing hospital costs and long-term care rather than outpatient services; (2) there are limited funds available for home care, especially for children; and (3) there are limited prevention expenditures for children.

Currently, 2% of the U.S. population uses 60% of all the health care dollars, with the cost of care for the chronically ill rising faster than other expenditures. Not only can families not afford to pay the costs of care for chronic illness, but they also face a circumstance in which there are tremendous variations in support for different conditions. For example, if one can access community residential and other care for the mentally retarded, it is often generously supported by public funds, but care for mental illness is less endowed.

Complicating matters further are the enormous variations in insurance coverage and even in public programs from state to state. Optional services that are used by children and adults with special needs are not uniformly paid for by Medicaid, a federal-state funded program. For example, in 1986 there was no Medicaid coverage for physical therapy in 28 states, for occupational therapy in 26 states, and for speech and language therapy in 21 states. Furthermore, coverage by private policies was enormously variable. This pattern has generally continued, and poor families can hardly afford to pay for these services out of pocket.

HEALTH CARE FINANCING STUDY FOR SEVERE DEVELOPMENTAL DISABILITY

Because of the concern about the adequacy of financing for children and young adults with severe developmental disabilities, three federal agencies provided support for a study[3] in which the two authors of this chapter participated. Components of the study focused on children with severe mental retardation and autism. This study collected data in 1985 and 1986 from a national sample of individuals under age 25 who were residing within 13 urban, suburban, and rural school districts in 9 states. Districts selected were a composite of the national population's socioeconomic status, ethnicity, and access to medical resources. The population studied included 308 individuals with autism and 326 with severe or profound mental retardation.

The study produced some interesting findings and noted several important contrasts concerning the costs of medical and health care, its financing, and the utilization of services. The highlights included the following:

1. At that time and within the group studied, only one of the children had expenditures in excess of $50,000, and very few reached the upper $20,000s.

2. For children with autism the average annual health care expenditure was about $1000 and $1700 for young adults as compared with the $414 average for all American children. The children with autism had an average of four physician visits annually, slightly above the national average for children. Hospitalizations accounted for one-third the health care expenditures among children with autism but for two-thirds among young adults.

3. For children and young adults with severe retardation the average expenditure on health care was about $4000, primarily related to costs resulting from the physical limitations in two thirds of the children. They averaged about 12 physician visits annually, falling to about 8 among young adults. Children were hospitalized about eight times the national rate for all children and young adults and about twice the national rate for their age peers.

4. For both groups studied there was little use of preventive or habilitative services, and consequently these services were but a tiny fraction of health care expenditures. For individuals whose primary physicians judged that they would benefit from physical or speech therapy, less than one quarter were receiving these interventions.

5. Inequities abounded in the financing of health care. Almost 20% of the parents of children with severe or profound mental retardation and 10% of the parents of autistic children had experienced refusals or limitations in the health insurance that they could buy for their child. In both disability groups about 15% of those with private insurance had policies that specifically excluded coverage for some of the child's health care. Some of the exclusions of families were from health maintenance organizations (HMOs), apparently based on concerns relating to the potential cost to the HMO of including a child with a severe disability on their roster.

6. The study group's samples of autistic individuals from higher-income families were twice as likely to be covered by private insurance than were severely or profoundly mentally retarded individuals. Seven percent of the autistic and 4% of the severely and profoundly mentally retarded surveyed had no insurance coverage. As a consequence, the percentage of the uninsured who did not visit a physician in the 12-month study period was three times higher than for insured individuals.

7. Only 60% of all children surveyed had routine dental examinations within the 12-month study period, a worse record than the average American child.

8. Income differences between the two groups of families were dramatically revealed when out-of-pocket expenses were compared. For families of autistic children the average out-of-pocket medical expenses were almost $1000, about 3% of family income, but very few families, about 2%, had medical expenses greater than 15% of their income. Families with a child who had severe or profound retardation typically spent almost $2000 out of pocket on medical expenses, an average of 7% of their income, but as many as 10% spent more than 15% of their total income. Medical debts over $2000 burdened 1% of the families with autistic children and 5% of the families with children who had severe or profound retardation. Additionally, mothers whose children with disabilities lived at home were less likely to work than those whose children were in residential care.

9. Families of children with severe mental retardation had average out-of-pocket medical expenses in excess of similar average expenditures for entire families sampled in the 1987 Health Care Utilization and Expenditure Survey. Out-of-pocket expenditures for health services for each autistic child followed were slightly less than half of the average for all

American families, including parents and children. There are also hidden costs for related services. These services include personal care expenses, travel costs for extra medical visits, and home modifications; and when they are added to direct medical care costs, the total family payments increased for the population with autism to 2.8 times the national average for health-related expenditures and 2.4 times for those with severe mental retardation. These related services are rarely covered in strict indemnification insurance policies or in HMOs. Yet these services support home-based family care for a child with a disability and reduce the need for costly long-term residential care outside of the home.

10. Health insurance coverage varied with the child and parent's ages, parents employment status, and location.

11. Children with disabilities were overrepresented on the public insurance rolls (e.g., Medicaid) disproportionately to their families' social class background. This was apparently due to their being excluded from private insurance and the tendency to spend down family assets to then qualify for relatively generous Medicaid coverage.

12. The inability of all young adults with severe or profound mental retardation and most adults with autism to engage in paid employment results in a substantial indirect cost that can be calculated in lifetime earnings foregone. Caring for dependent children and adults at home involves loss of economic opportunities via employment or self-employment. Defined as *opportunity costs*, these constitute a major indirect cost for the family. Because they are primary caretakers, mothers found holding a job poses special hardships. Current Labor Department Statistics found mothers with young children working full-time at a rate at least 12% higher than the rate for mothers of severely retarded children. Nationally, among mothers whose youngest child is between ages 6 and 13, 48% are in full-time paid employment and another 18% are in part-time employment. By contrast, mothers whose mentally retarded children are in residential placement are likely to be working full time and are not far below the national average of working mothers. The indirect costs in lost income due to mothers foregoing work are substantial. Finally, the paucity of support services for young adults in their parents' homes exacerbates the burden on the families. Fewer families used overnight respite care than placed their child in a permanent residence.

Third Party Coverage and the Uninsured

These last three summary statements (10, 11 and 12) require some amplification. Health insurance in the United States is very much tied to employment. It is common in the United States for both parents to be in the work force. Table 5-1 illustrates how, in the study population, the parents' employment status

TABLE 5-1. Private Health Insurance Coverage Among Individuals Living at Home

Characteristic	Percentage Covered	
	Autism N = 284	Severe Mental Retardation N = 254
PARENTS' WORK STATUS		
2 full-time	98%	90%
1 full-time	80	75
Part-time or unemployed	20	25
AGE		
Under 28 years	70	60
18-24	50	40
RACE		
White	70	60
Black	50	30

From Birenbaum A, Guyot D, and Cohen HJ: *Health care financing for severe developmental disabilities,* Washington, DC, 1990, American Association on Mental Retardation.

Note. Results are rounded for presentation.

related to the coverage of children and young adults living at home. When both parents had full-time employment, private health insurance covered almost 100% of the children with autism and almost 90% of the children with severe retardation. However, in families where only one parent was working full-time, the proportions for both disabilities dropped by approximately 15%. There is even more concern for the one fifth of the children whose parents had only part-time employment; roughly one third of these children had private coverage. About 20% had private insurance when no parent was employed.

Does the age of the disabled person make a difference? About 70% of children with autism had private insurance, whereas only about 50% of young adults were insured. A similar drop, from about 60% to about 40%, occurs between childhood and adulthood for people with severe mental retardation. This pattern is similar to the situation of all young adults in America, in that they age out of family insurance coverage and do not acquire their own insurance. For the study population the type of parental employment combined with minority group status strongly influences retarded African-American children and young adults covered by private health insurance, half the rate of whites. The difference for African-American children compared to white children did not change even when taking into account whether or not a parent was working full time and whether or not family income was above $15,000. Among children with autism, at least, racial disparity was not as pronounced. However, some strong regional differences emerged, with fewer children in the South covered by any insurance, compared with those in the northern and western states.

Medicaid is the most common public program serving these children with autism and severe mental retardation. Next in coverage is the Social Security Act's Title V program, Services for Children with Special Health Care Needs, formerly known as Crippled Children Services. Marked inequities exist in public coverage by place of residence. In states where there are restrictive financial eligibility rules for gaining access to Medicaid, fewer children have public health insurance coverage. Among the scattering of state and local programs, the one that is available to all children with autism and mental retardation is the Michigan family supplement of $225 per month for the parents to use as they choose.

Racial disparity in private insurance is generally compensated for by public coverage; minority families were the neediest of all those in the study population. For both white and black families Medicaid and other public programs bring coverage to more than 90% of children with autism and to more than 95% of children with severe mental retardation.

Discontinuity of insurance coverage for children is a serious problem when parents change jobs and move in and out of eligibility for Medicaid. Relying on parents' recall about events for the past 11 months, the authors found that roughly 5% of the study population lacked insurance for part of the year. However, because this question was only asked at one point in time, this result may be an underestimate.

Insurance coverage produces more physician contacts. Children without health insurance are likely to have fewer physician visits. About one quarter of the autistic children lacking insurance had no physician visits as did about 15% of the children with severe retardation.

HEALTH CARE FINANCING REFORM AND FAMILIES OF CHILDREN WITH SPECIAL HEALTH CARE NEEDS

In the current era of reform and cost containment and following the initial unsuccessful attempt by the Clinton administration to overhaul the health care payment system, families of children with special needs represent a vulnerable population. The first concern is whether existing coverage or benefits will be terminated or limited. The second problem is to eliminate financial barriers to care through affordable insurance for children with serious chronic illnesses or developmental disabilities. From an optimistic standpoint at least most proposed reforms recommend eliminating the exclusion for pre-existing conditions from any form of insurance coverage.

The next key issue is what shall be covered by insurance programs for children with special health care needs? While identified by experts on maternal and child health as a population requiring family-centered community-based services, we do not know if health care financing reform will reduce or increase the burden of expenses for families of children with severe developmental disabilities. Will families have the opportunity to choose plans that increase access to appropriate care at reasonable cost or will they encounter greater difficulties in obtaining specialized services for their children? This is of particular concern to families who are increasingly being forced into or solicited to join managed care systems. Most serious are the efforts by many states to reduce Medicaid costs by requiring that Medicaid recipients be enrolled in managed care systems. At least 15 states have submitted what are called *1115 Medicaid Waiver Requests* that will require managed care participation, though some "carve out" care for populations with special needs will be permitted so that access to special services may not be restricted.

What is known about the experiences of families with children with disabilities enrolled in cost-conscious HMOs? Reports on consumer experiences with HMOs for families of children with special needs are rare. Still, a recent survey of five HMOs serving state employees in two urban counties in Wisconsin found high levels of satisfaction based on good relationships with physicians and other providers, overall low costs, and reduced paperwork.[6] A few families had difficulties with HMOs in "...determining which specialty services were covered, obtaining and maintaining referral authorization for specialized services, and a lack of choice of specialty providers."[6] HMOs need to reinsure or enter into contractual arrangements with appropriate providers to manage the rare but costly specialty care required by children with special health care needs.

Central to satisfaction with services in the Wisconsin study was the establishment of a good relationship with the primary care physician. Referrals for specialty care were not a problem under this circumstance. The HMOs studied did not seem to ration care, nor did they have and established policy on standards of care for each serious chronic illness or disability. However, a primary care physician needed to provide case management for managed care to work. Future expansion of HMOs would need to take into account parents' views as to what constitutes good care and would need to investigate to what extent this matches up to professionally developed standards (e.g., monitoring and follow-up visits at a specialty care source; the provision of appropriate therapeutic services).

The American Academy of Pediatrics (AAP)[1] recommends physician-directed case management programs for seriously chronically ill or developmentally disabled children to attain coordination of specialty care, compatibility of drug therapies, and identification of families in need of counseling or health-education services. This AAP plan eliminates cost sharing for preventive care to encourage the use of periodic health monitoring and screening services. This type of managed care could control costs and provide needed services to vulnerable populations—so long as there is a strong emphasis on case management and on selection of appropriate therapeutic interventions based on the evidence of effectiveness and the assessments of assistance they may provide.

CONCLUSION

The system for delivering health care, in general and to children with special needs specifically appears to be at a critical juncture as the federal government, the states, employers, and advocates make proposals and try to reform the health care system and determine how health care will be paid for.

Children and adults with special health care needs, especially those with severe chronic disabilities, represent a vulnerable and more expensive population for whom to provide care. In the past this group of citizens has been discriminated against in private insurance systems and is also being excluded from HMOs or having their services rationed or limited in managed care systems. Persons with disabilities are overrepresented in public insurance programs, such as Medicaid, but are subjected to enormous variations from state-to-state in terms of eligibility for reimbursable therapeutic services. This is true not only for Medicaid but also for private insurance policies. The concerns about access to specialized services, especially for those eligible for Medicaid, have escalated with the growing number of states attempting to impose managed care membership on all persons on the Medicaid rolls. Capitated rates are likely to lead to rationing of specialty services except when these have been categorically excluded from the capitation requirements.

In addition, the social consequences of lack of access are important; we must consider the stress and other possible adverse effects of inadequate healthcare financing on families of children and young adults with special health care needs. The vulnerability of these families to dissolution will likely be enhanced by the financial strain. Therefore, assisting families with non-medical expenditures and permitting caretaking members to avoid opportunity costs appears to be as important a policy goal as access to services. A full analysis of what it means financially to care for a children with severe or profound handicaps within the home requires paying attention to these hidden costs. We propose that (a) personal care and family support are necessary related services that should be included in health care requirements, (b) family-centered care should be promoted, (c) appropriate programs and care should be provided for young adults no longer in school, (d) financing and organizing of family supports and subsidies should be administratively simple, (e) Medicaid should be expanded to increase use of home- and community-based services, and (f) direct financial support should be provided to needy families. The current proposals to limit SSI payments run counter to what is required to support families in their attempts to keep a child with disabilities at home.

Future health care delivery must guarantee equal and easy access to primary care and to a reasonable range of specialty and support services for all persons with disabilities. If services must be limited in some manner, then this should not be based on who the person is or what is the nature of his or her disability may be, but rather on a determination of whether or not the intervention is effective.

REFERENCES

1. American Academy of Pediatrics' Committee on Child Health Financing: Financing health care for the medically indigent child, *Pediatrics* 80:957-960, 1987.
2. Birenbaum A: *Putting health care on the national agenda*, Westport, Conn., 1993, Praeger Publishing.
3. Birenbaum A, Guyot D, and Cohen HJ: *Health care financing for severe developmental disabilities*, Washington, DC, 1990, American Association on Mental Retardation.
4. Cartland J: More children on Medicaid, but uninsured problems still growing, *American Academy of Pediatrics Child Health Financing Report* 10(3):4, 1993.
5. Center for the Future of Children: U.S. health care for children, *The Future of Children 2*, 1992.
6. Karson TA, Sumi MD, and Braucht SA: *The impact of health maintenance organizations on accessibility, satisfaction and cost of health care for children with special needs*, Madison, Wis., 1990, Center for Health Systems Research and Analysis and Center for Public Representation.
7. Levit KR et al: National health expenditures. In Cooper BS, editor: *Health Care Financing: Review* 16(1):247-294, Baltimore, 1993, U.S. Government Printing Office.
8. McManus MA and Newacheck P: Health insurance differentials among minority children with chronic conditions and the role of federal agencies and private foundations in improving financial access, *Pediatrics* 91:1040-1047, 1993.
9. Newacheck PW, McManus MA, and Gephart JJ: Health insurance coverage of adolescents: a current profile and assessment of the trends, *Pediatrics* 90:589-596, 1992.
10. Oberg CN: Medically uninsured children in the United States: a challenge to public policy, *Pediatrics* 85:824-833, 1990.
11. Pear R: Gaps in coverage for health care, *New York Times*, D23, March 29, 1994.
12. Rowland D et al: Update: a profile of the uninsured in America, *Health Affairs* 13Spring II:283-302, 1994.
13. Schieber GJ, Poullier J, and Greenwald LM: Data watch: health system performance in OECD countries, 1980-1992, *Health Affairs* Fall:100-112 1994.
14. U.S. Bureau of the Census: *Persons without health insurance, by state.* Pub No 170, Washington, DC, 1995, U.S. Government Printing Office.

PART TWO

FUTURE DIRECTIONS

The development of community-based systems of services for children with special health care needs and their families that are comprehensive, coordinated, family-centered, and culturally competent is now a widely accepted national goal. The subject of the three chapters in Part Two is future directions of services for special-needs children and their families in light of this national goal.

Chapter 6 discusses what is being done to achieve the national goal of community-based systems of services for special needs children and their families with particular emphasis on the health component of such systems. It then discusses the development of community-based systems of services given the dramatic growth of managed care organizations and integrated health systems that are fundamentally altering the delivery and financing of health services.

Chapter 7 builds upon the preceding chapter by exploring the crisis that is occurring in the allocation of health resources because of the ever increasing costs of health services and responses to this crisis. It specifically explores prioritization—that is the allocation of scarce health care resources using established criteria in a visible, explicit process—and its effect on children with special needs.

Chapter 8 explains the important role that the federal government historically has played in improving the care and status of children with special health care needs through numerous federally funded programs. It further explains that it is unclear whether the federal government will continue to play this role because of efforts to limit federal spending and to shift responsibility for programs affecting these children and their families to states and localities.

CHAPTER 6

Future Directions of Community-Based Service Systems for Children with Special Health Care Needs and Their Families

JOHN C. MACQUEEN
JOSEPHINE GITTLER

There is an emerging consensus calling for the development of community-based systems of services for children with special health care needs and their families. Systems development entails the creation of organizational infrastructures at the community level for the delivery of health services and other types of services to these children and their families, and the systems to be developed should provide community-based, comprehensive, coordinated, family-centered, and culturally competent services.[5,7,10]

The Office of the U.S. Surgeon General and the Federal Maternal and Child Health Bureau proclaimed development of such systems of services a national goal in the late 1980s.[5,7,11] Subsequently, the U.S. Public Health Service's national health promotion and disease prevention objectives for the year 2000 called for such systems development.[10]

This chapter presents an overview of why systems development has become a national goal, what must be done to achieve this goal, and what effect governmental health care reforms and market-driven reforms may have on efforts to achieve this goal. In particular, this chapter focuses on future directions of the health component of community-based service systems.

POPULATION IN NEED OF SERVICES AND SERVICES NEEDED

Systems of health services and other services must be developed for a broad population of children with special health care needs. Children with special health care needs have been defined as children who have health problems requiring something beyond routine or basic care. More specifically they are children who require specialty and subspecialty medical services and other specialized health services.

Traditionally the population of children with special health care needs has been composed of children with physical disabilities that limit ability to function. Over time it was realized that the ability of children to function also could be limited by a chronic or recurring systemic illness not necessarily resulting in a physical disability. Another segment of the population of special-needs children that increasingly has received recognition is children with "new morbidity" problems, which include health-related developmental, learning, and behavioral problems. Although a great deal of progress has been made in the provision of health services to children with disabilities and chronic illnesses, most health care professionals have not been heavily involved in serving children with the "new morbidity" kinds of problems.

The population of children with special health care needs has evolved and will continue to evolve. Medical science and technology has a large effect on the nature and extent of this population. Advances in medical science and technology (e.g., vaccines for diseases like poliomyelitis) have eliminated or substantially reduced some child health problems requiring specialized health services. Such advances also have made possible the survival of children with once-fatal congenital anomalies, illnesses, and injuries. However, some of these children who survive need long-term specialized health services.

It is difficult to generalize about the health service needs of children with special health care needs. The health services sector has steadily expanded its focus to encompass not only a child's physical status but also a child's cognitive, emotional, and social status. Consequently, the parameters of the health care system, as opposed to the parameters of other systems, (e.g., the educational system, the mental health system, and the social services system), have become increasingly blurred. The population of children with special health care needs is heterogeneous and includes children with many different health problems, and even children with the same medical diagnosis may vary widely in their health care needs.

Nevertheless, it is clear that children with special health care needs, as a group, should have available and accessible a continuum of health care, consisting of different *levels* of care that reflect different degrees of specialization of physicians and other health professionals. These levels of care are the following: 1) primary care, consisting of basic health services for routine health problems and medical monitoring and management of complex/unusual health problems; 2) secondary care, consisting of specialized consultant and direct services for unusual/complex problems; and 3) tertiary care, consisting of highly specialized consultant and direct services for unusual/complex problems.

Children with special health care needs, as a group, also should have available and accessible a continuum of health care consisting of different *types* of health services. By definition this population of children needs specialized health services and health-related habilitation and rehabilitation services. As with the population of children as a whole, this population of children also needs health services for acute illnesses, primary health care, and health promotion activities.

ORGANIZATION OF NEEDED SERVICES
Centralization of Care and Tertiary Children's Hospitals

Specialized health services for children have been highly centralized in tertiary level children's hospitals, which are often located within university-affiliated medical centers and health science centers. When a primary care physician identifies a child as having or being at risk for a health problem requiring specialty or subspecialty medical care, the physician typically refers the child to such a hospital.

The last several decades have witnessed a tremendous expansion in large tertiary centers. This expansion is intertwined with the ever-increasing specialization of physicians and the ever-increasing sophistication of health services.

Although the importance of large tertiary medical centers in providing high-quality and up-to-date medical care to children with special health care needs cannot be over stressed, the predominance of such centers in care of these children is not without drawbacks. These centers are relatively few in number and are usually located in large urban areas. Children living in communities where these centers are located have ready access to the excellent care that they provide. However, there are a significant number of children whose home communities are quite far from these centers, and it is not unusual for a child to receive care at a center and then to return home to a community some distance from the center.

In some cases where the child's home community is distant from the tertiary medical center, the child and the child's family must travel to the center for follow-up care. They may find it difficult to comply with a frequent appointment schedule. Even if they are able to comply, the travel required can be disruptive, create hardships, and at the very least be inconvenient. Moreover, the child's family must bear the cost of transportation, and family members accompanying the child can incur loss of income because of absence from work. In addition, the child and the child's family may experience insecurity because of a fear that the child, while at home, may need care for an emergency or some other event related to the chronic condition or disability.

In other cases where the child's home community is distant from the tertiary medical center, the child is referred back to a community physician or other community professional for follow-up care. This distance can produce difficulties in the transfer of information related to the child's special health care needs from the tertiary center to the community physician and other community health professionals. This distance also can produce difficulties in the transfer of information related to the child's primary health needs, care coordination needs, and community service needs from community health professionals to the center.

Community-Based Secondary and Primary Care

The development of tertiary care in large medical centers and health science centers has received a great deal of attention, but the development of community-based secondary level care, which can and should be provided by community physicians and other community health professionals, has received relatively little attention. Some children with specialized health needs should be referred to a tertiary center for a complete evaluation and then receive ongoing, long-term secondary level services in their home communities. Other children have specialized health needs that can and should be met through the provision of secondary level care in the community and do not necessarily have to be referred to a tertiary center. It must be emphasized that standards for the provision of quality secondary care must be formulated, that community physicians and other community health professionals must receive the education and training required for the provision of such secondary care, and that mechanisms must be established to facilitate communication between tertiary medical centers and community physicians and other community health professionals providing secondary care.

Children with special health care needs require primary level care as well as tertiary and secondary level care. Unfortunately, the primary care needs of these children are often neglected. Many children with special health care needs, particularly low-income children in urban areas, do not have access to private sector primary care. These children receive primary care, if at all, largely in public health clinics. These clinics have limited resources and frequently have difficulty in providing children with personalized care, continuity of care, and extensive care coordination.

The population of children with special health care needs should receive primary care in the private sector from pediatricians and to a lesser extent from family practitioners. The American Academy of Pediatrics has long advocated that every child should have a "medical home." This means that a child with special health care needs should have a personal physician who provides comprehensive primary care to the child, who coordinates the child's medical care, and who provides day-to-day monitoring and management of the child's medical condition. However, community pediatricians often are reluctant to assume the responsibility for children with major special health care needs because of a lack of education and training that prepares them for this role, lack of strong linkages with tertiary medical centers, lack of reimbursement for primary care and care coordination commensurate with the time and effort involved, and lack of mechanisms for coordination with other community service providers.

Linkages Between Tertiary, Secondary, and Primary Care Providers

To create a continuum of health care consisting of different types of health services and different levels of care for children with special health care needs, strong links must be forged between the medical centers providing tertiary health care and other facilities and individuals that are providing or may provide secondary and primary care. These may include public health programs, regional and community hospitals, private sector community physicians, early intervention programs, and special education programs in the public schools and voluntary agencies.

In fact, programs that incorporate such a continuum of care are becoming more common. Under these programs the medical center physician and other members of the center's health care team are responsible for evaluating the child, formulating a plan for specialized health services that normally includes the establishment of a protocol for the provision of these services, and identifying the follow-up care to be furnished by a community physician. The community physician is responsible for monitoring the child's response to medical treatment and providing day-to-day medical management of the case. Communication between medical center personnel and the community physician is as frequent as necessary to ensure that the care plan is effectively carried out. Such arrangements decrease the number of follow-up visits the child must make to the medical center and thereby decrease the costs and inconvenience associated with these visits for the child and his or her family.

Coordination of Health Services and Other Types of Services

Children with special health care needs and their families often may have multiple service needs that extend beyond health services, including early intervention services, special education, vocational rehabilitation, social services, mental health services, and family support services. They usually receive services from different service providers affiliated with different agencies, institutions, and organizations in different service sectors. Many public and private providers serving these children and their families have overlapping or inconsistent mandates, eligibility requirements, policies, and practices. This leads to gaps and duplications in services for these children and families and makes it difficult for them to obtain comprehensive and coordinated services. Hence the call for the establishment, expansion, and upgrading of community-based service systems—organizational infrastructures at the community level for the delivery of health services and other types of services in a coordinated manner.

Community Plan of Services and Case Management

The prevailing pattern has been for the community service providers with whom a child and family comes into contact to create their own care plan. It is not unusual for a community service provider to have little or no information about the care plans of other service providers and for these plans not to be compatible. This situation is compounded by the fact that if a family receives services from multiple providers, the family may have to deal with multiple case managers whose function it is to implement different care plans. Therefore, a key to the provision of comprehensive, coordinated services is the development of a community plan of services for a child and his or her family by community health service providers and other community providers of services and the implementation of the plan by an identified community service team, one of whom functions as a case manager.

Table 6-1 summarizes the elements of the health component of the community-based system of services discussed in the preceding pages. It indicates what services are to be provided, who is to provide the services, where services are to be provided, and how services are to be provided.

However, there are many different models for community-based service delivery systems involving collaboration between providers of health services and involving collaboration between the health service sector and other service sectors at both community and state levels.[12] The community-based service systems actually developed will vary from community to community within a particular state, and they will vary from state to state because of differences between communities and states with respect to their service system needs and resources.

EFFECT OF HEALTH CARE REFORMS ON SYSTEMS DEVELOPMENT

In the future the organization of the health component of community-based service systems will be shaped, if not determined, by health care reform efforts. These reforms can be characterized as governmental reforms and market-driven reforms.

TABLE 6-1. Health Component of System of Services for Children with Special Health Needs

	Level I (primary)	Level II (secondary)	Level III (tertiary)
What services are provided	• Health promotion activities and preventive services • Services for routine problems • Ongoing monitoring/management of non-routine problems • Family/child education and counseling • Case management • Family support services	• Specialized/complex services • Consultation • Family/child education and counseling • Development of community service plan • Education and training for Level I and Level II health care providers and other community service providers	• Highly specialized/complex services • Consultation • Family/child education and counseling • Development of hospital discharge plan • Development of innovative care programs • Education and training for health care providers at all levels and for other professionals • Clinical research
Who provides services	• Primary care physicians including pediatricians and family practitioners • Other primary health care providers • Providers of home health care services • School personnel • Child's family	• Specialty physicians, including pediatricians with special interest practice • Other specialty health care providers	• Subspecialty and specialty physicians • Hospital-based health care providers and support personnel
Where services are provided	• Offices of physicians and other health care providers • Local public health units and clinics • Community hospitals (Emergency rooms) • Child's school • Child's home	• Regional/district specialty centers and clinics • Regional/community hospitals • Regional/district special education agencies	• Academic medical centers • Academic health centers • Children's hospitals
How services are provided	• By community team in or near child's home community in accordance with community service plan	• By regional/district interdisciplinary team	• By medical health center or hospital interdisciplinary team in centralized fashion as determined by child's hospital record

From MacQueen JC: Health component of community-based service systems in U.S. public health service. In *Developing community-based systems of services for children and their families: an overview*, Iowa City, Ia, 1991, National Maternal and Child Health Resource Center.

Note: Facilities may sometimes be the site for more than one level of care.

Governmental Reforms

Recent federal and state health reform legislation and legislative proposals are primarily a response to two related but distinct problems. One problem is the lack of universal coverage—that is, a sizeable proportion of the American population, including children with special health care needs, has either no health insurance or inadequate health insurance. The other problem is the inflation in health care costs—that is, the large and persistent increases in expenditures for health services for Americans, including services for children with special health care needs. Both of these problems are especially significant for children with special health care needs because they frequently require high-cost services over a considerable period of time.

In 1993 the Clinton administration submitted a sweeping health care reform proposal to Congress, which in turn generated numerous proposals by congressional committees and individual members of Congress. None of these proposals were enacted, and the prospects for comprehensive, as opposed to incremental, federal health care reform are not good, at least in the short term. However, health care reform legislation has been enacted in some states, and state reform efforts may accelerate because of the failure of comprehensive federal reform efforts.

Market-Driven Reforms and Growth of Managed Care

While debates raged over federal and state health reform legislation, reforms in the health care marketplace were fundamentally transforming American health care. These market-driven reforms are the product of the economics of the health care marketplace and the drive to contain health care costs by those who actually pay for health services.

To understand market driven reforms it is necessary to understand traditional health care financing methods. The most important source of payments for health services is the "third party" arrangement under which a party other than the patient pays for the services. For example, Blue Cross and Blue Shield plans and commercial insurers are private, third-party payers, and the Title XIX Medical Assistance (Medicaid) program and the Medicare program are public third-party payers. Historically most health insurance plans, called indemnity insurance plans, have allowed patients freedom of choice of provider and have reimbursed providers retrospectively on an undiscounted fee-for-service basis.

However, market-driven reforms have led to the growth of managed care organizations. Managed care has been defined as: "Health care systems that integrate the financing and delivery of appropriate health care services to covered individuals by arrangement with selected providers to furnish a comprehensive set of health care services."[6]

A confusing alphabet soup of acronyms is used to describe different types of managed care organizations (MCOs). The best known and most prevalent types of MCOs include the health maintenance organization (HMO), the preferred provider organization (PPO), and the point of service (POS) plan. The box on p. 66 describes different types of MCOs.

Although the hallmark of the first generation of market-driven reforms is the growth of managed care organizations, the hallmark of the second generation is a wave of mergers, acquisitions, and consolidations, involving physician group practices, hospitals, and managed care organizations. This has facilitated and led to the emergence of organizational entities for health care delivery and financing, variously known as integrated delivery systems, integrated health systems, and organized systems of care.

These organizational entities are vertically integrated as well as horizontally integrated, and they provide a full spectrum of health services ranging from ambulatory services by physicians and other health professionals to inpatient hospital services and from preventive and primary care to tertiary care.[2] Some experts anticipate that a limited number of such organizational entities eventually will be an exclusive or primary source of health services to most of the population within a given geographic area.

Managed care plans and integrated health systems are rapidly becoming the dominant mode for the delivery and financing of health services. In 1994 two thirds of individuals with employment-based private insurance benefits were enrolled in an HMO or some other type of managed care plan, and during the period 1983 to 1994 enrollments in HMOs alone increased from 12.5 million to 50 million.[13] There likewise has been a dramatic rise in the enrollment of publicly insured individuals in managed care plans under the Title XIX Medical Assistance (Medicaid) Program. Since 1985 an estimated increase of 200% in the number of Medicaid recipients enrolled in managed care plans has occurred.[9]

The enrollment of children with special health care needs in managed care plans and integrated health systems is increasing. A recent study, based on 1992 data from the National Health Interview Survey, indicates that a significant number of such children are enrolled in HMOs.[3] Moreover, the study found that most children in HMOs are more likely than children in indemnity plans to have a limitation in a major activity. Table 6-2 sets forth the number of selected reported chronic conditions among children enrolled in indemnity plans and in HMO plans.

Managed Care and Development of Community-Based Service Systems

It remains to be seen what the impact of changes in the delivery and financing of health service will be on the development of community-based systems

Forms of Managed Care

Health Maintenance Organization (HMO)

A managed care plan that provides a wide range of comprehensive health care services to an enrolled population of patients for a fixed periodic payment (called a *capitation rate*). In addition to the four key elements of managed care plans enumerated above, HMOs typically employ some form of capitation payment to providers and provider risk sharing, and many deliver care through integrated medical facilities.

Four models of HMOs have been identified
1. Staff model HMOs provide services directly through physicians who are salaried employees of the plan.
2. Group model HMOs contract with an independent group of practitioners to provide services.
3. Network HMOs contract with two or more group practices. Under both the group and network models, physicians may be paid on a fee-for-service, salaried, or capitated basis.
4. Independent practice association (IPA) HMOs contract directly with individual physicians in private practice. Physicians are paid on either a discounted fee-for-service or capitation basis.

Preferred provider organization (PPO)

An arrangement by an insurer to provide medical services through a panel of preferred providers who contract to deliver services at lower-than-usual fees in exchange for prompt payment and a certain volume of patients. The PPO usually also provides some utilization review services. Enrollees are not restricted to the panel of providers but incur lower out-of-pocket costs if they use participating providers.

Point-of-service (POS) plan

Combines characteristics of both HMOs and PPOs to balance cost control with freedom of choice. Enrollees select a primary care physician gatekeeper from a network of physicians contracted to the plan. The cost to the enrollee for care provided by a network provider is very low or nothing. Enrollees may obtain care from out-of-plan providers but with significantly higher cost sharing.

Primary care case management (PCCM)

A form of managed care for Medicaid enrollees under which a specific person or agency (typically a clinic), called a gatekeeper, is responsible for coordinating the medical care of an enrollee and for arranging for necessary referrals to consultants, hospitals, or special services. Prior approval of the gatekeeper for specialty or hospital care is typically required except in true life-or-death emergencies.

Single service or targeted managed care

Managed care applied to specific services, such as mental health and substance abuse services, prescription drugs, and dental care. Plans may include utilization review, networks with gatekeepers, case management services, and discounted prices from network providers.

From Freund DA, Lewit EM: Managed care for pregnant women: promises and pitfalls, *The Future of Children* 3:92-122, 1993.

Table 6-2. Selected Chronic Conditions per Thousand Persons Under 18 in Indemnity Plans and HMO Plans

Type of Chronic Conditions	Indemnity	HMO
Selected skin and musculoskeletal conditions		
Arthritis	1.7	1.8
Selected impairments		
Visual impairment	9.5	4.3
Hearing impairment	13.4	8.0
Speech impairment	17.6	16.0
Orthopedic impairment/deformity	36.9	35.3
Selected conditions of the genitourinary, nervous, endocrine, metabolic or blood systems		
Diabetes	—	2.0
Epilepsy	2.0	1.5
Selected heart conditions		
Heart rhythm disorders	14.2	10.2
Congenital heart disease	1.6	4.5
Other heart disease	1.6	3.0
Selected respiratory conditions		
Chronic bronchitis	65.1	53.8
Asthma	58.9	67.0

From National Health Interview Survey (NHIS), 1992, Insurance Supplement; Fama T, Fox PD and White LA: Do HMOs care for the chronically ill? *Health Affairs* 14:234, 238-239, 1995.

of services for children with special health care needs. Managed care plans and integrated health systems have some features that incorporate essential elements of the health component of community-based service systems for this population, but they have other features that are problematic in terms of these essential elements.

It has been pointed out that these service systems should offer a continuum of different levels of health care, including community-based primary care. It also has been pointed out that a child should have a primary care physician, in or near the child's home community, who coordinates the child's medical care and provides day-to-day monitoring and management of the child's medical condition.

Managed care plans and integrated health systems do in fact place priority on the provision of primary care to enrollees. Such plans and systems employ primary care physicians, who are responsible for direct provision of patient care, and who, together with nonphysician case managers, are responsible for the coordination of overall patient care. Because such plans and systems generally have service sites in or near the home communities of their enrollees, delivery of this care can be characterized as community based.

However, as stated earlier, community-based service systems should offer a continuum of health services that consist of secondary and tertiary level care as well as primary care. This care includes specialty and subspecialty physician services and inpatient hospital services. Managed care organizations and integrated delivery systems have in common financial incentives and utilization management features aimed at reducing the costs of services provided by reducing utilization of services, particularly high-cost specialty and subspecialty physician services and inpatient hospital services. The box on p. 69 summarizes these financial incentives and utilization management features.

These financial incentives and utilization controls have given rise to concerns that children with special health care needs may encounter barriers and impediments to necessary and appropriate secondary and tertiary level care.[1,4,8] The validity of these concerns is unclear. There is a paucity of systematic empirical studies about the effect of these features on children with special health care needs. In addition, generalizations are suspect because of differences in the structure, operations, and quality assurance and grievance mechanisms of managed care organizations and integrated delivery systems.

Another distinct problem is the continued vitality of university-affiliated medical and health science centers in view of the growth of managed care organizations and integrated health systems. These centers are the source of much of the specialized health care that children with special health care needs receive and that is unavailable elsewhere. Equally important, these centers have been the source of research leading to advances in medical science and technology and innovations in health care delivery that have benefited these children. Yet in a more cost-conscious health care environment, in which managed care organizations and integrated health systems dominate, the survival of these high-cost centers, at least in their present form, is questionable.

As stated earlier, the health component of services systems for children with special health care needs should offer a continuum of different types of health and health-related services. There are concerns that managed care organizations and integrated delivery systems will not offer benefits packages that are comprehensive enough for children with special health needs, because they either do not cover or furnish only limited coverage of certain types of services, such as habilitation and rehabilitation services.

Finally, as stated earlier, in service systems for children with special health care needs there must be organizational infrastructures at the community level for the delivery of not only health services but also early intervention, educational, vocational services, mental health, social, and family support services in a coordinated manner. Here again there are concerns, namely

Financial Incentives and Utilization Management

FINANCIAL INCENTIVES

Capitation

An all-inclusive payment to a physician or hospital to provide all specified health care services to an enrollee during a designated period of time. Places most of the financial risk for utilization on the provider.

Discounted charges and fee schedules

Managed care plans use their purchasing power to negotiate fee schedules or percent discounts from contracted providers' usual charges for services provided to enrollees.

Performance incentives

Financial incentives paid to physicians to encourage cost savings which may include allowing physicians to keep the difference between the capitation rate and actual patient costs, a return of an amount withheld from fee-for-service reimbursement to cover potential cost overruns, and/or a bonus or share in the profit of the organization.

UTILIZATION MANAGEMENT

Precertification, concurrent review, and discharge planning

Programs designed to reduce the use of inpatient services by requiring a review of the reasons for an elective admission prior to the admission (precertification), monitoring the progress of the patient after admission (concurrent review), and providing for the expeditious discharge of the patient (discharge planning).

Gatekeeper (case management)

Typically a primary care physician whose role is to refer and authorize payment for specialty, emergency, and hospital care, and other special services.

Preauthorization

A procedure that requires permission from the insurer or gatekeeper physician before a patient can use a service (specialist referral, emergency room visit, hospital admission) for which the plan will pay.

Physician practice profiles

Profiles of individual physicians' practice patterns created from claims data, which may be used by plan medical directors to "educate" providers with divergent patterns and by plans to purge from their networks physicians who appear to deliver poor quality or excessively expensive care.

High-cost case management

Coordination of health care and sometimes other support services from a variety of providers for individuals with complex and lengthy or chronic illnesses. Used to facilitate cost-effective care; may facilitate home care and reduce overall costs of expensive illnesses.

From Freund DA, Lewit EM: Managed care for pregnant women: promises and pitfalls, *The Future of Children*, 3:92-122, 1993.

whether managed care organizations and integrated delivery systems have the capacity and interest in participating in the establishment and maintenance of such infrastructures.

CONCLUSION

Some progress has been made in achieving the national goal of developing community-based systems of comprehensive, coordinated, family-centered, culturally competent services for children with special health care needs and their families, but much remains to be done. The organization of the health component of such systems, which provides a continuum of health services with strong linkages between providers of health services and with coordinated provision of needed health services and other types of services, presents very real challenges in the context of the large and rapid restructuring of the delivery and financing of health care that can be seen in the growth of managed care organizations and the emergence of integrated delivery systems.

A focus and locus for the organization of the health component of community-based service systems is essential. Public health programs, by virtue of their mandates, experience, and resources, are better positioned and equipped than private health providers to assume a leadership role in organizing the health component of community-based service systems. It is therefore significant that 1989 amendments to the Federal Maternal and Child Health Block Grant legislation redefined the mission of the State Programs for Children with Special Health Care Needs, to encompass this role. Other public programs must assume a leadership role in organizing other components of community-based systems of services.

REFERENCES

1. Berman S, Gross RD, Lewak N, editors: *A Pediatrician's guide to managed care*, Elk Grove Village, Ill, 1995, American Academy of Pediatrics.
2. Boland P, editor: Organized delivery systems, *Managed Care Quarterly* 2:1-49, 1994.
3. Fama T, Fox PD, and White LA: Do HMOs care for the chronically ill? *Health Affairs* 14:234-243, 1995.
4. Freund DA, Lewit EM: Managed care for children and pregnant women: promises and pitfalls, *The Future of Children* 3(91):109-111, 1993.
5. Gittler J: *Community-based service systems for children with special health care needs and their families*. U.S. Surgeon General's Conference, Campaign '88, Iowa City, Ia, 1988, National Maternal and Child Health Resource Center.
6. Health Insurance Association of America (HIAA): Source book of health insurance data, Washington, DC, 1990, The Association.
7. National Maternal and Child Health Resource Center: *A National goal: building service delivery systems for children with special health care needs and their families, family centered, community-based, coordinated care*, Iowa City, Ia, 1989, National Maternal and Child Health Resource Center.
8. Newcheck DW et al: Children with chronic illness and Medicaid managed care, *Pediatrics* 93:497-500, 1994.
9. US General Accounting Office: States turn to managed care to improve access and control costs, 1993, Washington, DC.
10. U.S. Public Health Service: Healthy people, national health promotion and disease prevention objectives, Washington, DC, 1990, U.S. Government Printing Office.
11. U.S. Public Health Service: Surgeon general's report, children with special health care needs, Campaign '87. Washington, DC, 1987, U.S. Government Printing Office.
12. U.S. Public Health Service, Maternal and Child Health Bureau, Division of Services for Children With Special Health Needs, Maternal and Child Health Bureau: Developing community-based systems of services for children with special health needs and their families: an overview, National Maternal and Child Health Resource Center, 1991, Iowa City, Ia.
13. While Congress remains silent, health care transforms itself, *New York Times*, p 1,24, December 18, 1994.

CHAPTER 7

Allocation of Health Care Resources

TINA CIESIEL KITCHIN

Health care costs have skyrocketed. In the past decade national health expenditures have more than doubled from $249 billion in 1980 to $671 billion in 1990—an annual rate of increase of 10.4%.[6] Health care is consuming a greater percentage of resources. The health care portion of the gross national product increased from 9.1% in 1980 to 12.2% in 1990.[6] States spent 10% of their budgets on Medicaid in 1985, 14% of their budgets in 1990, and are projected to spend 22% of their budgets in 1995.[3] Private health insurance premiums for large employers increased by an average of 37% between 1988 and 1990.[5] These rapid increases in costs—combined with the growing realization that Americans have not had similar increases in health and fueled by the growing fear that fewer Americans will be able to afford insurance—have increased interest in exactly how these resources are being spent and how to allocate them fairly.

HEALTH CARE RATIONING VERSUS
PRIORITIZATION OF HEALTH SERVICES

Rationing

Health care rationing has been proposed as a partial solution to the current health care crisis. *Rationing* (as it is used here) is a method of allocating health care resources that results in some health care services being limited or unavailable to some people. Because of such limitations, this process demands close scrutiny. The idea of controlling the cost of health services is justifiably of great concern to children with special health care needs (CSHCN), their families, and those who provide services for these children.

They are concerned because CSHCN require some of the most expensive forms of long-term habilitative services (e.g., services for children with spina bifida, muscular dystrophy, and cystic fibrosis) and some of the most expensive procedures requiring new technologies (e.g., organ transplants, cancer care, and long-term ventilator support care).

Rationing restricts the availability of health services by determining who pays for what services and which persons will receive what services. Although the current health care delivery system in the United States has no stated policy that health care is to be rationed, rationing does currently occur. It occurs in the sense that different segments of the population have varying access to health services. Those with adequate personal resources or adequate public assistance have had almost unlimited access to a vast array of health services, while others have had very limited access to restricted resources. For example, hospitalized people receive different levels of treatment based on their insurance status.[2] People with health insurance who consider themselves in poor-to-fair health visit their physicians twice as often as those without insurance.[1]

Although no state government currently has a policy of rationing health services, state governments, in managing their Medicaid programs, currently decide how poor is poor enough to qualify for state support. In addition, certain categories of people are eligible or not eligible for medical payment programs. For example, a single woman or man without children cannot qualify for Medicaid unless she or he has a disability. States delineate the number of hospital days or physician visits that will be covered by Medicaid, and states have been forced to eliminate certain categories of services such as home oxygen, dental services, and even medication because of the amount of state funds that are appropriated. Rationing occurs even in the way health care is delivered; health care dollars can be used to pay for rehabilitation services to correct an adult's speech problem caused by an injury, but cannot be used to pay for the education of a young child who has the same speech problem caused prenatally. Thus it must be recognized that rationing does exist, and that the decisions that are now being made are based on poorly organized and irrational reasons.

Prioritization

Prioritization is another method that has been proposed as a partial solution to the current health care crisis. *Prioritization* (as it is used here) is a method of allocating health care resources using established criteria. In contrast to rationing, prioritization is a visible, explicit process that involves rational choices and, when done well, emphasizes fairness and the good of the community.

This chapter briefly describes the experiences of the state of Oregon in creating a health care system that includes prioritization of health services within the Medicaid program. The decision on the part of Oregon to create a method of prioritizing health services was based on the acknowledgment that resources are not sufficient to provide every health service to everyone who desires it, that the distribution of and access to health services are often inequitable, and that the problem is growing and appears to be uncontrollable. With that acknowledgment came the realization that it was necessary to make tough choices about what services should be provided and who should receive them.

CRITERIA USED IN THE PRIORITIZATION PROCESS

Prioritization or rationing of health services can be achieved using different methods and different criteria—at a society level by policy makers or at the personal level by the providers of health care. Socialization of medical care tends to shift the rationing process from a personal basis using market forces to a society basis using bureaucratic and political forces. It is also important to recognize that when a society makes certain major societal policy decisions about health care, they are forced to ration personal health services. For instance, when the British National Health Services capped global spending, it became necessary to limit the number of dialysis machines, which in turn forced physicians to decide which persons with kidney failure should receive dialysis.

Numerous criteria can be used to prioritize health care. All have been discussed and most have been used. They generally fall into two categories—patient-centered criteria and resource-centered criteria.

Patient-Centered Criteria

Patient-centered criteria are based on characteristics of the person requesting services. At best they are used to determine which person will benefit most from a resource; at worst they determine which person is most worthy of treatment. Typically, most patient-centered criteria are used by a health care provider during the delivery of services to determine who receives a specific health service.

Patient-centered criteria include the following:

- **Age**-In Great Britain the elderly (i.e., those over 50) are much less likely to receive renal dialysis than those who are younger.
- **Ability to pay**-This is the most widespread form of rationing in the United States.
- **Place of residence**-A person whose income is at 60% of the federal poverty level qualifies for government-sponsored medical care in Michigan but not in New York.

- **Life expectancy**-People with terminal cancer are not currently considered for unrelated solid organ transplants, such as kidney or heart.
- **Needs**-In 1965 the U.S. government established Medicare/Medicaid to pay for the health care of three high need groups—the elderly, children, and people with disabilities.
- **Past or future contributions**-Should a mother with small children receive a scarce organ transplant before an unemployed worker?
- **Life-style choices**-Individuals who smoke pay more for health insurance.
- **Race or other social characteristics**-Despite the fact that end-stage kidney disease is more common among racial minorities than whites, fewer blacks than whites undergo kidney transplants.

Resource-Centered Criteria

Resource-centered criteria are based on the features of the services to be delivered and ignore differences in the people who receive the services. Typically, these criteria are used by the policy makers of a society—legislators, state and federal governments, insurance providers, and purchasers—to determine which services should be funded.

Resource-centered criteria include the following:

- **High technology**-In the United States, the bias is for high technology—insurance will pay for a coronary-artery bypass operation using a heart-lung machine, but will less often pay for childhood immunizations or well-child check-ups.
- **Service categories**-Insurance carriers provide a benefit package defined by service categories such as dental care, therapy services, or durable medical equipment like wheelchairs.
- **Basic vs. nonbasic services**-It is easy to achieve consensus that basic or essential services should be provided. The problem is that there is no agreement on what is basic.
- **Cost-benefit ratio**-Despite development of a methodology to measure benefit, lack of accurate data and current methods make it impossible to accurately prioritize health services.
- **Type of practitioner**-Traditional insurance packages usually pay for services provided only by certain practitioners such as psychologists vs. psychiatrists, or nurse midwives vs. obstetricians.
- **Service delivery setting**-Health services may or may not be paid, depending on the site of delivery, such as hospitalization vs. outpatient services.
- **Class of service**-Is the service preventive or curative, palliative or rehabilitative?

PRINCIPLES FOR PRIORITIZING SERVICES AND RESOURCES

The decision that the resources to pay for health services should be rationed makes it necessary to determine the priority given to each health service, which, in turn, makes it essential to establish criteria for determining the priority given to each service. The outcome of the prioritization process determines that certain people will have access to certain services and others will not, which makes it necessary to carefully create principles to use in the prioritization decision-making process.

Some of the principles that should be considered include the following:

- **Justice/fairness**-Are the resources distributed in an equitable manner?
- **Common good**-Does the allocation protect the collective needs of the community?
- **Respect for the dignity of people**-Is the individual worthiness of each person respected?
- **Protection of the most vulnerable people**-Are the people least able to help themselves protected?
- **Protection of the caring relationship between patient and health care professional**-Do health care professionals remain in a position where they can speak in the best interests of the patient?
- **Visibility of the process**-Is the method by which health care resources are allocated publicly explained?
- **Equal voice**-Do the people affected by the decisions have input into the decision-making process?

PROBLEMS ASSOCIATED WITH THE PRIORITIZATION PROCESS

Prioritization is a situation in which there are competing needs and limited resources and in which it is impossible to totally satisfy everyone. Some of the competing needs include the following:

- **Individual benefit vs. community benefit**-Individuals experiencing a condition or disease have a very different perspective of the worth of a treatment compared to the community as a whole.
- **High-incidence disease vs. low-incidence disease**-In a prioritization process there is a tendency to give preference to diseases that are familiar. However, this evaluates society's knowledge of the disease rather than the effect of the disease.
- **Visible people vs. invisible people**-There is a tendency to approve the use of unlimited resources for a few people who happen to become visible in the press and might have unusual diseases, while denying resources to faceless thousands.

- **Current benefit vs. future benefit**-It is difficult to fund services that will save unknown people from diseases in the future and not fund services to treat people with current diseases.
- **Acute life-threatening diseases vs. chronic disabling diseases**-In the prioritization process there is a tendency to give preference to acute, life-threatening diseases over diseases that are chronic and require long-term services.

THE OREGON HEALTH PLAN: PRIORITIZATION IN ACTION

In 1989 and 1991 the Oregon legislature enacted a series of laws known collectively as the Oregon Health Plan.[4] Although the prioritized list of health services that are paid for under the plan has received the most publicity, the plan also includes a series of insurance reforms and business mandates that will virtually eliminate preexisting-condition exclusions and expand insurance coverage to all permanent employees. The plan has also expanded by 420,000 the number of Oregonians who are eligible for services or insurance, while still containing the cost of health services. The plan addresses the problem of cost containment from several directions—emphasis on preventive services, reliance on managed care, the establishment of a separate commission to examine the distribution of high technology services and practice guidelines, and the establishment of a prioritized list of health services.

Based on the premise that not all health services are equal in value and effectiveness, the legislature established an 11-member commission consisting of a public health nurse, a social worker, five physicians, and four consumers who reviewed existing data about the known reported outcome of health services and received expert clinical testimony. Community meetings and public hearings were used to elicit the values that Oregonians believe should guide health care spending decisions. The purpose was to produce a prioritized list of conditions and diseases matched to their treatments that was rational and based on the values expressed by the public.

After rejecting a list based on a pure cost-benefit method, the commissioners established a more comprehensive method that ranked 17 general categories of health care (e.g., Category 1 includes acute fatal conditions in which treatment prevents death and promotes full recovery; Category 2 includes maternity care; and Category 17 includes fatal or nonfatal conditions in which treatment causes minimal or no improvement in a person's quality of life), assigned each condition-treatment pair (the grouping of a medical condition or disease with its appropriate treatment) to a category, and then ranked each pair within the category using the net benefit of each pair as defined by a formula comparing a condition's progress with and without treatment. The measurements of treatment benefits took into account the presence or absence of symptoms and measured their severity by their effect on functioning. The symptoms were assigned weights or levels of importance by Oregonians in a random, digit-dialed telephone survey. For the final step in the process the commissioners adjusted the ranking of condition-treatment pairs, based on the values expressed by the public and to correct the situation when the data did not appear to adequately reflect the benefit of a treatment.

1993 Oregon Prioritized List of Health Services

Top Three
  1. Severe/moderate head injury
     Treatment: medical and surgical
  2. Insulin-dependent diabetes mellitus
     Treatment: medical
  3. Peritonitis (infection of the abdomen)
     Treatment: medical and surgical

Last Three
694. Tubal dysfunction
     Treatment: In vitro fertilization
695. Hepatorenal syndrome (a fatal, untreatable condition in which both the liver and kidneys fail)
     Treatment: medical
696. Spastic dysphonia (uncontrollable voice fluctuations)
     Treatment: medical

Criteria for Adjustment

  A. General preventive services
  B. Comfort care
  C. Maternity care
  D. Family planning services
  E. Prevent a condition before treatment
  F. Medical ineffectiveness
  G. Prevent additional complications
  H. Prevent future costs
  I. Cosmetic services
  J. Self-limiting conditions
  K. Congruent conditions
  L. Public health risk

In response to federal concerns that this method might violate the Americans with Disabilities Act (ADA), the commissioners developed a final process which prioritized the condition-treatment pairs using cost of treatment and the probability of preventing death to produce the 1993 prioritized list. This process eliminated the use of all symptoms and relied heavily on adjustments by the commissioners using preestablished criteria. (See the boxes on p. 78.)

THE POTENTIAL EFFECT OF THE OREGON PLAN ON THE PROVISION OF SERVICES FOR CSHCN

One strong concern throughout the entire Oregon prioritization process was how people with disabilities would be affected. In 1991 the Oregon legislature established a commission subcommittee on the blind and disabled to address these issues. The subcommittee recommended two groups of changes. The first group dealt with an adjustment of certain medical conditions in which the treatments have a different effect on people with certain disabilities than they do on the general population. As an example, esophagitis usually causes only mild heartburn in the general population but can be life threatening in someone with severe spastic quadriplegia (a form of cerebral palsy). In the list before 1993, medical treatment of esophagitis was the last covered benefit, and surgical treatment of the problem was not on the list. The subcommittee recommended a higher placement for medical treatment and the creation of a surgical treatment line.

The second group of changes addressed two other concerns. One of those concerns was that of using effectiveness as a criterion to prioritize health services. Most people with disabilities have conditions that are not curable; thus treatments for their conditions are not considered "effective" and most of these conditions could be ranked low. However, in the list, most conditions causing disabilities actually were ranked fairly high because the commission recognized the value of services that prevent deterioration for conditions causing disabilities.

The second concern was that multiple diseases can cause the same disability (e.g., a disability in mobility can be caused by a head injury, a prenatal event [cerebral palsy], or an infection around the brain [meningitis]). Each disease is found in a different condition-treatment pair—some funded and some not — but each results in the same pattern of disability and has the same need for treatment. In response to both dilemmas, the subcommittee and then the full commission adopted a series of dysfunction lines (such as line 311—dysfunction of posture and movement—to pay for durable medical equipment, therapy services, orthopedic procedures, doctor visits, etc. to keep people mobile).

Although it will take time to understand its full effect on the health of children with disabilities, the Oregon Health Plan has taught several lessons. One is that using categories of service to determine what services should be funded places children with disabilities at a disadvantage. Currently, the optional categories of Medicaid services for which states are allowed to refuse payment include several categories that are used extensively by people with disabilities, such as physical therapy services, durable medical equipment like wheelchairs and braces, and home oxygen. The Oregon Health Plan solves this problem by including payment for all ancillary health services within a condition-treatment pair so people with disabilities will have greater access to ancillary services.

By prioritizing health services, not people, it is believed that the Oregon Health Plan should prevent the rationing on people-based criteria that sometimes occurs for people with disabilities. Furthermore, the public manner of conducting the prioritization process allows individuals to be fully aware of the reason for denial of services and allows a mechanism for appeal.

Because resources shrink, all health care delivery systems have methods to decrease services. In the current Medicaid system, states have the option of removing people from coverage or limiting or eliminating categories of services. The services that are most commonly limited are those heavily used by people with disabilities, and therefore those people are more heavily affected by budget cuts. The Oregon Health Plan provides a mechanism to share the effect of budget cuts among a greater percentage of the population and in a manner that is more visible and accountable.

CONCLUSION

This chapter provides an abbreviated description of an example of the complex societal planning that is needed to prioritize health services for the purpose of controlling the cost of health care and assuring that health services are provided equitably and wisely. The Oregon Health Plan provides a process by which to prioritize health services in an equitable and visible manner and has brought the debate of allocation of public health care resources to the attention of the nation.

REFERENCES

1. Freeman HE: Uninsured working-age adults: characteristics and consequences, *Health Services Research* 24:819, 1990.
2. Hadley J, Steinberg EP, and Feder J: Comparison of uninsured and privately insured hospital patients, *Journal of the American Medical Association* 256:374-379, 1991.
3. National Governor's Association: *A healthy America: the challenge for states,* 1991.
4. Oregon Health Services Commission: Prioritization of health services: a report to the governor and legislature, Salem, Ore, 1991, State of Oregon.
5. Swoboda F: Health care costs climb 21.6% in '90, *Washington Post*, p D5, Jan 29, 1991.
6. Weiner JM: Rationing in America, overt and covert. In Strogsberg et al, editors: *Rationing America's medical care: the Oregon plan and beyond*, Washington, DC, 1992, The Brookings Institution.

CHAPTER 8

Federal Legislation for Children with Special Health Care Needs and Their Families: Past, Present, and Future

HELEN M. WALLACE
JOSEPHINE GITTLER

HISTORICAL BACKGROUND

Early efforts to develop services for children with special health care needs* began in the United States in the 1880s through the provision of institutional care, most of it private. The 1930s marked the first overt commitment on the part of the federal government to large scale assistance of the disadvantaged and the vulnerable. In the face of the suffering caused by the Great Depression, and the inability of the private sector, states, and localities to substantially alleviate this suffering, President Roosevelt launched the New Deal. A hallmark of the New Deal was the 1935 enactment of the Social Security Act, and Title V of that Act made available to the states federal funding for State Crippled Children's Services Programs to improve access to diagnosis, treatment, and rehabilitative services for children with physical disabilities.

The 1960s witnessed President Johnson's proclamation of the Great Society and his declaration of the War on Poverty, which brought into being fed-

---

*As used in this chapter the term *children* refers to young persons of all ages—infants and toddlers at one end of the spectrum and adolescents and young adults at the other end of the spectrum.

eral legislation expanding existing programs and creating new programs of importance to children with special health care needs and their families. From the 1960s to the beginning of the 1990s, the expansion and creation of such programs continued.

These programs both contributed to and reflected a series of changes in the care of children with special health care needs. These changes may be summarized as follows:

- Children with all types of chronic illnesses such as diabetes and asthma received more attention.
- Clinicians increasingly treated not only high-severity, low-prevalence problems but also low-severity, high-prevalence problems, such as learning disabilities and attention deficit disorders.
- Interdisciplinary, multidisciplinary team care, including case management or care coordination, for children with special health care needs became the norm rather than the exception.
- An emphasis on inpatient care was replaced by an emphasis on ambulatory care and community-based services.
- More focus was placed on the prevention of disabilities and chronic illnesses.
- It was recognized that children with special health care needs required not only health services but also psychological, social, educational, and vocational services, and that their families required support services.
- Special-needs children increasingly remained in the community, either in the home or in independent living arrangements, rather than being institutionalized.
- Special education and related services were developed for school-age children with disabilities.
- Early identification and intervention services were developed for infants, toddlers, and preschoolers with or at risk of disabilities.
- Transition services were developed for adolescents and young adults with disabilities to help them with matters such as employment and independent living arrangements.
- Parents of special-needs children formed networks and groups for the exchange of information and mutual support, and they organized politically to become effective advocates for their children.
- Development of community-based systems of comprehensive, coordinated, family-centered, culturally-competent services became a widely accepted goal.

FEDERAL LEGISLATION FOR CHILDREN WITH SPECIAL HEALTH CARE NEEDS AND THEIR FAMILIES

In the last several decades there has been a proliferation of federal laws that directly or indirectly affect children with special health care needs and their families and under which many different programs are authorized and funded.[8] One recent compendium of major legislation related to persons with disabilities lists more than 60 federal statutes and it does not purport to be a full listing of such statutes.[8] As Table 7-1 indicates, much of this legislation falls into one or more of the following subject areas: health, income maintenance or assistance, education, vocational rehabilitation, social services, and civil rights.

Health Legislation

Children with special health care needs, by definition, require health and health-related services. The federal health legislation of the greatest importance to these children and their families is Title V of the Social Security Act and Title XIX of the Social Security Act.

Table 7-1.   Typology of Legislation Affecting Children with Special Health Care Needs with Selected Examples

---

HEALTH

- Maternal and Child Health Services Block Grant (Title V of the Social Security Act)
- Medical Assistance Program (Medicaid) (Title XIX of the Social Security Act)

INCOME MAINTENANCE

- Supplemental Security Income (Title XVI of the Social Security Act)

EDUCATION

- Individuals with Disabilities Education Act

VOCATIONAL REHABILITATION

- Rehabilitation Act of 1973

SOCIAL SERVICES

- Developmental Disabilities Assistance and Bill of Rights Act
- Head Start Act

CIVIL RIGHTS

- Americans with Disabilities Act

Title V, originally enacted in 1935, was amended in 1981 to consolidate the State Crippled Children's Services Programs and State Maternal and Child Health Programs with other programs into the Maternal and Child Health Services Block Grant.* Subsequent amendments renamed the State Crippled Children's Services Programs and redefined their mission. They are now called the State Programs for Children with Special Health Care Needs, and they have a threefold mission: 1) the provision and promotion of family-centered, community-based, coordinated care for children with special health care needs; 2) the development of community-based systems of services for these children and their families; and 3) the provision of rehabilitation services for blind and disabled children who meet certain eligibility requirements.

Title XIX, enacted in 1965 as part of the Johnson administration's War on Poverty, established the Medical Assistance (Medicaid) Program.† Medicaid finances health services for poor and low-income individuals, and it has become the largest source of public financing of health services for special-needs children.

Income Maintenance Legislation

There are costs, besides the costs of health services, that are associated with caring for children with special needs that are beyond the financial means of their families, particularly poor and low-income families. The enactment of the Social Security Act in 1935 and subsequent amendments to the Act created several income maintenance programs, among which is the Supplemental Security Income (SSI) Program for the Aged Blind and Disabled.‡ Title XVI of the Social Security Act that established the SSI Program authorizes income supplements to poor and low-income blind and disabled children as well as adults who meet Title XVI eligibility requirements. A link exists between receipt of SSI payments and access to Medicaid because in most states children eligible for SSI are eligible for Medicaid.

Education

Children with special health care needs, like all children, have a right to education. The landmark federal law in this area is the Individuals with Disabilities Education Act (IDEA), formerly known as the Education of the

---

*Social Security Act (Title V), Maternal and Child Health Services Block Grant, 42 U.S.C. §§701-709 (1988 ed; Supp. V 1994).

†Social Security Act (Title XIX), Grants to States for Medical Assistance Programs, 42 U.S.C. §§1396a-1396v (1988 ed; Supp V. 1994).

‡Social Security Act (Title XVI), Supplemental Security Income for Aged, Blind, and Disabled, 42 U.S.C. §§1383(d) (1988 ed; Supp V. 1994).

Handicapped Act, and in part, the Education for all Handicapped Children Act, which was originally enacted in 1975.* Part B of IDEA requires participating states to furnish all children with disabilities a free, appropriate public education; it provides for grants to the states for special education and related services for school-age children and separate allotments to the states for special education and related services to children ages three to five. Part H of IDEA provides for grants to states for the development of a coordinated, comprehensive, statewide network of early services for infants and toddlers ages birth to two with or at risk of disabilities.

Vocational Rehabilitation

As children with special health care needs reach adolescence and enter adulthood, they must begin to make the transition from school to work. Federal vocational rehabilitation legislation, at least in part, addresses problems that may occur in connection with this transition. Although there are several federal statutes dealing with vocational rehabilitation, the chief statute is the Rehabilitation Act of 1973, as amended.† This act's purpose is to foster and facilitate full-time, part-time, or supported employment of individuals with mental and physical disabilities in the regular labor market. This is accomplished through provision of federal funds to states to support vocational rehabilitation services and federal grants for demonstration, training, and research activities.

Social Services

Children with special health care needs and their families frequently require a wide array of what are usually referred to as social services or support services. There are a number of federal laws serving this population that are generally classified as social service or support programs. One example is the Developmental Disabilities Assistance and Bill of Rights Act and another is the Community Services Act.

The Developmental Disabilities Assistance and Bill of Rights Act evolved from the Mental Retardation Facilities Construction Act of 1963 and has been extensively amended over the years.‡ It authorizes four grant programs: 1) basic grants to states for state developmental disability councils and for the planning and coordination of services for persons with developmental disabilities; 2) grants to university-affiliated programs used to provide interdisciplinary training for personnel that work with persons with disabilities;

---

*Individuals with Disabilities Education Act, 20 U.S.C. §§1400-1485 (1988 & Supp V1993).
†Rehabilitation Act of 1973, 29 U.S.C. §§718-797b (1988 & Supp V1994).
‡Developmental Disabilities Assistance and Bill of Rights Act, 42 U.S.C. §§6000-6083 (1988 & Supp V1994).

3) grants for programs of national significance to expand opportunities and provide assistance to persons with developmental disabilities; and 4) grants to states for protection and advocacy systems to ensure that persons with developmental disabilities receive appropriate services and benefits.

The Community Services Act* authorizes the Head Start program, which was another outgrowth of the Johnson administration's War on Poverty. Head Start provides comprehensive child development services to preschool children from poor and low-income families and involves their parents in program activities. The authorizing statute for the program requires that children with disabilities constitute at least 10% of Head Start enrollees in each state and that they receive the full range of Head Start services.

Civil Rights

In addition to federal laws designed to provide or fund services or furnish income maintenance to children with special health care needs and their families, there are a series of federal laws designed to protect the civil rights of individuals with disabilities. The most recent and far-reaching of these laws is the American with Disabilities Act of 1990.† This act addresses all forms of discrimination against individuals on the basis of disability and prohibits discrimination in employment, public services, public accommodations (defined as privately operated settings that are open to the public), transportation, and telecommunications.

THE FUTURE OF FEDERAL LEGISLATION

The future of federal legislation affecting children with special needs and their families is uncertain. A series of interrelated developments may have the effect of drastically limiting federal funding for programs established pursuant to such legislation and dramatically shifting responsibility for these programs from the federal government to state and local governments. These developments include actions to balance the federal budget, consolidate federal programs into state block grants, and restrict unfunded federal mandates.

Balancing the Federal Budget

It is probable that, in the coming years, actions to balance the federal budget will place a severe constraint on federal programs of significance to children with special health care needs and their families. Since the 1960s there has been

---

*Community Services Act, Head Start Program, 42 U.S.C. §§9831-9848 (1988 ed, Supp V1994).

†Americans with Disabilities Act of 1990, 42 U.S.C. §§12101-12113 (Supp V1993).

an imbalance between the federal government's spending and its revenue, the product of which has been the federal budget deficits.[1] These deficits must be covered by federal government borrowing and their aggregate constitute the national debt.[1] Beginning in the 1960s there was a steady rise in federal deficit spending, and in the 1980s federal deficit spending rapidly accelerated. The result was a ballooning federal debt. In 1980 the federal debt was almost $1 trillion, and it has been projected that by the year 2000 the federal debt will approach $7 trillion.[1]

Successive congresses and presidents have grappled unsuccessfully with the upward spiral in federal budget deficits and the national debt. The advent of the 104th Congress in January of 1995—Republican-controlled for the first time in 40 years—has signaled a fundamental change in congressional support for balancing the federal budget. This Congress passed the Fiscal Year 1996 Budget Resolution aimed at balancing the budget by the year 2002 through unprecedented reductions in projected rates of spending for federal programs, many of which are of importance to children with special health care needs and their families.[2,*]

A budget resolution, which sets forth overall targets for levels of spending for broad functional categories rather than specific programs and specifies overall targets for levels of revenues, must be passed by both houses of Congress but does not require the signature of the President. Therefore, a caveat regarding the Fiscal 1996 Budget Resolution is that it is only a blueprint of legislation regarding spending and revenues that eventually must be passed by Congress and signed into law by the President over the next 7 years. Although the Budget Resolution does not guarantee that the reductions in projected spending will actually take place, it does make it likely that some, if not all, of these reductions will become a reality.

From the standpoint of children with special health care needs and their families, a troubling aspect of the fiscal 1996 Budget Resolution is that the spending reductions for which it calls are likely to fall disproportionately on domestic spending for the so-called "social programs." Under the Budget Resolution large reductions must be made in discretionary spending for programs such as Title V Maternal and Child Health Services Block Grant, which is determined annually through appropriations of a specific amount. The Budget Resolution contemplates even larger reductions in spending for entitlement programs, such as the Title XIX Medicaid program, which require the government to pay specified benefits to anyone who meets specified eligibil-

---

*House Concurrent Resolution 67, 104th Congress, 1st Session (1995).

ity requirements. The expenditures for the former are "capped" by the amount of their appropriations, whereas expenditures for the latter grow automatically if the number of individuals qualified for and seeking benefits grows. Under the Budget Resolution spending cuts for both types of programs may take the form of cuts either in current levels of funding or in projected growth in levels of funding.

State Block Grants

Efforts by the Republican-controlled 104th Congress to restructure federal programs is another development that may have a negative effect upon federal legislation affecting children with special health care needs and their families. These efforts have centered on creating state block grants involving the consolidation of federal programs and the removal of the federal government's restrictions on how states and localities can use program funds.

The concept of state block grants is not new. In 1981 President Ronald Reagan proposed to consolidate almost 90 federal programs into three block grants; ultimately, nearly 60 programs were consolidated into nine block grants and approved.[5,6] It was at this time that the State Crippled Children's Service Programs were consolidated with other programs into the Maternal and Child Health Services Block Grant under Title V of the Social Security Act. Historically, block grants have consolidated similar discretionary spending programs. What distinguishes the block grant proposals of the 104th Congress is that they are directed at converting entitlement programs into block grants as well as consolidating discretionary spending programs.

Medicaid, a major source of funding for health care for children with special needs, is among the entitlement programs targeted for conversion into a block grant by Replication majorities in the Senate and House of Representatives. Thus in late 1995 the 104th Congress passed a massive budget recondiliation package containing provisions under which Medicaid would become a block grant and the states would have broad latitude in determining who receives health insurance coverage and what level of coverage is received. These provisions were aimed at ending Medicaid's entitlement status that results in a federal guarantee of coverage to any individual who meets federal eligibility requirements. In addition these provisions reduced the projected rate of Medicaid spending. President Clinton vetoed the budget reconciliation bill, and one of the reasons for the veto was his objection to its Medicaid provisions. The dispute between President Clinton and the Republicans in the 104th congress over the shape and size of Medicaid is a component of a larger and ongoing impasse between them over a 7-year balanced budget plan. As of the spring of 1996 no agreement had been reached between them on a balanced budget plan that would include turning Medicaid from an entitlement program into a capped block grant program.

To some extent state block grant creation is a natural outgrowth of the existence of multiple overlapping programs providing or funding particular services for particular populations. As it has been pointed out, there has been a proliferation of federal laws affecting children with special health care needs and their families. Likewise, there has been a proliferation of laws affecting other populations. The programs established by these laws are administered by different agencies or components of agencies at the federal, state, and local levels, and they have different sources of funding, eligibility requirements, policies, and practices. It is well documented that as a consequence, there are gaps in and duplication of services and that all too often the delivery of services is uncoordinated and fragmented. The consolidation of programs into block grants can be seen as at least a partial solution to problems in service delivery arising from multiple overlapping programs.

Nevertheless, the solution of these problems is not the primary rationale for the drive of the 104th Congress to create state block grants. This drive is fueled by the many members of Congress who have adopted and adhere to the goal of devolution of power to the states—that is the transfer of responsibility for the design and implementation of federally funded programs from the federal government to the states.[6] The debate over block grants increasingly revolves not so much around whether they should be created as around what federal strings should be attached to receipt of block grant funds by the states.

Proponents of state block grants take the position that the states need flexibility to tailor federally funded programs to state-specific priorities based on state-specific conditions. However, opponents take the position that the federal government should set national standards for program eligibility, benefits, and services of federally funded programs and monitor program administration by the states to ensure that their expenditure of federal funds is appropriate. They also believe that some state legislatures, governors, and administrative agencies lack the capacity and experience to assume the responsibilities for these programs. Proponents take the position that states can more efficiently and effectively operate federally funded programs than the federal government. However, opponents, assert that a significant number of state legislatures, governors, and administrative agencies lack the capacity and experience to assume the control of and responsibility for these programs. In the abstract it is difficult to evaluate the validity of arguments pro and con regarding block grants. Rather, what is needed and what is generally lacking is an identification of the principles and considerations that should govern the allocation of power between the federal government and the states in the context of particular types of programs.[4]

In the case of the numerous programs serving children with special health care needs and their families, their incorporation into state block grants raises several concerns. One concern is that programs for these children and their families will be unable to successfully compete with other programs for state block grant funds. Underlying this concern is the fear that the needs of these children and families will be neglected and overlooked because they constitute a relatively small proportion of the total population and they often require a variety of long-term and high-cost services. A related concern is that the result of block grants will be variations, perhaps great variations, from state to state in the eligibility of these children and families for benefits and services and in the nature and extent of the benefits and services provided because of the absence of federal standards and monitoring.

The actual effect of the creation of state block grants upon children with special health care needs depends upon what programs are consolidated. For example, a block grant consisting of several health programs, including programs targeted to special needs children, programs serving other populations such as the elderly, and programs aimed at the general public is more problematic than a block grant consisting of a variety of programs (health, income maintenance, education, vocational rehabilitation, social services) specifically targeted to special needs children or both children and adults with special needs stemming from disabilities and chronic illnesses. It is likely that far fewer resources will be allocated to special needs children under the first type of block grant than the second type.

The effect of state block grants upon children with special health care needs and their families also depends upon the degree to which federal requirements with respect to the use of state block grant funds are contained in authorizing legislation. For example, the Title V Maternal and Child Health Services Block Grant legislation mandates that a certain proportion of state block grant funds be allocated to children with special health care needs, specifies the activities for which these funds are to be expended, and conditions receipt of funds upon an annual state application setting forth a plan for expenditure of funds.

Finally it must be emphasized that the state block grant proposals of the 104th Congress are not fiscally neutral. Rather they are instruments for balancing the budget.[3,6] It is anticipated that, under the Fiscal 1996 Budget, the consolidation of nonentitlement programs into state block grant programs would be accompanied by reductions in current or previously projected levels of federal funding. Even more importantly, it is anticipated that the conversion of entitlement programs, such as Medicaid, into state block grants would limit federal budgetary exposure by ending their entitlement status. In short, open-ended federal funding for these programs will be replaced by a fixed amount of funding for these programs for each state.

In theory the creation of block grants will lead to a lessening of federal bureaucracy and regulation that will in turn save administrative costs and allow states more freedom to experiment with cost-effective program design and implementation. However, it is doubtful that the cost-cutting potential of block grants, even if realized, will compensate for anticipated substantial reductions in federal funding for block grant programs. During the Reagan administration many states contributed state revenues to make up for the loss of federal funds accompanying the creation of block grants, but the ability and willingness of states to do so again is open to question.

Federal Unfunded Mandates

Still another development that may have a negative effect upon federal legislation related to children with special needs and their families is the enactment of the Unfunded Mandates Reform Act of 1995.* This act makes it more difficult for Congress to impose expensive mandates on states and localities and the private sector without paying for the costs of compliance with the mandates. It requires the Congressional Budget Office to conduct cost-benefit analyses of unfunded mandates in proposed legislation; it creates procedural barriers to congressional passage of legislation with unfunded mandates that would cost states and localities more than $50 million annually and the private sector more than $100 million annually; and it requires federal agencies to conduct cost-benefit analyses when promulgating regulations in connection with unfunded mandates.

In recent years unfunded federal mandates have become the subject of mounting criticism.[7] Supporters of unfunded mandates cite the value of national standards in some areas to achieve goals that benefit the nation as a whole. However, unfunded mandates have generated opposition among state and local officials on the ground that they place undue fiscal burdens on states and localities that have limited resources and they substitute the priorities of the federal government for the priorities of state and local governments. Opposition to unfunded mandates is also part of a larger regulatory reform movement directed at lessening federal regulation of a variety of public- and private-sector activities.

Some federal statutes affecting children with special needs and their families contain unfunded federal mandates. The Americans with Disabilities Act,

*Unfunded Mandates Reform Act of 1995, Public Law 104-4, 109 Stat. 48 (1995).

prohibiting discrimination on the basis of disability, is frequently pointed to as containing federal unfunded mandates because it requires expenditures on the part of states and localities and privately operated businesses to make buildings, facilities, transportation systems, and telecommunications services accessible to the disabled. The Individuals with Disabilities Education Act, requiring participating states to furnish children with disabilities a free, appropriate public education, is also sometimes cited by state and local officials as containing a federal unfunded mandate because the federal government pays for a relatively small share of the costs of educating these children.

The actual effect of the Unfunded Mandates Reform Act on federal legislation of significance to children with special health care needs and their families may be less than its sponsors initially intended because the act does not apply to mandates in existing legislation and exempts civil rights and antidiscrimination mandates. Nevertheless, the act will constitute a restraint on the ability of Congress to pass legislation or revise existing legislation imposing unfunded mandates. Perhaps equally important is that the enactment of this act reflects a fundamental change in the political environment that has in the past produced so many federal statutes benefitting children with special health care needs and their families.

CONCLUSION

Beginning with the Roosevelt administration's New Deal, continuing through the Johnson administration's Great Society and War on Poverty, and extending to the present day, a number of federal laws affecting children with special health care needs and their families have been enacted. As a result of these laws, the federal government has played a critical role in the improvement and expansion of health, education, vocational rehabilitation, social services, and other services for special needs children; the federal government has played a critical role in a movement away from the isolation, segregation, and institutionalization of these children toward their full inclusion in the lives of their home communities; and the federal government has played a critical role in the recognition of the right of these children to be legally protected from discrimination.

It is unclear whether the actions initiated by the 104th Congress to limit funding for federal programs and shift responsibility for these programs from the federal government to state and local governments are first steps in the dismantling of programs that have their roots in the New Deal and the Great Society or simply represent a reform and downsizing of these programs. Thus, it remains to be seen whether the federal government will continue to offer leadership in assisting children with special health care needs and their families.

REFERENCES

1. Concord Coalition: *A primer on the debt and the deficit,* Washington, DC, 1995, The Concord Coalition.
2. Concord Coalition: *The Fiscal Year 1996 Budget Resolution, issue analysis (95-1),* Washington DC, 1995, The Concord Coalition.
3. Peirce NR: Block grants—the inevitable fix? *National Journal,* 35:2178, 1995.
4. Peterson PE: Who should do what? *The Brookings Review,* Spring: 6-11, 1995.
5. Peterson GE et al: *The Reagan block grants: what have we learned?* Washington, DC, 1986, Urban Institute Press.
6. Stanfield RL: Devolution: will the states be left holding the bag? *National Journal,* 36:2206-2209, 1995.
7. St. George JR: Unfunded mandates: balancing state and national needs, *The Brookings Review,* Spring: 12-15, 1995.
8. U.S. Department of Education, Office of Special Education and Rehabilitative Services: *Summary of Existing Legislation Affecting People with Disabilities,* Washington, DC, 1992, U.S. Government Printing Office. (This report was prepared for the Office of Special Education and Rehabilitative Services by the National Association of State Mental Retardation Program Directors.)
9. U.S. Department of Health and Human Services, Assistant Secretary for Planning and Evaluation: *Task II Federal Programs for Persons with Disabilities,* Washington, DC, 1990, Office of Assistant Secretary for Planning and Evaluation. (This report was prepared under contract for the Office of the Assistant Secretary for Planning and Evaluation by System Metrics/ McGraw-Hill and Mathematical Policy Research.)

PART THREE

ISSUES

Successful community-based programming for children with special health care needs requires broad, multidimensional thinking that goes beyond individual disciplinary boundaries. Yet, how many professionals have taken coursework in health care financing, cultural competency, sexuality, or public policy advocacy?

This section provides an overview of issues that do not have a single theme but that professionals confront each day. Insufficient financial resources, for example, perennially plague families of children with disabilities or chronic illness and impede progress that might be achieved if recommendations for services were fully implemented.

Several chapters in this section deal with legal or legislative issues including individual rights, confidentiality, and advocacy. Recent laws such as the American with Disabilities Act and the Individuals with Disabilities Education Act provide new impetus for progress in comprehensive services for children and youth with disabilities and chronic illness, if they are used to greatest advantage.

With these new laws emphasizing coordination of care and effective use of financial and personnel resources, an understanding of how services can and should be organized most efficiently is paramount. Years of tradition, entrenchment, and territorialization must be overcome. The chapters on systems of care, interorganizational collaboration, and needs assessment provide a framework and strategy for meeting this challenge.

Finally, we now recognize that the preservation and support of the family in our society is imperative. While the definition of family may have changed over the years, still a stable, nurturing, personal environment is essential to the optimal physical, emotional, and cognitive development of every child. Although the chapter on family roles is embedded in a mass of other important issues in this section, it should not be seen as a component but rather the cornerstone of all other considerations.

CHAPTER 9

Legal Rights of Children With Disabilities

JOSEPHINE GITTLER

Historically, individuals with disabilities have been socially, educationally, and economically disadvantaged. The disability rights movement has waged a decades-long struggle to secure the enactment, interpretation, and application of laws to bring this population into the mainstream of American life. The product of this struggle is a large and complex body of disability rights law. This body of law is an amalgam—at times a somewhat confusing one—derived from federal and state constitutional provisions, statutes, administrative regulations and guidelines, court decisions, and opinions of administrative agencies.

This chapter is intended to furnish the reader with a brief introduction to the legal rights of children with disabilities. (For a comprehensive analysis of the laws related to children with disabilities, the reader should consult the bibliography at the end of this chapter.) The chapter specifically describes the three main federal statutes that provide legal protections for children with disabilities: (1) the Rehabilitation Act of 1973, (2) the Americans With Disabilities Act of 1990 (ADA), and (3) the Individuals With Disabilities Education Act (IDEA).

THE REHABILITATION ACT OF 1973

The Rehabilitation Act of 1973 was the first major federal statute furnishing protection against discrimination to individuals with disabilities. The portion of the act of most relevance to children with disabilities is Section 504, prohibiting federal agencies and any program or activity that receive "federal financial assistance" from discriminating "solely on the basis of his or her disability" against an "otherwise qualified" individual who has a "disability."*

*29 U.S.C. §794(1988 & Supp. V 1993).

Section 504 uses a three-part definition of an individual with a disability. According to this definition, such an individual is

> any person who (i) has a physical or mental impairment which substantially limits one or more of such person's major life activities, (ii) has a record of such an impairment, or (iii) is regarded as having such an impairment.*

"Major life activities" refers to the activities of "caring for one's self, performing manual tasks, walking, seeing, hearing, speaking, breathing, learning, and working."†

Section 504 protects an individual with a disability only if the individual is also "otherwise qualified" for participation in a covered program or activity. In the context of services or benefits, this requirement means that an individual with a disability must meet essential eligibility criteria for benefits and services that are applicable to all applicants. In the employment context the "otherwise qualified" requirement means that an individual with a disability must be able to perform the essential functions of the job. However, if an individual with a disability is unable to meet essential eligibility requirements for benefits or services or is unable to perform essential job functions, reasonable accommodation must be made to enable individuals with disabilities to meet such requirements or perform such functions.

In general, Section 504 covers the population of children who are the subject of this book. The Section 504 prohibition against discrimination is applicable only to recipients of federal financial assistance, and there are a number of organizational entities that conduct programs and activities of benefit to children with disabilities and their families and that are recipients of federal financial assistance. Examples are hospitals that receive federal funds under the Title XIX Medical Assistance (Medicaid) program and the Title V Maternal and Child Health Services Block Grant and local school districts that receive federal funds for special education under IDEA.

AMERICANS WITH DISABILITIES ACT OF 1990

Seventeen years after the enactment of the Rehabilitation Act, Congress passed and the president signed the Americans with Disabilities Act of 1990 (ADA).‡ The ADA has been called the Emancipation Proclamation for people with disabilities. The purpose of the ADA is to establish a national mandate for the elimination of discrimination on the basis of disability and to ensure a central role for the federal government in the enforcement of standards addressing such discrimination.

---

*29 U.S.C. §706(8) (Supp. V 1994).
†45 C.F.R. §84.3(j) (2) ii (1994).
‡42 U.S.C. §§12101-12113 (Supp. V 1993).

The ADA builds upon the protections against discrimination on the basis of disability as set forth in the Rehabilitation Act of 1973. Thus, the ADA's definition of disability is taken directly from the Rehabilitation Act's three-part definition of disability. Although the persons protected are essentially the same under the ADA and the Rehabilitation Act, the protections provided under the ADA are greater than under the Rehabilitation Act because the ADA antidiscrimination mandate is not restricted to recipients of federal financial assistance.

Public Entities

One title of the ADA deals with discrimination on the basis of disability by public entities. The ADA defines a public entity as a state or local government and its instrumentalities. Most public entities are already covered by the antidiscrimination ban of Section 504 of the Rehabilitation Act by virtue of their receipt of federal financial assistance, but the ADA basically extends this ban to all public entities regardless of whether they receive federal financial assistance.

The ADA protection of individuals with disabilities against public sector discrimination, like that of Section 504, is significant for children with disabilities because there are a host of public sector programs, activities, and services of importance to them. They include programs, activities, and services of state and local health departments, community health centers, municipal hospitals, public schools, state and local child social-service agencies, public swimming pools, public libraries, and public zoos.

Public Accommodations

Another title of the ADA deals with discrimination in public accommodations. By applying protections against discrimination to public accommodations, the ADA fills a major gap left by Section 504 of the Rehabilitation Act.

The ADA defines public accommodations as private entities that affect commerce. The ADA enumerates the following categories of public accommodations: service establishments (e.g., hospitals and professional offices of health care providers), places of education, social-service center establishments (e.g., day care centers, adoption agencies, food banks, and homeless shelters), places of lodging, establishments serving food or drink, retail or sales establishments, places of exhibition or entertainment, places of public display or collection (e.g., museums or libraries), places of exercise or recreation, and places of public gathering (e.g., auditoriums).

From the standpoint of children with disabilities, it is significant that the ADA prohibition of discrimination in public accommodations applies to privately operated entities that furnish health, educational, social, and support services of the kind that these children need. Moreover, this prohibition applies to other privately operated entities to which these children must have access in order to enjoy normal patterns of daily living.

Moreover, the public accommodations coverage of the ADA goes beyond individuals with disabilities to individuals with whom they have a relationship or association. As a result, parents of children with special health care needs, other family members and persons who live with and care for them are protected against discrimination in public accommodations. For example, a sibling of a child with HIV infection cannot be excluded from a day care center because of the sibling's relationship with the child.

Employment

Still another title of the ADA deals with employment discrimination on the basis of disability. Although Section 504 of the Rehabilitation Act protects individuals with disabilities from employment discrimination, its reach is limited to the recipients of federal assistance. In contrast, the ADA extends to all private as well as public employers who employ 15 or more employees.

The ADA employment discrimination provisions are extensive and detailed. In general, the ADA prohibits employers from discriminating in the hiring, promotion, or discharge of an individual with a disability who is qualified for an employment position with or without reasonable accommodation. A qualified individual is one who can perform the essential functions of the position—that is, meet necessary job-related requirements (e.g., education, training, work experience, skills, etc.). An employer must provide reasonable accommodation (e.g., job restructuring, part-time or modified work schedules, acquisition or modification of equipment, etc.) to an individual with a disability.

As children with disabilities reach the point of transition into adulthood and seek to obtain or retain employment, the ADA prohibition of employment discrimination on the basis of disability becomes significant to them. The ADA employment discrimination prohibition is significant to parents of children with disabilities, other members of their families, and unrelated persons, who live with or care for them, because the prohibition extends to persons who have a relationship with or association with someone who has a known disability.

The ADA employment discrimination prohibition is obviously important to individuals with disabilities and their families because employment carries with it a salary or wages that promote economic self-sufficiency. This prohibition is also important to this group because employment may carry with it private health insurance for which those with disabilities, including children, are likely to have a pressing need.

The ADA employment prohibition is applicable to the provision and administration of employment-based health insurance. Therefore, employees with disabilities must be furnished with the same health insurance coverage as other employees. However, the ADA allows employers and administrators of health insurance benefit plans to provide health insurance coverage in a manner not inconsistent with state law so long as what is done is not a "subterfuge" to evade the provisions of the ADA. Accordingly, an employer may offer health insurance plans that limit coverage for preexisting conditions, limit coverage for certain procedures, limit particular treatments to a specified number per year, and/or limit reimbursements for certain types of procedures or drugs, even though such exclusions and limitations may adversely affect individuals with disabilities unless these limitations are being used as a subterfuge to evade the purpose of the ADA.

Architectural, Transportation, and Communications Barriers

In addition to the aforementioned provisions, the ADA contains a series of provisions directed at the elimination and reduction of architectural barriers to the access and use of facilities and buildings by individuals with disabilities. The ADA imposes obligations upon public accommodations that are most stringent with respect to new construction and least stringent with respect to existing structures. Under the ADA new construction must be "readily accessible" and "useable," whereas changes must be made to existing structures only if they are "readily achievable," which means "easily accomplishable and able to be carried out without much difficulty or expense." The ADA imposes obligations upon state and local government as well as public accommodations that are similar to but greater than those imposed upon public accommodations.

The ADA also contains a series of provisions, the thrust of which is to assure that individuals with disabilities can access and use public transportation that is both publicly and privately operated. These provisions enunciate fairly complicated requirements for different types of ground transportation systems, services, and facilities.

Finally, the ADA contains a series of provisions designed to promote and facilitate access to and use of telecommunications by hearing-impaired and speech-impaired individuals. Thus, the ADA requires telephone companies to furnish services known as telecommunications relay services that permit hearing-impaired and speech-impaired individuals to communicate with hearing people.

The ADA requirements for removal of architectural, transportation, and communications barriers are obviously of particular assistance to children with mobility impairments, children with hearing impairments, and children with speech impairments. The ability of these children to take advantage of the ADA antidiscrimination mandates in public accommodations, in state and local government programs and activities, and in employment, ultimately depend to some extent on the ADA requirements relating to removal of architectural, transportation, and communications barriers. More broadly, these requirements make it possible, at least in theory, for these children to engage in the same activities of daily living as other children.

INDIVIDUALS WITH DISABILITIES EDUCATION ACT

The Individuals With Disabilities Education Act (IDEA), a federal statute formerly known as the Education of the Handicapped Act and in part the Education for all Handicapped Children Act, was originally enacted in 1975.* Its purpose is:

> [T]o assure that all children with disabilities have available to them . . .
> a free appropriate public education which emphasizes special education
> and related services designed to meet their unique needs, to assure that the
> rights of children with disabilities and their parents or guardians are pro-
> tected, to assist States and localities to provide for the education of all chil-
> dren with disabilities, and to assess and assure the effectiveness of efforts
> to educate children with disabilities.[†]

Part B of the IDEA is its core; it establishes a program under which each state receives a federal grant conditioned upon the state's development and implementation of a state plan to assure a free appropriate public education (FAPE) to all children with disabilities who are state residents.

There is an overlap between Part B of the IDEA and Section 504 of the Rehabilitation Act and the ADA, but the scope of the former is different from that of the latter. Section 504 and the ADA prohibit discrimination against children with disabilities as defined in those acts. Part B of the IDEA, unlike Section 504 and the ADA, is a funding statute providing federal assistance to states for the free and appropriate education of children with disabilities and establishing substantive and procedural rights related to such education. However, the population of children covered by Section 504 and the ADA is broader than the population of children covered by Part B of the IDEA.

*20 U.S.C. §§1400-1485 (1988 & Supp. V 1993).
†20 U.S.C. §1400 (c) (Supp. V 1993).

To be entitled to a free and appropriate public education under the IDEA, a school-age child must have one or more disabilities as enumerated by the IDEA and must need special education by reason of a disability and the related services as may be required to assist the child to benefit from special education. A disability is defined so as to encompass "mental retardation, hearing impairments . . . visual impairments . . . serious emotional disturbance, orthopedic impairments, autism, traumatic brain injury, other health impairments or specific learning disabilities."* If a child has one or more of the enumerated disabilities but does not need special education, the child does not fall within the purview of the Act. For example, a child amputee has an orthopedic impairment, which is defined as a disability under the IDEA. Nevertheless, the child will not be IDEA eligible because the disability does not create a need for special education. Similarly, as a general rule a child who needs related services but not special education does not fall within the purview of the Act.

The IDEA specifies that a free and appropriate public education may have two components: special education and related services. The IDEA defines special education as "specially designed instruction . . . to meet the unique needs of a child with a disability."† The IDEA defines "related services" as:

> transportation, and such developmental, corrective, and other supportive services (including speech pathology and audiology, psychological services, physical and occupational therapy, recreation . . . social work services, counseling services . . . and medical services, except that such medical services shall be for diagnostic and evaluation purposes only) as may be required to assist a child with a disability to benefit from special education.‡

The IDEA's central principle is that special education and related services provided for children with disabilities must be appropriate. However, the term *appropriate* is not precisely defined in the act and has been the subject of much interpretation. A related IDEA principle is that every child with a disability must be educated in the least restrictive environment (LRE) appropriate to meet his or her needs. This principle creates a presumption in favor of inclusion or integration of children with disabilities in a regular educational setting, albeit the presumption is rebuttable. Another related IDEA principle, known as the "zero reject" principle, is that all children, regardless of the severity of their disabilities, are entitled to receive a free and appropriate public education.

*20 U.S.C. §1401 (a) (1) (A) (Supp. V 1993).
†20 U.S.C. §1401 (a) (16) (Supp. V 1993).
‡20 U.S.C. §1401 (a) (17) (Supp. V 1993).

Under the IDEA, the Individualized Education Program (IEP) is the vehicle for assuring that a particular child identified as having a disability receives a free and appropriate public education through a program of special education and related services. The IEP is a written statement describing the child's present educational performance, the specific educational services and placement designed to meet the child's needs, annual goals with instructional objectives, and a plan to assess whether those objectives are being achieved. The IDEA requires the process of IEP development to be collaborative and to involve both educational personnel and the child's parent or guardian.

In addition, the IDEA requires educational agencies to follow certain procedures designed to safeguard the rights of children with disabilities. Among these procedural safeguards is a due-process hearing, conducted by an impartial hearing officer, that may be initiated by a parent or an education agency if they are not in agreement regarding the identification, evaluation, placement, or provision of a free and appropriate public education for a child with a disability or suspected disability.

The IDEA does not apply only to school-age children. Part B of the Act authorizes grants for programs for children with disabilities, ages three through five, and Part H of the Act furnishes federal assistance to the states for programs providing early intervention services for infants and toddlers, from birth to 2 years of age.

CONCLUSION

Upon passage of the ADA by the United States Senate, Senator Harkin, a leading sponsor of the legislation, declared:

> All across our Nation mothers are giving birth to infants with disabilities. So I want to dedicate the Americans With Disabilities Act to these, the next generation of children and their parents. With the passage of the ADA, we as a society make a pledge that every child with a disability will have the opportunity to maximize his or her potential to live proud, productive, and prosperous lives in the mainstream of our society.*

Laws have a major role to play in making this promise a reality through prohibiting discrimination against individuals with disabilities and promoting equality of opportunity for them. However, the existence of such laws does not automatically mean that this promise will become a reality. Rather, the existence of such laws must be viewed as part of a larger, multifaceted effort to assure that children with disabilities are able to live their lives in the mainstream of society.

*Statement of Senator Tom Harkin, 136 Cong. Rec. 5, 9684, 9689 (daily ed. July 13, 1990).

BIBLIOGRAPHY

Gittler J and Robinson J: *The Americans With Disabilities Act and children with special health care needs and their families*, Iowa City, 1995, National Maternal and Child Health Resource Center.

Gostin LO and Beyer HA, editors: *Implementing the Americans With Disabilities Act, rights and responsibilities for all americans*, Baltimore, 1993, Paul H. Brookes Publishing Co.

Rothstein LF: *Special education law*, edition 2, New York, 1990, Longman Publishers U.S.A.

Tucker BP and Goldstein BA: *Legal rights of persons with disabilities: an analysis of federal law*, Horsham, Penn, 1992, LRP Publications.

Wehman P: *The ADA mandate for social change*, Baltimore, 1993, Paul H. Brookes Publishing Co.

CHAPTER **10**

Family Roles: The Most Relevant Aspect of Family-Centered Care

JOSIE THOMAS
BEVERLEY H. JOHNSON

Families who have children with chronic illnesses and disabilities face many challenges, including a world of complex and possibly frightening emotions, multiple health encounters, involvement with numerous health, educational, and social service professionals, and at times, difficult ethical decisions about the care and treatment of their children. Many families struggle as they attempt to weave together the array of services and supports their children and family need. These families describe the sense of disempowerment, confusion, and isolation they experience as they work to find services for their children.[6,8,14]

FAMILY-CENTERED CARE

During the last 50 years there have been enormous gains in the physical treatment of childhood chronic and acute conditions. Unfortunately, the systems of care that evolved have too often fostered dependency in families and excluded them from full participation in the delivery of care for their children. Beginning in the 1980s, however, a profound shift in the organization and delivery of care and services to children "redefined relationships between families and professionals, fostering partnership and mutual respect; refocused programmatic efforts to enable and empower families; and renewed belief in the power of families and communities to effectively advocate for social change."[9] These changes reflect a new approach, called family-centered care, to providing care and services. The family-centered philosophy is based on the belief that all families are deeply caring and want to nurture and support their children. "Family-centered policies, programs, and practitioners seek to build on the strengths of families, both collectively and individually, to follow the family's lead in designing and delivering care, and to foster respectful, dynamic partnerships between families and professionals."[9]

In 1987, Surgeon General C. Everett Koop articulated the eight elements of family-centered care; a ninth element was added in 1990 (see the box on p. 108). These elements are the essential components of family-centered practice. While these concepts have been most widely discussed in the health care field, parallel movements in the fields of early intervention, developmental disabilities, and family preservation reflect similar values and beliefs. Family-centered care is creating a common language among professionals from many disciplines and between families and professionals. It is building bridges and forging relationships across agencies and organizations and between families and service providers.

Family-centered care is recognized as the best practice in the provision of services to children with special health care needs and their families. Federal legislation now requires that state Title V programs reflect the principles of family-centered care. Part H of the Individuals with Disabilities Act of 1991 mandates statewide, comprehensive, family-centered systems of early intervention for infants and toddlers with special needs and their families.

FAMILY ROLES

> In putting together a national health policy . . . we have learned from families. They told us that they want to work with us in different ways. They wish us to recognize that they are the constant in their child's life, and that we are the Tuesday morning clinic. And, they told us that they need to be partners in very different ways because they have that 24-hour responsibility.[13]

Family-centered care is built on collaboration. In family-centered service delivery, families are involved at all levels of care—at the level of care of the individual child, at the program level, and at the policy level. Collaboration between families and professionals is the foundation on which many of these roles are built. Recognition that both families and professionals have expertise and bring something to the table based on their experience is essential to the development of mutually respectful, collaborative relationships. As the practice of family-centered care becomes more widespread, families and professionals alike are recognizing that these collaborative relationships provide a means for bringing about changes in the system of care, making it more responsive and more respectful of family priorities.

Key Elements of Family-Centered Care

- Recognizing that the family is the constant in a child's life, while the service systems and personnel within those systems fluctuate
- Facilitating parent/professional collaboration at all levels of service delivery:
  - care of an individual child
  - program development, implementation, and evaluation
  - policy formation
- Honoring the racial, ethnic, cultural, and socioeconomic diversity of families
- Recognizing family strengths and individuality and respecting different methods of coping
- Sharing with families, on a continuing basis and in a supportive manner, complete and unbiased information
- Encouraging and facilitating family-to-family support and networking
- Understanding and incorporating the developmental needs of infants, children, and adolescents and their families into service delivery systems
- Implementing comprehensive policies and programs that provide emotional and financial support to meet the needs of families
- Designing accessible service systems that are flexible, culturally competent, and responsive to family-identified needs

Modified from Johnson BH, Jeppson ES, and Redburn L: *Caring for children and families: guidelines for hospitals*, Bethesda, Md, 1992, ACCH.

These collaborative relationships are new roles for providers as well as for families and bring with them new sets of challenges for families and providers alike. Dunst, Trivette, and Deal[5] say that family-centered care requires professionals to assume new roles—that of empathetic listener, teacher/therapist, consultant, resource enabler, mobilizer, mediator, and advocate. These challenging new roles may require professionals to learn new attitudes and skills, allowing them to recognize and build on family competence and resourcefulness. Families also may need to learn new skills as they assume more collaborative roles in their interactions with service providers.[3]

There is no one role that is right for all families. Families differ in the strategies they adopt to realize their dreams for their children and themselves. Understanding, respect, and support from professionals for family choices and priorities is fundamental to the practice of family-centered care and the realization of family priorities.

The descriptions that follow are some of the roles that families are assuming in the development, implementation, and evaluation of care for their children with special needs. They are by no means complete, but serve only as a small sample.

Families as Experts in the Care of Their Children

Families play a pivotal role in the lives of their children. "Families are the constant in their children's lives while the service systems and personnel within those systems fluctuate."[15] Because they are the only ones who see their children over time in different settings, parents are finely tuned to their child's needs as well as their responses to the care given them.[2]

As the primary providers of their children's care, parents are the repository of key information about their children. The information they have to offer about their child is often essential to that child's care. Listening to families and providing an array of opportunities for families to share this information is an important role for professionals. For example, in developing an Individual Family Service Plan (IFSP) for a family who has a baby with special needs, listening carefully to a family's concerns and priorities for their child and themselves is the basis for the development of outcomes and identification of service needs for the child and family.

Sharing information with parents helps them make better decisions, conveys respect, and changes the relationship with professionals.[7] Providers can share information with families through informal conversations, formal meetings, and written reports. Providing a family with information about their child's diagnosis and treatment alternatives, offering access to medical records and charts as well as the medical library and family resource library, and offering information about family-to-family support groups and other family-support resources in the community are all essential pieces of information that a family may require to make the best possible choices in the care their child needs and to function as an equal partner on the child's care team. "Frequent, accurate, and thorough information about their child's condition helps empower parents as protectors, supporters, and decision makers for their child."[10]

Families as Coordinators of Their Children's Care

Involvement with multiple service providers and agencies is often the rule rather than the exception for families of children with special needs. Because families find that no one person, professional, or agency can meet all of their children's or family's needs, they must interface with multiple service providers and agencies and sometimes even multiple care or service coordinators. Lack of coordination between health, education, and social services is a common and especially difficult problem. A family is then not only coping with the overwhelming demands of caring for their child but also with having to organize and coordinate services. Service systems that require their own coordinators are operating in the bureaucratic interests of the system, not in the best interests of families.

When care coordination across agencies and services exists and functions well, parents still provide overall coordination because, by necessity, all services must pass through the family.[1] As one foster parent stated, "Trying to coordinate teachers, doctors, dentists, mental health professionals, maternal visitation, and caseworkers into a planned treatment of care is a full-time job."[11]

Some families choose to serve as their child's care coordinator. While this choice should be respected, families must receive the necessary support to carry out this role. At a minimum, families must have access to all information and records; authority to coordinate appointments, convene service plan meetings, and prioritize goals; and practical supports, such as copies of community-resource directories and agency personnel lists. Ideally, families should be reimbursed for their time as care coordinators and have access to photocopying equipment, computers, telephones, and fax machines.

It is a tenet of family-centered care that families be able to determine the exact role they want in coordinating their child's care. Whatever choice they make should be honored and supported.

Families as Consultants and Advisors

Families have come to be acknowledged not only as experts in the care of their children, but also as experts in the way services are planned, delivered, and evaluated. Families can speak first hand about the services that they receive and to help guide policies. Parents can also help providers see the need for change and bring up important but sensitive issues that others may find difficult to discuss. Family members can offer suggestions to improve services, can comment on plans and programs, and most importantly, using their expertise as family members, can answer the question, "Would this work for the children and families I know?"

Families, working in collaboration with professionals, are changing policies and practices in federal and state agencies, professional training programs, hospitals, and community-based health, education, and social-service programs and organizations. Parents of children with special needs review state and federal grant proposals, serve on advisory committees to state and federal agencies, direct federally funded projects, and are hired as staff in key positions at the state level. State Title V Children with Special Health Care Needs (CSHCN) programs are actively seeking family expertise in the policy development and evaluation of services. A 1992 survey of CSHCN programs by the Federation of Children with Special Needs revealed the shift to family involvement.[17] Every state CSHCN program was surveyed and each reported that families were involved as advisors. The CAPP report also made recommendations for a variety of ways in which families can be involved in these state programs. These recommendations include the development of the following roles for families:

- participants on committees and task forces
- participants in inservice training as planners and teachers
- participants in Title V block grant preparation
- participants in the selection process for Title V staff
- paid consultants or staff to Title V programs

The report further recommends that programs should facilitate parent and family involvement by offering preparation and support for these roles.

The CSHCN program in the Department of Public Health in Michigan has developed a comprehensive approach to ensure the involvement of families as consultants and advisors in their programs.

- CSHCS implemented the Parent Participation Program to strengthen the relationship between the department and families. Directed by the parent of a child with special needs, the primary goals of the program are to provide a mechanism for parental input in CSHCS policy development and program implementation and to develop a network of parent-to-parent support statewide.
- The Family Support Network of Michigan was established. This network has a central office within CSHCS and is staffed by volunteers and paid staff all of whom are themselves parents of children with special needs
- CSHCS and the Parent Participation Project successfully sought private and public funding for Project Uptown. The goal of the project is to increase social and emotional support for families from the many cultural and ethnic groups in Detroit and to ensure their active involvement in CSHCS policy and program development.
- The department established a family/professional CSHCS Advisory Committee to advise the department chief and to act as a resource in training and education activities. This committee comprises representatives of consumers, provider agencies, professional disciplines, and human-service agencies. Parents of children with special needs are significantly represented and hold key positions.
- The department also appointed a task force of more than 2 dozen statewide organizations to update the policies and procedures by which provider eligibility is determined. Key health care professionals as well as family members, universities, hospitals, and other consumer groups were represented.

Although involvement of family members as consultants and advisors has led to major changes in many programs, hospitals, and agencies, families continue to struggle to be recognized as experts and to be included as partners in the development of programs and policies. Even where families are serving in significant numbers as consultants and advisors, they are primarily from the dominant culture and middle-class and not reflective of the racial, ethnic, cultural, and socioeconomic diversity of the community or state. Efforts to include these families are just beginning at the local, state, and national level. The Institute for Family-Centered Care, with funding from the federal Maternal and Child Health Bureau, has recently developed for policy makers, program planners, federal officials, and families a guidance publication, *Essential Allies: Families as Advisors*, on the participation of families, as consultants and advisors.

Families as Teachers of Professionals

Children and families have long been teachers of professionals on an informal basis. Recently, however, the importance of systematically involving families as teachers has been recognized. In preservice professional education, such as medical schools, parents of children with special needs are developing curriculum, teaching, and sharing life experiences with students.

The Medical Education Project at Parent to Parent of Vermont is one such example. Begun in 1985, the Medical Education Project is a collaborative effort of Parent to Parent of Vermont and the University of Vermont College of Medicine and department of psychology. In lectures and discussions jointly taught by university staff and parents of children with special needs, third-year medical students explore feelings and personal biases that influence their diagnosis, treatment, and prognosis of people with disabilities. Home visits where medical students spend time with families in nonclinical settings are mandatory. At the end of their pediatric rotations, students reevaluate their attitudes through discussion of home visiting experiences, and significant changes in the attitudes of medical students who have completed the course have been documented.

Family members are also providing training on a variety of topics at grand rounds, inservice programs, continuing education activities, conferences, and seminars. For example, Parents Helping Parents in San Jose, California, has developed a training program for practicing physicians, residents, and students on delivering diagnostic news to a family. The training program includes media, lecture, discussion, and resource display. These training workshops are contracted by the local hospital on a 5-year rotation schedule. The hospital pays a fee to Parents Helping Parents and arranges space, time, and other logistics.

These are not isolated examples. Replication of these and other similar models is occurring in medical education programs, in schools of nursing and social work, and in the training of child-life workers.

Families as Providers of Support

> When I first started out with this I was alone on the mountain top ... feeling alone and isolated ... then I went to group and found I wasn't alone .

The mother of a child with HIV
speaking of her family-to-family support network

Because their own experiences in accessing information, support, and resources to care for their child can be frustrating, parents are often highly motivated to help other people. One of the most effective ways to provide support and develop coping skills has been parent- and family-support groups and networks. Such networks can provide a nonthreatening, supportive environment that encourages families to help others, establishing a two-way process that is both therapeutic and empowering. By reaching out through meetings, phone networks, visitation programs, and parent-to-parent programs where veteran parents are matched with parents whose children are newly diagnosed, families provide mutual support, develop friendships, gather and share important information, and find ways to improve the system.[12]

Although organized parent-to-parent support has existed since the mid 1970s and is gaining strength, it is still not broadly available in many communities. Organized parent-support networks for families who have children with special needs are especially missing in low-income communities as well as in communities where families are not from the dominant culture. Typically, families who are struggling with poverty, especially families of color who are poor, have been underrepresented in parent-to-parent programs. A national survey of parent-to-parent programs across the country reports that 96% of parents involved in such programs are from the dominant culture and a large majority (61.5%) are middle income or above.[4] Many program planners and service providers continue to believe that these kinds of parent and family activities are only for well-educated, middle-class, white families. Often referrals are not made or programs are not developed for low-income and minority families. The recent development of both local and national networks and organizations for families caring for children with HIV or AIDS has shown, however, that these families are both willing and able to participate in and lead parent support activities.[18]

Families as Advocates and Visionaries

Having a vision is not just planning for a future we already know how to get to. It is daring to dream about what is possible.

Janet Vohs[16]

The persistent voices of families have created a watershed in the development of services for individuals with disabilities and chronic illnesses. In pursuing their dreams for their children and themselves, families have led the way for what is possible for all children.

Strong grassroots advocacy efforts have led to the passage of landmark legislation to protect the rights of children and individuals with disabilities. Since the early 1970s legislation has ensured the rights of children with disabilities to be educated with their peers who are not disabled. Because of the passage of the Americans with Disabilities Act in 1990, the civil rights of individuals with disabilities are now protected from discrimination at work, in the community, and in recreational activities.

Today grassroots efforts by families to ensure full inclusion of their children with disabilities in educational settings and to ensure that access to health care is right for all Americans are at the forefront of the parent movement. Because health care is still not considered to be a right, individuals with disabilities and chronic illnesses are the most vulnerable when cuts are made in health care financing; they are the first dropped when they become ill, and they are the first excluded because of preexisting conditions. The voices of families are rising up during this time of health care reform discussions to ensure that the needs of children and individuals with disabilities and chronic illnesses are included in the debate.

CONCLUSION

There is no one role that is right for all families at all times. Families move in and out of roles over time and as their children's and family's needs change and evolve. Family-centered care enables and empowers families to choose roles that are meaningful to them. The role of the professional is to respect, support, and work in partnership with families in their chosen roles.

REFERENCES

1. Allen DA and Hudd SS: Are we professionalizing parents? Weighing the benefits and pitfalls. In Hanft B, editor: *Family-centered care: an early intervention resource manual, Rockville, Md, 1989, The American Occupational Therapy Association, Inc.*

2. Anderson B: Parents of children with disabilities as collaborators in health care, *Coalition Quarterly* 4:2-3, 15-18, 1985.

3. Bailey DB: Building positive relationships between professionals and families. In McGonigel et al, editors: *Guidelines and recommended practices for the individualized family service plan, Bethesda, Md, 1991, ACCH.*

4. Beach Center on Families and Disability: *Parent to parent national survey project,* Lawrence, Kan, 1992, The University of Kansas.

5. Dunst CJ, Trivette CM, and Deal AG: *Enabling and empowering families: principles and guidelines for practice,* Cambridge, Mass, 1988, Brookline Books.

6. Featherstone H: *A Difference in the Family,* New York, 1980, Basic Books.

7. Hanson J: A journey with parents and infants: rethinking parent professional interactions, Washington DC, 1989, The George Washington University.

8. Hartman AF, Radin MB, and McConnell B: Parent-to-parent support: a critical component of health care services for families, *Issues in Comprehensive Pediatric Nursing* 15:55-67, 1992.

9. Johnson BH et al: The process of change. In Hostler S, editor: *Family-centered care: implementation in tretiary care settings,* Charlottesville, Vir, 1995, Kluge Children's Medical Center.

10. Kasper JW and Nyamathi AM: Parents of children in the pediatric intensive unit: what are their needs? *Heart and Lung* 17(5): 574-581, 1988.

11. Mayer J: Advocacy: one family's story, *Focal Point* 6(1): 14-15, 1992.

12. Nathanson M: Organizing and maintaining support groups for parents of children with chronic illness and handicapping conditions, Washington DC, 1986, ACCH.

13. National Center for Family-Centered Care: *Physician Education Forum Report,* Bethesda, Md, 1990, ACCH.

14. Schulz JB: Heroes in disguise. In Turnbull A et al, editors: *Cognitive coping, families, & disability,* Baltimore, 1993, Brookes.

15. Shelton TL, Jeppson ES, and Johnson BH: *Family-centered care for children with cpecial health care needs,* Washington DC, 1987, ACCH.

16. Vohs J: On belonging: a place to stand, a gift to give. In Turnbull A et al, editors: *Cognitive coping, families, & disability,* Baltimore, Md, 1993, Brookes.

17. Wells N, Anderson B, and Popper B: Families in program and policy: report of a 1992 survey of family participation in state title V programs for children with special health care needs. Boston, Mass, 1993, CAPP National Parent Resource Center, Federation for Children with Special Needs.

18. Wiener LS et al: National telephone support groups: a new avenue toward psychosocial support for HIV-infected children and their families, *Social Work with Groups* 16(3), 1993.

BIBLIOGRAPHY

Advances in Family-Centered Care. Semiannual newsletter of the Institute for Family-Centered Care, Bethesda, MD.

Dunst, C.J. (1990). Family support principles: Checklists for program builders and practitioners. *Family Systems Intervention Monograph*, 2, Number 5. Morganton, NC: Family, Infant, and Preschool Program, Western Carolina Center.

Edelman, L. (Ed.) (1991). *Getting on board: Training activities to promote the practice of family-centered care.* (Available from Project Copernicus, Kennedy Krieger Institute, Baltimore, MD).

Edelman, L., Elsayed, S.S., & McGonigel, M.J. (1992). *Overview of family-centered service coordination.* (Available from Project Copernicus, Kennedy Krieger Institute, Baltimore, MD).

Edelman, L., Greenland, B., & Mills, B.L. (1992). *Family-centered communication skills* and *Building parent/professional collaboration.* (Training activities available from Project Copernicus, Kennedy Krieger Institute, Baltimore, MD).

Gerteis, M., Edgman-Levitan, S., Daley, J., & Delbanco, T.L. (Eds.). (1993). *Through the patient's eyes: Understanding and promoting patient-centered care.* San Francisco, CA: Jossey Bass Publishers.

Harrison, H. (1993). The principles for family-centered neonatal care. *Pediatrics, 92,*643-650.

Hanson, J.L., Johnson, B.H., Jeppson, E.S., Thomas, M.J., & Hall, J.H. (1994). *Hospitals moving forward with family-centered care.* Bethesda, MD: Institute for Family-Centered Care.

Hunter, R. (1995). *Parents as Policy-Makers: A handbook for effective participation.* Portland, OR: Research and Training Center on Family Support and Children's Mental Health.

Jeppson, E.S., & Thomas, J. (1995). *Essential Allies: Families as advisors.* Bethesda, MD: Institute for Family-Centered Care.

Johnson, B., Jeppson, E., & Redburn, L. (1992). *Caring for children and families: Guidlines for hospitals.* Bethesda, MD: Association for the Care for Children's Health.

Singer, G.H. & Powers, L.E. (1993). *Families, disability, and empowerment: Active coping skills and strategies for family interventions.* Baltimore, MD: Paul H. Brooks.

Wells, N., Anderson, B., & Popper, B. (1993). *Families in program and policy: report of a 1992 survey of family participation in state Title V programs for children with special health care needs.* Boston, MA: Federation for Children with Special Needs.

CHAPTER **11**

Cultural Competency

RICHARD N. ROBERTS
JOHN E. EVANS

As communities continue to develop family-centered, community-based, coordinated systems of care for children with special health needs, they must ensure that these programs are also culturally competent. If programs are to serve families within local communities, they must do so in a way that draws upon and respects the cultural strengths, interaction patterns, beliefs, and customs of families who make up the community. Programs that do so are more likely to be effective in reaching all of the families of children with special health needs. Though culture is only one of the forces that shapes a community, it is an important one because it provides a context for much of the social interaction that goes on between community members.

This chapter gives a brief introduction to the rationale for including cultural competency as a central cornerstone in building effective systems of care. First, the construct of cultural competency is defined, followed by a discussion of the reasons why programs must become more culturally competent over time. Some of the problems that are encountered in providing services in a culturally competent manner are discussed along with principles that must be understood to create solutions to these problems. Finally, the work of the Maternal and Child Health (MCH) National Resource Center on Cultural Competency is used as an example of the efforts needed to assist states and local health care systems in creating programs that address the cultural differences among clients.

DEFINITION OF CULTURAL COMPETENCE

The Maternal and Child Health National Resource Center on Cultural Competency for Children with Special Health Care Needs has developed a working definition of cultural competence as follows:

> *Cultural Competency* is a set of behaviors, attitudes, and policies that come together on a continuum to enable a system, agency, and/or individual to function effectively in transcultural interactions. The word *cultural* is used because it implies an integrated pattern of human behavior that includes thought, communication, action, customs, beliefs, values, and institutions of a racial, religious, socioeconomic, educational, occupational, or geographical group. The word *competence* is used because it implies having the ability to function effectively. Cultural competency is a goal which a system, agency, and/or individual continually aspires to achieve.[3]

There are several points within this definition that should be emphasized. First, it places the responsibility on service providers to become culturally competent by creating systems of care responsive to the cultural needs of families. Families should not be forced to change their cultural expectations and norms or their ways of interaction and practices to meet the demands of the agency. Second, the definition moves beyond the constructs of cultural diversity, cultural sensitivity, and cultural responsiveness in that it provides for action as well as belief. It is insufficient to be aware of cultural differences without integrating awareness and sensitivity into action. Finally, cultural competence exists along a continuum and is not a static state. Cross et al[3] describe a continuum of cultural competence that moves from cultural destructiveness to cultural proficiency. The continuum provides the opportunity for both self-assessment and training as individuals and programs continue to grow toward cultural proficiency.

THE NEED FOR CULTURALLY COMPETENT SYSTEMS OF CARE

Demographic Considerations

As the United States continues to become more culturally and ethnically diverse in its population, the concepts of minority and majority cultures become less meaningful. Different ethnic and cultural groups continue to represent a higher percentage of the entire U.S. population, and the number of children within each group who require special services continues to grow. Agencies must become equipped to provide appropriate services to children whose families have cultural roots and practices outside of the mainstream white population.

In addition, children below age 19 make up increasingly larger percentages of the population for specific ethnic groups other than white. Within

African-American, Latino/Hispanic, and Native American populations, the percentage of children below age 19 within each group ranges from about 40% to 50%. It is estimated that by the year 2020, children of ethnic and cultural minorities will increase to 40% of the child population in the United States.[2] For these reasons there is both a demographic and moral imperative to provide services in a culturally competent manner.

Lack of Culturally Diverse Service Providers

The increasing percentage of children of ethnic and cultural minorities who require services is coupled with a scarcity of service providers from the same cultural and ethnic groups. Because these families have a higher representation in populations that are poor and less educated, it is less likely that they are represented in professional groups that provide services to families. Most service providers in the U.S. continue to be white and are frequently male. Thus, the cultural differences between the service providers and those who are receiving services will remain a factor in the service delivery models for some time to come.

Need for Outreach Efforts

One may wonder why it is necessary to establish models of cultural competence when the field has been moving toward family-centered, community-based, coordinated care already. It is our position that though the concepts of family-centered, community-based care are highly relevant and serve as building blocks for culturally competent care, they are insufficient. Service providers can be very family centered in their efforts to provide services but may only provide those services to families who are like themselves. Programs that are culturally competent seek out families who would not normally avail themselves of services because of cultural barriers and differences; services are provided to such families in a manner consistent with the cultural practices of the different cultural groups they represent. Thus, culturally competent programs create proactive outreach efforts to ensure that they are reaching the needs of all children with special needs within their catchment areas. It is this distinction that makes cultural competence a logical next step for programs seeking to provide services within a family-centered, community-based context.

PROBLEMS IN CREATING CULTURALLY COMPETENT SYSTEMS

There are a number of barriers that may systematically deny services to families from minority cultures who have children with special health needs, but these barriers are not insurmountable. It must first be recognized that these

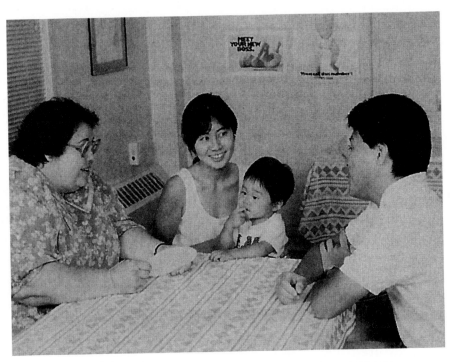

From Clemen-Stone, Eigsti, McGuire: Comprehensive Community Health Nursing, ed 4, St Louis, 1995, Mosby–Year Book.

problems exist at every level within the health service system (from federal to local service providers) in policy, training, and practice. We will concentrate on six major areas including lack of community ownership, racism, lack of knowledge by key personnel, lack of funding, imbalance in staffing, and insensitivity to the issues of cultural competence by policy makers.

Lack of Community Ownership

For programs to become culturally competent there has to be a shared sense of responsibility for the program between the community in which it functions and the program staff. Without this shared sense of responsibility the dominant culture tends to impose its programs on other cultural groups within the community.

Racism

Earlier views of racial integration in the U.S. suggested that legal mandates for integration would be sufficient to solve some of the deep-seated issues of racism that exist within the U.S. However, experience has not borne out this assumption; institutional and individual racism continue in many of the programs and communities across the country.

Racism within the construct of culturally competent programs means that programs systematically exclude children of racial and ethnic minorities from services for any of several reasons including lack of an outreach program, services that denigrate and insult family members, services that do not allow cultural practices to be included within the treatment regimens, active discouragement for including nonwestern healing practices within the program, and services that are not accessible or acceptable to families who represent different cultural values. Thus racism as a policy can be subtle, in a sense that programs do not actively seek to have a negative effect on families of color, or it can be active, in that programs systematically seek to destroy cultural beliefs and practices. It is critical, however, that as we move along the continuum of cultural competence, we address the issue of racism in a forthright manner in order to move beyond it.

Lack of Knowledge

Many health care providers are not knowledgeable about the cultural practices, beliefs, and customs of patients who come from cultures different from their own. Relatively few training programs across the country emphasize such kinds of training, and it has only been recently that national organizations have advocated inclusion of cultural materials and curricula into training programs for health care providers. This is not to say that there is not a tremendous interest on the part of some health care workers in the area of cultural differences and cultural values. We have found in our own work that when opportunities are provided for training in this area they receive a very enthusiastic response.

Lack of Time and Money

Most health programs, whether privately or publicly funded, are already busy. There are too few health care providers for the many families and children in need of additional health care services. Many early intervention programs, for example, are desperately understaffed with respect to qualified professionals across the range of services needed. In most cases funding is fairly low, and it becomes an ethical and logistical conundrum to actively seek clients who will make waiting lists longer when many of the legal mandates require that a waiting list cannot even be developed. Thus health care workers who seriously address outreach as part of their effort to become more culturally competent will find that their program will expand in the number and type of services they provide. In these days of constricted budgets, this is a serious issue.

Imbalance of Staffing

Most health care programs throughout the country are staffed with a higher percentage of Caucasian professionals than minority professionals. When ethnic diversity is found, it is more within paraprofessional groups. Even with aggressive recruitment programs for professionals from minority cultures, the number of qualified professionals across the country who are from ethnic and cultural minorities remains much smaller than needed for the foreseeable future. This places a strong mandate on training programs to continue to recruit minorities into the health care field. Meanwhile, health care program managers must ensure that their staff receive training on cross-cultural issues and that cultural concerns are raised suppositions.

Insensitivity of Policy Makers

Only recently have policy makers taken seriously the issue of cultural competence in developing guidance for programs and making it part of their mandate for family-centered, community-based, culturally competent, coordinated care for children with special needs. Even with the best of intentions programs face formidable institutional and financial barriers in creating culturally competent systems. Unless there is a clear, consistent written policy from the federal to the local level, it is very difficult for individual programs to overcome existing institutional and financial barriers to become truly culturally competent.

PRINCIPLES THAT SHOULD DRIVE CULTURALLY COMPETENT PROGRAMS

1. Culturally competent services must also by definition be family centered and community based. Much of the discussion above has addressed this principle.
2. Staff should be aware that each family is unique and must be treated as such. It is as culturally insensitive to assume that all families within a given cultural group will react the same way as it is to ignore the fact that culture is an important variable in determining how we behave.
3. Care must be taken in separating cultural issues from the effects of poverty and discrimination experienced by many minority groups within the United States. Families that have few options and resources at their disposal are often forced to resort to the most economical methods of providing health care. For instance, the economics of being poor may require families of minority groups to obtain health care for their children from programs that are not culturally preferred.
4. Program staff should have the capacity and opportunity to assess for themselves their own cultural values and understand the effect of their

backgrounds on their ability to provide culturally competent services. This cultural self-awareness is an ongoing discovery process and can be a valuable tool in defining new program and training needs.

5. It is not necessary to be of a culture to provide services to members of that culture. However, it is important that staff understand the dynamics of the inherent tension caused when two or more cultures interact to provide a service or solve a problem. It is critical to ensure that members of the cultural group being served are able to effect decisions concerning practice, training, hiring, and policy.

6. Good programs are the product of hard work in developing personal relationships and networks across agencies and communities. Even so, mechanisms are needed to ensure that components of a program have been institutionalized and are not dependent on one person from the institution and one person from the community to maintain them over time. The commitment needs to be at the institutional level with sufficiently broad-based involvement that the institutional commitment survives staff turnover and changing interests.

7. The development of programs such as these requires a paradigm shift on the part of service providers to share ownership and decision making. As with many shifts of this nature, once program staff and administrators make that shift it becomes a very natural way of viewing the world. However, such a shift is not without risk. It requires a higher tolerance for ambiguity as programs, parents, and community leaders map a course together. However, those who enter into the process have the potential to create programs with a high degree of community and family satisfaction., which leads to higher staff morale and a higher caliber of service.

EFFORTS TO CREATE MORE CULTURALLY COMPETENT SYSTEMS OF CARE

In the spring of 1990 the Children with Special Health Care Needs (CSHCN) Division of the Maternal and Child Health (MCH) Bureau, Health Resources and Services Administration of the Public Health Service, U.S. Department of Health and Human Services solicited plans from state Title V CSHCN programs to deliver statewide, culturally competent services. This initiative was not only indicative of the federal recognition of the need to establish culturally competent methods of service delivery, but was also an integral component of the Year 2000 health objectives established at the U.S. Surgeon General's Conference in 1987. As a result of the solicitation for plans, six states were selected to form a work group consisting of parents and representatives from MCH Special Projects of Regional and National Significance (SPRANS).

This work group served in an advisory capacity for cultural competency to the MCH Bureau and as a consortium to promote the establishment of culturally competent service delivery among its member states and projects.

The work group led to the establishment in October, 1992 of a National MCH Resource Center on Cultural Competency. The new center's mission, to "improve the quality of care and effectiveness of leadership in state CSHCN agencies by creating culturally competent systems of care through policies, decision-making, staff training, and service delivery," is based on the need to establish objective methods to assure definitive and measurable levels of cultural competency in the provision of community-based services.

This effort can assist states and communities as they move toward more culturally competent systems. However, as with any national center, it cannot do the job alone. As programs from the federal to the local community levels engage in systems development, they must ensure that they have created comprehensive, coordinated, and family-centered systems of care that are accessible and acceptable to all families in this country.

REFERENCES

1. Child Welfare League of America: *Cultural competence self-assessment instrument*, Washington DC, 1993, Author.
2. Children's Defense Fund: *A vision for America's future: an agenda for the 1990s—a children's defense budget*, Washington DC, 1989, Children's Defense Fund.
3. Cross TL et al: *Towards a culturally competent system of care: a monograph on effective services for minority children who are severely emotionally disturbed*, Washington DC, 1989, CASSP Technical Assistance Center, Georgetown University Child Development Center.
4. Gonzalez VM et al: *Health promotion in diverse cultural communities*, Palo Alto, Cal, 1991, Health Promotion Resource Center.
5. Isaacs MR and Benjamin MP: *Towards a culturally competent system of care*, vol 2, Washington DC, 1991, CASSP Technical Assistance Center, Georgetown University Child Development Center.
6. Nelkin VS: *Improving services for culturally diverse populations: division activity 1990-1991*, St. Paul, Minn, 1991, Pathfinder Resources.
7. Nelkin VS: *Improving state services for culturally diverse populations: focus on children with special health needs and their families*, St. Paul, Minn, 1991, Pathfinder Resources.
8. Randall-David E: *Strategies for working with culturally diverse communities and clients*, Washington DC, 1989, The Association for the Care of Children's Health.
9. Roberts RN et al: *Developing culturally competent programs for families of children with special needs: monograph and workbook*, ed 2, Washington, DC, 1990, Georgetown University Child Development Center.

CHAPTER **12**

Confidentiality Requirements in Integrated Programs

LOLA J. HOBBS

There is an inherent tension between an individual's right to privacy and the more general social good. Each of us subscribes to both of these values when we consider them singly. However, when we consider the values together, and we must do so as both program administrators and direct-service providers, we sense feelings of ambivalence and uncertainty. We know the public good must be served, but at what cost to the privacy of the individuals who are the public? Given this state of affairs it is no surprise that normative rules and practices have arisen around the question of what constitutes an appropriate exchange of confidential records and information between and among various service providers.

The problems associated with negotiating those rules and practices have become known as the *confidentiality barrier*. This chapter is intended to provide guidance on managing integrated health and human service programs to assure there is an appropriate exchange of confidential information and records. A clear distinction is made between legal barriers and other barriers to the successful exchange of confidential information and records in interagency settings. This distinction is critical to understanding which rules and practices require legal reform.

The central theme of this chapter is that confidentiality laws do not prevent the exchange of confidential information among providers serving the same patients/clients; it is the institutions providing the services that erect the major barrier. The law both anticipates and provides guidance for exchanging confidential information and records among practitioners and across program lines. As one might expect, the law attempts a neat balancing act wherein the right to privacy and the general public good are placed in a just relationship. The two principal legal requirements that direct and control such exchanges are: (1) to assure that any release of confidential information and records is based on informed consent; and (2) to prevent wrongful rerelease of confidential information obtained through proper release procedures. Various methods for complying with these requirements in interagency program settings are described and discussed in this chapter.

THE NEED TO OVERCOME CONFIDENTIALITY BARRIERS TO INTEGRATED SERVICES

Health and human service providers have extensive files on the needs, treatment plans, and outcomes of services to children and their families. These vast repositories of personal information on millions of individuals can serve as a resource for upgrading the level and quality of the care provided. Access to this information can reduce duplicate services, accelerate coordinated treatment planning and service delivery, and document service needs. These potential benefits are central to successful interagency programs. Without the ability to realize these benefits, the popular new notion of "seamless services" among agencies may become a utopian vision rather than a practical option.

Automation has given us an unprecedented ability to review and manage large volumes of personal information about our patients/clients as well as our neighbors and fellow citizens and there is a natural desire to access that information. However, personal information is private information. As such, it is protected and sequestered under federal, state, and local confidentiality statutes and regulations designed to protect the privacy of the individual. Correct and consistent interpretation of these rules is difficult as there are competing views on what must be done to manage and protect private or confidential information. Furthermore, there are many special rules as well as exceptions to the rules that mystify or confuse practitioners. This confusion and controversy has driven many practitioners and administrators to conclude that the safest answer to any interagency request for information from their records is to declare it confidential and unavailable.

Fortunately, there is a growing body of research on the role of confidentiality as a barrier to effective interagency services. New Beginnings, a San Diego County and City school-based, integrated family-service program, pioneered research on the confidentiality barrier[10] and methods to overcome the barrier.[5] Other authors have identified confidentiality as a barrier to integrated services. Prominent among them are Ooms and Owen,[11] Melville and Blank,[8] and Chaudry, Maurer, Oshinsky, and Mackie.[1] More recently, Greenberg and Levy[3] and Solar, Shotton, and Bell[13] published major works on various methods to effectively manage the exchange of confidential information in integrated services. Their research supports my view that laws and regulations on confidentiality are not in and of themselves barriers to effective interagency services. Rather, misunderstanding and misuse of the law are the most frequent causes for failure to exchange confidential information and records in a manner that is appropriate, consistent with the law, and supportive of integrated services. The other barriers to effective interagency services are discussed in the next section.

THE THREE ISMS: INSTITUTIONAL BIAS AND CONFIDENTIALITY BARRIERS

If clients/patients and professional colleagues wish to share confidential information and the law provides for such sharing, then why are there so many cases where confidentiality requirements seem to block coordinated and comprehensive interagency services? A number of variables are operative. In my view the three principal nonlegal sources of the confidentiality barrier are federalism, professionalism, and "turfism."

Federalism

Our federal form of government serves us well in many arenas. Certainly our founding fathers saw federalism as the cornerstone of democracy in a large and heterogenous nation. However, federalism also serves to make the technical rules on confidentiality more complex because it creates an opportunity for multiple interpretations at the federal, state, and local level of the meaning of fundamental privacy rights found in the Constitution. Those rights are described in two landmark federal laws: (1) the Freedom of Information Act* and (2) the Privacy Act.† These two laws form the foundation of all subsequent federal statutes and regulations, all enabling state laws and regulations, and all local policy ordinances and regulations that describe the privacy rights of individuals within the context of the best interests of the community.

The potential for diverse interpretations in our form of government grows more apparent when we examine the effect of federalism on administrative interpretation of confidentiality requirements. Federal law merely sets the parameters for privacy rights. These statutes must be elaborated upon by federal administrative agencies responsible for implementing the law as it applies to various programs. States are required to pass enabling

---

*Freedom of Information Act of 1966, 5 U.S.C. §552
†Privacy Act of 1974, 5 U.S.C. §552(a)

legislation to administer federally directed or funded programs. State agencies must interpret federal law and regulation as well as state statutes in the course of issuing program regulations. Local government agencies responsible for administering federal and state programs, must interpret, all federal, state, and local laws and regulations to implement local direct-service programs. There are many opportunities and/or necessities for administrators to interpret general rules and to add more rules relative to accessing and securing particular types of confidential information. Finally, at the program-delivery level, service providers view the rules through their professional and community "reality screens." It is no wonder that there are many versions of the confidentiality rules as public policy washes through multiple levels of government and through many agencies down to the service providers and their clients/patients.

Professionalism

Professional ethics guide the practice of organizations providing services to the public. For example, the National Association of Social Workers (NASW)[9] has issued a statement on ethics and confidentiality for school-based social workers to help guide them in handling confidential information in an inter-agency setting. However, professional ethics also reflect the particular world view and principal concerns of practitioners from each field of practice. There are real and legitimate differences in the views and concerns of various professionals serving the same clients. These differences affect interpretation of the standards for managing confidential records on services provided and/or the information provided by the client/patient who received the services.

Professional differences of opinion on confidentiality seem harmless enough until one begins to work across agency and program lines. At that point the professional ethic institutionalized in the agency's mission emerges as a potential barrier to the exchange of confidential information and records. We can gain some sense of the effect of this phenomenon by examining the role that institutional and professional norms play in casework service plans. The three institutions/professions we will examine are education (school), social services (welfare programs), and health services (doctors).

Education. Professionals in the field of education, grades K through 12, have special status because they provide a valued nonstigmatized public service and they act as substitute parents during the school day. However, they also work in an institutional context where parental privacy rights are held dear by law. They are keenly aware of the parent's right and responsibility to direct the education and the school records of their children, a right that is clearly spelled out in federal law* and by a Supreme Court decision.[4] At the same time school staff members are aware that regulation of public access to student records under the so-called directory information rule[†] is rather lenient as it permits release of basic student information without the consent of the parent. School staff members also know that an increase in incidents of student violence resulted in the expansion of their right and responsibility to release confidential information without parent consent under the need-to-know doctrine.[12] School staff do act *in loco parentis*, and school records can and do take on the appearance of a family album. They are full of confidential information on school performance and general family functioning, provided by the child, parent, and other professionals. All or some of that information may be accessible by the parents, reporters, policemen, and others because of the rights and rules noted above.

This set of circumstances sometimes causes professionals in other fields to think there is too little control of too much information in school records. These professionals decide they would rather not have confidential information from their agency included in open school records. These feelings initiate the desire to close the door to exchange of confidential information among education, social service, and health professionals serving the same children and families.

Social Services. Welfare programs, unlike public education programs, provide services to a segment of the population not necessarily valued in a society that places great emphasis on wealth and work. Program participants are frequently stigmatized. Consequently, federal and state laws on welfare records are very restrictive with respect to publishing information that will identify welfare clients. They specifically prohibit publishing lists of participants of Aid to Families with Dependent Children[‡] and food stamps.[§]

At the same time, welfare records contain massive amounts of personal information on program participants. Clients are required to provide accurate documentation of personal identity and family history, extensive information on income and resources, and supplemental information on the social, emotional, and physical health functioning of other family members. These records are seen as rich depositories of information by other professionals such as law enforcement officers and education staff counselors. These professionals frequently seek

---

*Family Education Rights and Privacy Act (FERPA) of 1974, 20 U.S.C. §1232g
[†]34 C.F.R. §99.30
[‡]45 C.F.R. §205.50; 45 U.S.C.A. §602(a) (9)
[§]7 C.F.R.S. §272.1(c); 7 U.S.C.A. §2020(E) (8)

a list of clients jointly served by welfare and the professional's own agency. Their typical reaction to the welfare policy of not publishing a list is that social service staff are nonresponsive and overly protective of the incredible data contained in their agency's records. This reaction increases the desire to close the door to interagency cooperation and appropriate exchange of confidential records.

Health. Health professionals provide services universally regarded as good and necessary on very personal matters and they are universally regarded as high-status professionals. Confidentiality laws and regulations for health services reflect these societal values and the high status accorded to health care professionals. Four distinct and seemingly conflicting sets of rules fall out of these circumstances: (1) The rules controlling access to and security of confidential health care records are the most restrictive of the three professions, education, social services, and health. (2) The rules are more permissive regarding exchange of information among health professionals than those for social service and educational professionals. (3) The rules in mental health service regarding the client's right to access their treatment records are exceptionally restrictive. (4) But the rules regarding the rights of minors to consent to their own health treatment and to control the records of that treatment are exceptionally strong.[2,6,7]

Other professionals tend to view health records and the complex, contradictory laws surrounding them as confusing and forbidding. They frequently express frustration about the reluctance of health professionals to share their records. After all, health records do contain information critical to developing complete case plans and assessing case outcomes. At times the natural reluctance of health professionals to share records is perceived as being based solely on their lofty professional status. When this final barrier is raised, the door closes to collaboration services among the three professionals, while the family and children are left poorly served.

Turfism

Turfism is a neologism for a certain kind of bureaucratic territorial behavior. It is not intended as a term of compliment when it describes the behavior of one professional toward another. Nonetheless, it is a behavior we all recognize. As Rapp, Stephens, and Clontz[12] point out, turfism explains the origin of much of the tension between professionals treating the same client. This behavior is politely called uncooperative when one professional speaks about the behavior of another professional. However, the *turfism* comes closer to describing the core problem because it focuses our attention on the underlying issue of power and control; information is power and the gatekeeper of information can exercise much power and control.

Turfism may not be a pretty word, but the condition it names needs to be recognized as a natural and somewhat inevitable problem in the delivery of interagency services. We all have a need for control in this complex and difficult world, and that need seems to go increasingly unmet. Collaboration requires us to give others an opportunity to participate in our planning process and invites them to have access to our confidential records. This invitation can accelerate a sense a loss of control over professional goals and personal job satisfaction. When that happens, maintaining one's turf becomes more important than effective and efficient services to clients/patients served by more than one program.

FOUR APPROACHES TO MANAGING
LAW-BASED CONFIDENTIALITY BARRIERS

There are a variety of methods to overcome the alleged legal barriers to the exchange of confidential information and records. Ironically, most of these solutions are already present in the law, so there is little need to seek major changes in the laws. These solutions can be identified by a resourceful practitioner, planner, or administrator. Four of the methods for exchanging confidential case information across program lines are briefly described in this section. All four comply with federal statutes and regulations and can be adapted to programs in other states with little or no change to state statutes.

Two of the four methods are relatively simple methods of exchanging case-specific and compiled confidential information and records. Method I involves developing a standardized informed consent form that will be accepted by all agencies to release case-specific information on a case-by-case basis. Method II permits agencies to share compiled confidential data through the use of statistical reports and/or narrative reports that contain no identifying information.

The other two methods involve more sophisticated procedures for the exchange of confidential records. Method III relies on special laws that permit the release of confidential information among a specified number of professionals, called members of multidisciplinary teams. The team uses one release form depending on the law. Method IV permits access to automated files on clients/patients served by more than one program by using individual releases for permission to access their files or by following statutory exceptions to legal requirements for informed consent. Method IV is the most favored method because it permits rapid exchange of information from personal records, quick preparation of statistical data based on confidential records, and quick production of authorized lists of patients/clients.

Method I—Informed Consent

As noted earlier, the law anticipates and provides direction for the release of confidential information and records. All confidentiality laws and regulations recognize procedures for informed consent from the individual who provides the personal information. With certain restrictions, individuals hold the authority to release their personal information to others. Agencies must ensure that their release procedures protect the individual's privacy rights and the integrity of their records.

Standards for informed-consent release forms are found in every program. They vary among health and human service programs, but there are more commonalities than differences among the rules for all service programs. One release form will suffice for almost all agencies if it contains nine (9) key elements. Those elements are: (1) the name of the individual whose record is to released; (2 and 3) the name and the signature of that individual or his or her legally authorized representative; (4 and 5) the name and address of the agency and the agency representative to whom and from whom the information is released; (6) the specific confidential information to be released; (7) the date the release was signed; (8) the date the authorization expires; and (9) a list of the specific privacy rights of the individual under the laws that govern the program(s).

A number of other writers have provided guidance on the proper language and citation of privacy laws by publishing model policies and procedures.[3,6,13] Generally speaking, the release form that complies with a state's standards for confidential health records will meet that state's requirements for their human service programs. A standardized informed-consent release form accelerates the exchange of information among agencies because it simplifies procedures and avoids the delays associated with acquiring a signature on each form from each agency. However, it will not resolve the issue of one release form signed once for all agencies that serve a client/patient. A method to accomplish that objective is discussed under Method III.

Method II—Compiled Data

Some professionals assume confidential information usually is unavailable to researchers and always unavailable to the public in any form. The first assumption overlooks the fact that laws and regulations do provide access for researchers under specified conditions. (One of the best examples of these rules is found in federal regulations detailing the researcher's right of access to confidential drug and alcohol information.*) The second assumption over-

*42 C.F.R., PART 2§2.50

looks the fact that statistical information based on confidential records can be printed by an agency if all personal information that might identify any individual is deleted from the reports. In sum, confidential narrative records or statistical reports may be accessed and published by agency staff and researchers so long as no identifying client-specific information is released by the researcher or the agency to the public.

Method III—Multidisciplinary Teams

California law permits release of confidential information to multidisciplinary personnel teams that use one or no release form for exchange of information or records within the team. This approach recognizes that professionals in education, health, human services, and certain other professions or roles frequently provide case-management services to the same clients. These case managers have special authority and responsibility for case planning/treatment under the law, and they are certified to carry out these responsibilities under professional or organizational standards.* In sum, the multidisciplinary personnel team, as a group, share confidential information and records while using one or no release form to carry out duties defined in the law that exempts them from standard informed consent requirements.

Developing a single informed consent form is the easiest task in implementing these laws. The harder task is developing procedures to properly secure the confidential information and records and guard them against inadvertent rerelease. The development of adequate security provisions requires use of interagency agreements, special training, and careful supervision of the quantity and specificity of the information released from or included in the case records. Appropriate record keeping for participants on multidisciplinary teams is different from the recording done by the team on casework at their home agency. Team members must limit confidential information placed in home agency records that is needed to document those services provided pursuant to their agency's administrative responsibilities.

Method IV—Automated Files

Today there is enormous capacity for rapid exchange of automated confidential records. We have reached a point in the age of technology where we rely heavily on automation to develop and store personal information records. Indeed, many practitioners are recognizing automated files as the principal resource to achieve efficient integrated interagency services. At the same time, there is growing recognition of the added risks to privacy rights.

*Cal. Welf. & Inst. Code §830, §5328, §5606.8. §19861. and §18986.40

Fortunately, a change in federal law, the Computer Matching and Privacy Act*, has provided added direction on procedural requirements for the release and the security of confidential information stored in automated records. Federal law now provides for the exchange of information in a manner that guards the privacy rights of the individual and protects the public good. More importantly, it also sets new standards to assure the integrity of the confidential records.

The simplest way to protect privacy rights and secure automated records is to use batch-match or tape-to-tape procedures. Batch-match procedures permit users to compile statistical data on confidential information and/or to produce authorized lists of jointly served clients/patients in a method that prevents inadvertent, wrongful rerelease. The actual confidential records are unseen by the individual who is compiling the statistical report or special list. This method also can assure that when personal data is released it is released from only those records where the other agency has a right to access it because of an exemption to the privacy laws or because there is a valid confidential information release form on file with the agency.

The right to gain online access to automated confidential records is also recognized in various laws. Online access entails greater risks of violation of privacy rights; therefore, the law has more specific requirements to secure the integrity of the records. Older computer programs were not designed for the secure exchange of information across program lines. However, new technology recognizes the value of proper releases of confidential information to other agencies and the need to organize the data in a manner that maximizes security. Generally speaking, this means building into the software extra security provisions and better organization of the records. It also means developing methods of access only to portions of the records, such as case-identifier information, that require less control of security-sensitive information than is required, for example, for information about the diagnosis and treatment of mental illnesses.

As technology advances emphasis is being placed on developing the so-called open-systems approach. Open systems allow for the communication of information across program lines and across different hardware and software. Open systems hold great promise for more effective integrated interagency service programs based on automated record exchange. At the same time they create more opportunities for misuse and/or inadvertent rerelease of confidential information.

*Computer Matching and Privacy Act of 1988, 5.U.S.C.§552a

CONCLUSION AND RECOMMENDATIONS

The belief that confidentiality laws and regulations absolutely prevent effective interagency programs is a myth. The law provides more than adequate direction on procedures for the exchange of confidential information among service providers working in various agencies. The challenge for administrators, direct-service providers, and other interested parties is to identify common requirements in the law. Those commonalities can be used to prepare standardized informed-consent release procedures and to write interagency agreements that will protect confidential information and records. The larger barriers to interagency cooperation and collaboration grow out of our federal form of government, our differing professional and institutional values, and our human proclivity toward turfism, provincialism, and resistance to change.

What are the implications of the finding that the law is not the primary source of failed interagency cooperation on matters related to confidentiality? The most obvious implication is that there is no need to launch a major campaign to change federal and state laws. We can and should look to other states for laws and procedures already developed to meet the special needs of interagency programs. One example is the recent change in California statutes to facilitate prompt exchange of confidential information among multidisciplinary personnel teams.

There are other actions we can take to mitigate the so-called confidentiality barrier. The three areas that seem to deserve the most attention are: (1) model policy and procedure, (2) better automated systems, and (3) special staff training. For the first area of concern we should continue to develop model policy and procedure for interagency programs because this type of service system is more complex to manage. It requires more direction on matters related to accountability, liability, and record security. To address the second area of emphasis we should continue to develop better methods to manage confidential information in automated records. The emphasis should be on designing software and hardware that maximizes opportunities to exchange confidential records across program lines and minimizes the risks of inadvertent release of the records. Finally, we should provide special training to policy makers and service providers who wish to develop or work in integrated interagency programs. The training should be designed to increase knowledge of the other agencies' missions and confidentiality rules and to enhance their collaborative management skills.

REFERENCES

1. Chaudry A et al: *Services integration: an annotated bibliography*, New York, 1993, National Center for Service Integration.
2. English A and Tereszkievicz L: School-based health clinics: legal issues, San Francisco, 1988, National Center for Youth Law and Center for Population Options.
3. Greenberg M and Levy J: *Confidentiality and collaboration: information sharing in interagency efforts*, Denver, 1992, Education Commission of the States Distribution Center.
4. Griswold v Connecticut, 381 U.S. 479, 495, 1965.
5. Hobbs LJ: *Tackling the confidentiality barrier: a practical guide of integrated family services*, ed 2, San Diego, 1993, San Diego County Department of Social Services, Office of the Director.
6. Legal Action Center: Confidentiality: a guide to the federal laws and regulations, New York, 1991, Author.
7. Medical Educational Services: Confidentiality: a guide to medical records in California, New York, 1991, Author.
8. Melaville A and Blank MJ: *What it takes: structuring interagency partnerships to connect children and families with comprehensive services*, Washington, DC, 1992, Center for the Future of Children.
9. National Association of Social Workers: *Commission on education position statement: the school social worker and confidentiality*. Silver Springs, Col, 1991, the Association.
10. New Beginnings Team: *New beginnings: a feasibility study of integrated services for children and families*, San Diego, 1990, San Diego City Schools, Office of the Superintendent.
11. Ooms T and Owen T: *Coordination, collaboration, integration: strategies for serving families more effectively*, Washington, DC, 1991, American Association for Marriage and Family Therapy, Research and Education Foundation.
12. Rapp JA, Stephens RD, and Clontz D: *The need to know*. Malibu, Cal, 1989, National School Safety Center.
13. Solar M, Shotton A, and Bell J: *Glass walls: confidentiality provisions and interagency collaboration*, San Francisco, 1993, Youth Law Center.

CHAPTER **13**

Child Abuse, Neglect, and Disabled Children

SUSAN REICHERT
RICHARD D. KRUGMAN

The abuse and neglect of children was described by the U.S. Advisory Board on Child Abuse and Neglect as a "national emergency" in 1990.[11] By 1993 the emergency was not ameliorated. More than 2.8 million reports of abuse and neglect translate to well over one million confirmed cases each year. No reliable data on the incidence or prevalence of abuse in children with disabilities exist. Studies that rely on information provided by child protective agencies are generally useless because most agencies do not have the time to evaluate properly such allegations in these children. Nevertheless, most professionals acknowledge that children with disabilities are probably at greater risk for physical, sexual and emotional abuse than children without disabilities.

LIMITS TO UNDERSTANDING

The acquisition of accurate data regarding the incidence of child maltreatment in the disabled population is hampered by the fact that child protective services reports, in most states, do not include any information about a child's disabling conditions. This omission thwarts efforts to determine to what extent children with disabilities are represented among the victims. Much of the research done to date supports the hypothesis that children with disabilities are more frequently maltreated than their normal-functioning peers. However, there are conflicting studies that suggest that the incidence of abuse among the disabled is the same as in the general population. Even if information about disabilities became available in reported cases of abuse and neglect, the true incidence of maltreatment of these children might never be known because of the difficulty in substantiating cases of abuse in children who may be unable to provide a reliable history.

Noncommunicative, severely or profoundly retarded persons, and those who never gain access to the world outside their care environment, may never have the opportunity to relay the mistreatment they may experience. This simple fact suggests that reports of abuse and/or neglect in this population are underestimates of the true incidence. Although nonhandicapped children may also have restricted access to reporting abuse, it is not so inherent a reality.

In the numerous research attempts to examine the occurrence of abuse among mentally retarded and otherwise disabled children significant difficulties have been encountered.[12] Many studies have methodologic flaws that make interpretation of results and extrapolation to larger groups unreliable. One of these shortcomings surrounds the definition of *disability*. The wide scope of conditions that may be included in this definition generates confusion. There is disagreement as to whether the same factors apply to children with mild versus severe disabilities, or to those with physical versus cognitive or psychiatric dysfunction, and it is unclear where children with visual deficits, communicative disorders, and learning disabilities fit in. Studies of large populations of children with all types of handicaps are needed before distinctions are relevant.

Other problems with some studies to date have been small sample sizes and a lack of appropriate control groups for comparison. It is noteworthy that even those researchers who have overcome these obstacles make a point of acknowledging the dangers of broadly generalizing from their results. Controversy has also been raised as to whether it is more pertinent to study groups of abused children and determine how many of them are disabled or more helpful to examine a sample of handicapped individuals and identify those among them who have been abused. In some cases it is difficult to separate victims whose first episode of abuse occurs after their disability is realized from those children whose very handicap may be the result of abusive treatment.

RISK FACTORS FOR ABUSE—IN CAREGIVERS, VICTIMS, AND SOCIETY

Abuse of children with disabilities occurs in various settings—home, school, residential institutions, and places in between. Abuse may be physical, sexual, emotional, neglect, or any combination of these. Certain characteristics of the disabled population increase the possibility that they will suffer maltreatment by family members, caregivers, or outsiders. Various factors must be considered.

The stress of parenting a child with a disability can be extreme. There are financial and physical burdens, and the emotional trauma may be marked and life long. Parents can be expected to feel guilt and grief about the fact that their child is not normal. Anger and resentment are commonly experienced. Families of children with disabilities may be isolated from usual social supports and sometimes feel ostracized because of their child's appearance or deficiency.

Children with disabilities not uncommonly develop cries that may be persistent and irritating. Some of these children have behavior problems that are very difficult to manage and that require extensive physical intervention by the parent or caregiver. All-consuming care requirements of some disabled children produce frustration and may become overwhelming for parents. Without adequate resources, parents' coping skills can become exhausted and the child may become the target of abusive stress relief.

Expectations seem to play a critical role in parental ability to cope with a disabled child. Although these data are somewhat controversial, it has been noted that incidence of abuse does not increase with increased severity of disability. In fact, the reverse appears to be true.[1,2,4]

Some researchers speculate that when it is known that a child's disability is profound, the parents adjust to that realization. They know what they are up against and tackle the problems as best they can. However, in less severe cases in which ability levels vary and assessment of functional possibility is unsure, parents may find greater frustration when their child does not live up to their hopes or when some capability is not achieved. There may never come the relief and resignation that actually reduces frustration and despair and, in essence, protects a child. Additionally, services and established support systems may not be as readily accessible to families of less-impaired youngsters, resulting in increased isolation and further stress.

Outside the home some of the same risk factors exist. Teachers and professional caretakers are also subject to frustration when dealing with demanding children. Selection processes should weed out individuals with short tempers, those prone to retaliation, and those with pedophilic tendencies, but this is not always achieved. Staff at some residential facilities are poorly paid; screening too carefully may not be possible given the limited pool of applicants. There are also positions that are not technically care providing roles, such as bus drivers, custodians, groundskeepers, and cooks, but that allow access to disabled children and often are not subject to screening criteria that examine abuse potential.[9]

Furthermore, children with disabilities have many characteristics that make them especially vulnerable to victimization. To varying degrees they are dependent upon others for their basic needs as well as for their social interactions and sense of well-being. This fact results in relationships in which the disabled individual is at a significant power disadvantage. The instructions of any person in authority are expected to be complied with implicitly. The disabled individual may rely upon his or her caregiver for a sense of self—behaving in such a way as to engender disapproval of the caretaker is self-destructive.

Children whose disability interferes with communication may be completely unable to disclose abuse they may experience. Those who try may not be understood. Whether they are believed is yet another hurdle for these victims. Deficits in communicability affect both the quality and quantity of contacts with others. Because of this, children with communication problems tend not to initiate discussion and would be unlikely to bring up abuse unless they were questioned directly about the subject.

The literature points out that children in the mild to moderate range of cognitive dysfunction are especially susceptible to coercion. Offers of rewards or capitalizing on the disabled person's need to feel that he or she will be fitting in or gaining affection may win a perpetrator access to sexual exploitation.[8]

A child's deficit may render him or her incapable of perceiving an act as sexually abusive. Lack of knowledge about sexual activity and proper conduct, not distinguishing between different forms of touching, being used to genital handling by caretakers, and not noticing the difference in abusive circumstances all contribute to an affected child's susceptibility to victimization. Furthermore, the confinement and isolation that may define the lifestyle of some disabled children make them more receptive to any form of attention or affection. And, although available data suggest that the most severely disabled children have the lowest incidence of abuse, one can argue that the facts will never be known because of the inability of these individuals to communicate their experiences.

In addition to the characteristics of the individuals who are victimized, there are far-reaching societal factors that make disabled children more likely targets of abuse and neglect. Our society projects a view of the abuse of healthy children as deplorable; applying this same standard, the maltreatment of unfortunate, disabled children should be even less tolerable. However, we are also a culture that devalues the infirm and actually dehumanizes individuals with disabilities. When handicapped persons are regarded as less worthwhile members of society, abuse of those members can also be minimized and subconsciously condoned.[3,12]

MANAGEMENT AND INTERVENTION

Just as is true in all situations of child abuse, maltreatment of disabled children cannot be diagnosed unless persons in authority and those providing care are willing to recognize the possibility. Clinicians who examine these individuals should be adept at differentiating patterns of accidental or self-inflicted trauma versus injuries caused by others. They must be skilled in genital examination to rule out sexual abuse and must be diligent about performing these brief but important exams on routine health care contacts.

Physicians must set aside extra time to handle the evaluation of disabled children most effectively. Assessing the individual patient's level of functioning and not stereotyping is critical to appropriately directing the interview and examination and allowing the child as much control as possible. The child's preferred method of communication should be utilized, with support persons or interpreters present to ease the child's relating and processing of information. One should not assume that the child with a disability experiences less emotion or that he or she cannot comprehend the abuse. Physicians should respect confidentiality and should place emphasis on recommending whatever intervention the disabled person will need to recover from the abusive experience. Reporting the abuse to authorities, initiating needed therapy, and advocating within the legal system and the community on behalf of the disabled victim are necessary steps clinicians must be willing to take.[6]

There is increasing precedence for validating disabled children's disclosures of abuse. Interviews done by professionals knowledgeable about the individual child's unique style of communication can reveal important details that may hold up well in court. Using facilitated communication has broken new ground in battling the isolation of victims who could not previously disclose details of maltreatment. Controversy surrounding the validity of disclosures made via facilitated communication has directed attention toward careful validation of information learned through this method.

Treatment of disabled children who have been abused has also seen recent progress. Instead of the standard limited offerings of behavior modification and medication, various forms of interactive psychotherapy are being tried. Family therapy, groups, and play modalities have met with some success. The client-therapist relationship may provide for some disabled children a healing experience of healthy intimacy with an adult whom they can trust.[10]

PREVENTION

As a culture we must make it clear that even our most debilitated children are precious. Children with disabilities are to be protected and carefully nurtured. Prevention of abuse and neglect in the families of disabled children should begin as early as possible in the affected child's life. The interruption in normal parental attachment that can occur when babies are premature or ill or less responsive should be recognized by medical staff who should set support systems into motion immediately. Ideally, such families should never leave the hospital without a safety net; a home-visitation arrangement, social services involvement, information about parent support groups, plans for ongoing follow-up, etc. should be considered.

Professionals should speak realistically with parents about their child's condition. They should discuss common reactions and difficulties and make a candid assessment of the particular family's coping strengths and abuse potential. In an effort not to raise false hopes for parents, clinicians often offer negative predictions of the things their child will never be able to do. However, a focus on the positive may be more beneficial—not candy-coating reality but helping parents see more than just the hopeless side of their particular circumstances. Again, realistic expectations should be fostered, but it may be consoling to advise that even the most severely disabled individuals also have abilities.

Physicians who, in their practices, care for disabled children should pay special attention to the coping skills of the parents and candidly discuss with them the difficulties they face. Being familiar with the signs and symptoms of abuse and neglect, the clinician, teacher, or other contacts of disabled children can act not only to report such concerns, but also to educated parents to identify abuse of their children that may be occurring outside the home.

Developmentally appropriate interventions must be undertaken to strengthen children with handicaps against violation. Programs to teach children about sexuality and sexual abuse prevention should be instituted—many good programs now exist, but they may not be accessible for many limited children. In schools where disabled children are mainstreamed, standard programs are not sufficient. The very deficits that make these children more vulnerable also inhibit their ability to comprehend the information relayed in general educational materials. Extra time and investment in disability-specific materials are warranted to ensure that these pupils adequately understand the important information being communicated to them.

Finkelhor[5] has described four preconditions for sexual abuse to occur: (1) the motivation to sexually abuse, (2) the overcoming of internal inhibitors, (3) the overcoming of external inhibitors, and (4) the overcoming of resistance from the child. Most strategies for the prevention of sexual abuse of children that have been developed over the last decade rely on building up the resistance of children. This approach teaches children about "good touch" and "bad touch," "red flags" and "green flags," and to tell an adult if anyone "touches them in their private parts." There have been relatively few studies to evaluate this approach, but those that have been done and that are methodologically sound indicate that building up the resistance of children works for some but not all children and those who are at greatest risk are those with the lowest self-esteem.

Other approaches, such as those developed over the last several years by the Boy Scouts of America[7], have focused on the external inhibitor precondition. With this strategy the responsibility for protecting children from sexual abuse rests with adults and other caretakers. Thus children should not be left alone for long periods of time or overnight with a single adult; other caretakers or other adults should be present to assist with and monitor the situation. There are no data to confirm that this approach is effective in reducing the number of cases of sexual abuse. However, because many children with disabilities are unable to provide resistance to an older child, adolescent, or adult who is interested in engaging them in sexual activities, it may be that the focus of a strategy that builds up external inhibitors holds the most promise for preventing sexual abuse among these children. There is a critical need for research on what gives motivation to sexual abusers. At this time, there is no predictive profile or psychologic screening, that can be done and appropriate vigilance is the best strategy.

For a field that is now more than 3 decades old, it is distressing to recognize how little has been learned about the recognition, treatment and prevention of sexual abuse in our most vulnerable children. Perhaps the next decade will be one in which more resources are spent on research, demonstration programs, and treatment.

REFERENCES

1. Ammerman RT and VanHasselt VB: Abuse and neglect in psychiatrically hospitalized multihandicapped children, *Child Abuse and Neglect* 13:335-343, 1989.

2. Benedict MI et al: Reported maltreatment in children with multiple disabilities, *Child Abuse and Neglect* 14:207-217, 1990.

3. Brookhouser PE et al: Identifying the sexually abused deaf child: the oto-laryngologist's role, *Laryngoscope* 96:152-158, 1986.

4. Chamberlain A et al: Issues in fertility control for mentally retarded female adolescents. I. Sexuality activity, sexual abuse and contraception, *Pediatrics* 73(4):445-450, 1984.

5. Finkelhor D: *Child sexual abuse: new theory and practice*, New York, 1985, Free Press.

6. Jaudes PK and Diamond LJ: The handicapped child and child abuse, *Child Abuse and Neglect* 9:341-347, 1985.

7. Potts Lawrence F: The youth protection program of the Boy Scouts of America, *Child Abuse and Neglect* 16:441-445, 1992.

8. Schor DP: Sex and sexual abuse in developmentally disabled adolescents, *Seminars in Adolescents Medicine* 3(1):1-7, 1987.

9. Sullivan PM et al: Patterns of physical and sexual abuse of communicatively handicapped children, *Ann Otol Rhinol Laryngol* 100:188-194, 1991.

10. Tharinger D, Horton CB, and Miller S: Sexual abuse and exploitation of children and adults with mental retardation and other handicaps, *Child Abuse and Neglect* 14:301-312, 1990.

11. U.S. Advisory Board on Child Abuse and Neglect: Child abuse and neglect: critical first steps in response to a national emergency, Washington DC, 1990, Government Printing Office.

12. Westcott H: The abuse of disabled children: a review of the literature, *Child: Care, Health and Development* 17:243-258, 1991.

CHAPTER **14**

Sexuality

MARILYN J. KRAJICEK
ELIZABETH A. CASSIDY

Children, adolescents, and young adults with developmental disabilities and chronic illness face sexuality issues similar to those issues faced by their peers who are not disabled. However, they often face some barriers not common among those peers who are not disabled, such as lack of socialization opportunities and or skills, lack of verbal language skills, and poor impulse control. For the most part, however, psychosexual development for people with developmental disabilities parallels that of children who are not disabled, although it is slightly delayed at times.[3] Education regarding sexuality for people with developmental disabilities and chronic illness is paramount.

The myth that people with disabilities are asexual and without sexual needs is sustained by parents and care providers who tend to focus their efforts on suppressing what they feel are inappropriate sexual behaviors. Although these behaviors are typically normal for the level of sexual development, reactions of care providers often communicate to individuals with disabilities and chronic illness a feeling of shame or guilt about their bodies thus contributing to their low self-esteem.

Many parents and care givers are poorly prepared to deal with their child, adolescent, or young adult's sexual development. This chapter addresses issues relevant to professionals working with people with developmental disabilities and chronic illness and their families. Sexuality education for individuals with developmental disabilities and chronic illness and their parents and care providers is particularly important because: (1) parents may be surprised upon finding their son or daughter developing sexual feelings although body changes have been observed, (2) people with developmental disabilities and chronic illness lack opportunities to acquire correct information from peers or other sources, and (3) people with developmental disabilities and chronic illness are at higher risk for unwanted pregnancies, sexually transmitted diseases, and abuse.[2,17]

A HELPFUL ORIENTATION

Professionals who are knowledgeable about disabling conditions and their implications for human sexuality are ideal candidates for sex-education counselors. Counselors must feel comfortable with their own sexuality and with people with disabilities and chronic illness as sexual beings. They may need to learn to be nonjudgmental because behaviors exhibited by persons with mental retardation, for instance, can be atypical depending on their socialization experiences.

Professionals counseling individuals with developmental disabilities about sexuality should have experience in both teaching children, adolescents, or young adults with disabilities and chronic illness as well as teaching human sexuality. A sex-education program can fail if the educator does not know enough about sexuality or is not familiar with the needs of children with disabilities or the techniques used to teach them.[4,22] Sex education needs to be presented to the child, adolescent, or young adult at a mental-age–appropriate level .

Assessment and Teaching

Both families and their children with developmental disabilities and chronic illness need to be educated about sexuality. First assessing the child's level of understanding of human sexuality is necessary. It is also helpful to find out if the parents of the child have any misconceptions, which may include the following: people with developmental disabilities have no sexual feelings; they should not marry; they are incapable of heterosexual or homosexual relationships; or they are sexually aggressive.[20]

Educators should involve parents and care providers by finding out what their expectations are for their child, adolescent, or young adult, what role they are willing to play, and what their concerns might be. Much of the teaching that is done with the individual can be done on a functional and experiential level within the context of everyday life and, in that case, parents play an essential role in the process.[16]

Using real-life situations, educators should address topics such as identification of body parts, growing up and biological changes, developing friendships, emotional feelings, reproduction, contraception, sexually transmitted diseases, marriage and parenting, masturbation, and sexual abuse. There are programs available specifically designed to address these topics with people with developmental disabilities and chronic illness and they may include videotapes, dolls, models, and illustrated books.[18] Sex education programs designed for these people with special educational needs should be documented, researched, and published so that future educational programs can benefit.[16]

SOCIALIZATION

Low self-esteem causes people with developmental disabilities and chronic illness to be at a greater risk for sexual abuse and exploitation. Therefore positive experiences in normal social situations should be created and encouraged. Often these individuals are denied such experiences because they are thought to be unable to acquire appropriate social skills or they are socially isolated.[16]

Skills that will help a person with developmental disabilities or chronic illness fulfill an adult sexual role are built on skills that are acquired in early childhood. Interpersonal skills are obtained through years of observation, discussion, practice, and constructive criticism. Experiential learning in home sit-

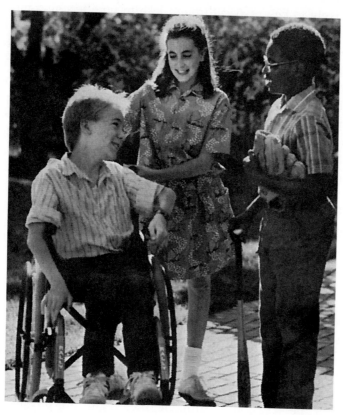

Copyright Jim Whitmer.

uations with parental or care-provider supervision and evaluation can help children, adolescents, or young adults with disabilities and chronic illness learn important aspects of socialization. Parents should be encouraged to allow their children to take part in entertainment and social situations. For example, having them greet guests and take their coats enables them to practice skills such as being polite, turn-taking in conversation, and maintaining eye contact, the social cues that are the basis for future social interactions. They should have opportunities to rehearse for these situations prior to the arrival of guests so they are able to experience success and gain self-esteem.[16]

Abstract concepts may create barriers to socialization for people with developmental disabilities and chronic illness. Two of the most common errors are recognizing the difference between strangers and friends, and public and private places. Stranger-friend errors occur when a child, adolescent, or young adult treats a stranger or acquaintance as a trusted friend. Public-private errors involve a child doing or saying something in public that society feels is unacceptable. Individuals with developmental disabilities and chronic illness are capable of learning to avoid these errors, but these concepts are not likely to be grasped through lecture-type teaching methods. Hands-on, experience-based learning, modeling, and explanation will help the individual with developmental disabilities to generalize to other situations.[2]

Building self-esteem early in childhood and continuing through adulthood by optimizing chances for success in social situations is the best way to protect individuals with disabilities and chronic illness from exploitation and to prepare them for their adult sexual roles. Experiential, concrete learning in real-life situations is the best medium to teach socialization skills. These skills should be addressed as early in childhood as possible to promote success in future relationships.

Masturbation

Masturbation is a normal behavior for both people with developmental disabilities and chronic illness as well as their peers who are not disabled. Although sometimes it can become a compulsive behavior, masturbation usually becomes a problem when it is done at inappropriate times and places. Making these public-private errors can create serious barriers to socialization.

Before deinstitutionalization began, masturbation was considered a rampant behavior for people with developmental disabilities and chronic illness. This was part of the myth that these people were promiscuous and sexually aggressive. Now it is believed that excessive masturbation within group-home settings is due to boredom, lack of social opportunities, segregation of the sexes, and stringent rules regarding physical contact with the opposite sex.[10]

People with developmental disabilities and chronic illness can be taught where, when, and how to masturbate. Harsh reactions to masturbation will only increase a feeling of guilt about one's body. Care providers and parents need to be comfortable with masturbation so that when they see the behavior in people with developmental disabilities they can accept it calmly. If these individuals are taught where, when, and how to masturbate, there may be fewer social errors and more positive associations with their sexuality. In the past, education only stressed appropriate versus inappropriate places to masturbate. Now, actually teaching individuals how to masturbate can be done using models.[17]

MARRIAGE AND FAMILY

There is a continuing trend for people with developmental disabilities and chronic illness to marry and as many as 50% of people in this population will likely do so.[15] It is not unusual for a person with developmental disabilities to desire having children. Parent training should be made available to those who express a desire to raise children. Education regarding contraception should also be made available to those who are not ready or are unable to manage the stress associated with marriage and raising a child.

Contraception

Contraception for people with developmental disabilities is controversial and yet a major concern; the disability itself may put a person at high risk for unwanted pregnancies. The decisions about whether to use contraception and what type of contraception to use should be made by the individual, with the guidance of care providers. Education regarding contraception should include responsibility for sexual actions, preventing pregnancies, and the mechanics of different kinds of contraception.

Choices of contraception should be dependent on the ability of the individual to use methods reliably. A care provider or parent may teach an individual how to use a condom, but the success rate for correct usage is questionable for a person who is more cognitively challenged or who has a physical disability.[12] Provision of models and graphic demonstration of the mechanics and logistics of obtaining and using a condom may supply them with the concrete experiences necessary for learning.[6]

The use of birth control pills is questionable for women who are severely mentally retarded as well as for women who take anticonvulsant medications for seizure disorders.[11] The success of birth control pills depends on a consistent regime. Alternatives for the daily birth control pill are intra-uterine devices and drugs such as Norplant and Depo-Provera. Norplant is surgically implanted into the upper arm and is effective for 5 years. Depo-Provera is injected into the muscle and is reported to be effective for 3 months. Both of these hormones are considered relatively safe, highly effective, and independent of compliance.[19] Because Depo-Provera and Norplant do not rely on a dependable user or mechanical insertion, they may be very useful for those identified as having a developmental disability or chronic illness.

Sterilization. Historically, sterilization was performed on nearly all of these individuals, regardless of consent. Until the mid 1950s leaving an institution was permitted only after sterilization was performed.[14] Today the decision to be sterilized is made by the individual with possible guidance from care providers and/or parents. Sterilization may be performed if it is in the best interest of the individual. If a person with developmental disabilities or chronic illness decides that he or she does not wish to have children, sterilization can be an option.

Controversy arises if the individual is unable to make an informed decision. In this case a multidisciplinary team may participate in the decision-making process, keeping in mind the best interests of the individual. Legal implications may accompany sterilization and may vary from state to state. It is important for the professional involved in sterilization decisions to be well informed and knowledgeable about the laws in their state and possible resources for individuals and their families who are considering sterilization.

SEXUAL ABUSE AND EXPLOITATION

People with developmental disabilities and chronic illness, including children, adolescents, and adults, often are at a greater risk for sexual abuse and exploitation than the general public. The following factors make them more susceptible: physical limitations that may make self-defense difficult; cognitive limitations that may make it difficult to determine safe and dangerous situations; lack of knowledge about sexuality; impulsivity; and low self-esteem from prior negative socialization experiences.[21]

Because people with developmental disabilities and chronic illness may lack social experience, they may be unaware that they are being taken advantage of or may not know that they have rights to self-advocacy. Underreporting of sexual abuse is more likely to occur within this population because of (1) lack of knowledge (i.e., good touch/bad touch), (2) poor communication, and (3) lifelong dependency on care providers, which makes them overly trusting or afraid that their care may be compromised.[21] It is important for caretakers to be alert for signs of abuse.

Abuse cannot be detected from a mere gynecologic examination. It has been found that women who are raped prior to being examined do not always show evidence of penetration.[5] It is suggested that there be a thorough baseline examination, including testing for sexually transmitted diseases, and that anogenital changes from examination to examination be documented and compared to look for discrepancies. A protocol for detection of abuse should be in operation at every group-home setting for people with developmental disabilities. A recommendation is that multidisciplinary teams, including gynecologists, mental health professionals, rape counselors, and care providers, be available for counseling and assisting with issues of abuse. There should also be a policy in place to determine how safety needs for individuals will be met.[5]

Because there is an increased incidence of psychiatric disorders among people who have developmental disabilities or chronic illness, it is likely that reactions to sexual abuse will be more severe than in the population not labeled. It is critical that a person interviewing a sexually abused person with a developmental disability establishes rapport, gains trust, diffuses anxiety and communicates at a mental-age–appropriate level about sexual and emotional issues.[21]

Sexually Transmitted Disease

Individuals with developmental disabilities or chronic illness are at potentially higher risks for contracting sexually transmitted diseases (STD) such as chlamydia, syphilis, herpes, and gonorrhea for the very same reasons that they are at a higher risk for exploitation and because of the difficulty they may have in using preventive measures such as condoms. Because STDs can be asymptomatic and a sign of sexual abuse, routine, complete gynecologic examinations are important.

Care providers should be aware of some of the symptoms of more prevalent STDs. Gonorrhea can cause pelvic inflammation, lower-right–quadrant pain, elevated temperature, problems in walking, and possible vaginal discharge or burning sensation in women, while in men there may be a puslike discharge and burning upon urination, or there may be no symptoms at all.[9] Herpes may appear on the lips, eyes, nose, or genitals as sores or blisters that may come and go; it can be spread by using another's glass, towel, or make-up and by lack of adequate hand washing.[8] Any kind of sexual play during the infected blister stage can spread the disease. Chlamydia is spread through sexual intercourse and can cause pelvic inflammatory disease. All STDs can be spread to an infant during childbirth. Because they may not be aware of the effects and symptoms of STDs, regular check ups for people with developmental disabilities and chronic illness are important.

People with developmental disabilities and chronic illness need to be informed that protection against pregnancy is not necessarily protection against STD. It may be more difficult to provide information about STDs to individuals with mental retardation. It will be harder for them to understand that someone can have a disease and still look healthy. It is important to present information in concrete ways (i.e., pictures of what symptoms may look like).

AIDS/HIV. Auto Immune Deficiency Syndrome (AIDS) and Human Immunodeficiency Virus (HIV) have serious implications for people with developmental disabilities. HIV and AIDS have been noted to cause developmental disability in children.[1] The vulnerability of people with developmental disabilities and chronic illness and their lack of self-esteem may place them at a higher risk for contracting HIV and having potential to contaminate sexual partners.

People with mental retardation may be a greater risk to others because they may not understand the implications and precautions that are a component of the disease. Deficits in social judgment and high-risk behavior put people with mental retardation at an increased risk of infection with HIV.[13] The single most effective method of fighting the spread of HIV is reducing at-risk behaviors.[7]

Controversy remains over whether someone who has contracted HIV/AIDS should be forced to disclose this information. This is especially controversial with the population of persons with developmental disabilities or chronic illness. Voluntary testing is recommended for all people, but they must give their informed consent.[13] In the case of people with developmental disabilities whether testing should or should not be voluntary is unclear; because there may be a lack of social judgment, the question remains whether their health status should be disclosed to potential sexual partners and their care providers. Agencies that serve this population of people should have a policy about AIDS testing.[13] In many cases people with developmental disabilities and chronic illness do not have a guarantee that they will still be served if they are identified as HIV positive or are diagnosed with AIDS.

As discussed earlier, education plays a key role in reducing the spread of AIDS. Programs should be concrete, simple, and brief to ensure attention and should be presented according to developmental level of understanding. All teaching personnel should be informed and should present accurate information.

THE ONGOING ROLE OF THE PROFESSIONAL

Professionals are involved with people with disabilities and chronic illness from early childhood throughout the life cycle. Issues of sexuality cannot be overlooked because of discomfort on the professional or care provider's part. These individuals with disabilities are sexual beings from birth on through adulthood just as are people without disabilities. If a child is prepared through building self-esteem and learning socialization skills he or she will be better equipped to handle issues about sexuality.

Overall goals for people with disabilities and chronic illness need to be documented from early childhood in the Individualized Family Service Plan (IFSP), during school years in the Individualized Educational Plan (IEP), and for transitions in life in the Transition Plan. Goals for learning and understanding human sexuality need to be addressed within the context of these plans to assure that sexuality issues for people with developmental disabilities and chronic illness will not be ignored and that individuals will be able to fulfill their roles as sexual beings. This continues to be a challenge for parents, professionals, and care providers.

REFERENCES

1. Bellman AL et al: Pediatric acquired immunodeficiency syndrome: neurologic syndromes, *Am J Dis Child* 142-29, 1988.
2. Chigier E: Sexuality and mental retardation, *Seminars in Neurology* 12:129, 1992.
3. David HP and Morgall JM: Family planning for the mentally disordered and retarded, *J Nerv Ment Dis* 178:385, 1990.
4. Dickman IR: *Sex education for disabled persons*, Pub No 531, 1985, Washington, DC, U.S. Government Printing Office.
5. Elvkin SL et al: Sexual abuse in the developmentally disabled: dilemmas of diagnoses, *Child Abuse Negl* 14:497, 1990.
6. Furman LM: Institutionalized disabled adolescents: gynecological care, *Clin Ped* 28:163, 1989.
7. Graham LL and Cates JA: To reduce the risk of HIV infection, *J Psychos Nurs Ment Health Serv* 30:9, 1992.
8. Gun T and Poore M: *The herpes handbook*, ed 5, Portland, Ore, 1984, The Venereal Disease Action Committee.
9. Harger D and Britton T: *Chlamydia and NGU*, Portland, Ore, 1984, Venereal Disease Action Committee.
10. Reference deleted in pages.
11. Information Services Bulletin, 320852, No. 14, Rockville, Md, 1980, National Clearing House for Family Planning.
12. Kaeser F: Can people with severe mental retardation consent to mutual sex? *Sexuality and Disability* 10:33, 1992.
13. Kastner TA, Hickman ML, and Belleheumer D: The provision of services to persons with mental retardation and subsequent infection with Human Immunodeficiency Virus (HIV), *Am J Public Health* 79:491, 1989.
14. Kempton W and Kahn E: Sexuality and people with intellectual disabilities: a historical perspective, *Sexuality and Disability* 9:93, 1991.
15. Koller H, Richardson SA, and Katz M: Marriage in a young adult mentally retarded population, *J Ment Def* 32:93, 1988.
16. Kupper L, Ambler L, and Valdivieso C: *Sexuality education for children and youth with disabilities*, 1993, Washington, DC, National Information Center for Children and Youth with Disabilities.
17. McNab WL and Birch DA: *Sexuality education for persons with developmental disabilities: a cooperative approach*, PALAESTRA 7:47, 1991.
18. Snow D: Teaching clients about sexuality, *Nursing Times* 87:66, 1991.
19. Sperffe L and Darney P: *A clinical guide for contraception*, Baltimore, Md, 1992, Williams & Wilkins.
20. Taylor MO: Teaching parents about their impaired adolescents sexuality, *Maternal Child Nursing* 14:109, 1989.

21. Tharinger D, Horton CB, and Milea S: Sexual abuse and exploitation of children and adults with mental retardation and other handicaps, *Child Abuse Negl* 14:301, 1990.

22. Torbett D: In Dickman IR, editor: *Sex education for disabled persons*, Pub No 531, 1985.

BIBLIOGRAPHY

Abramson PR, Parket T, and Weisberg SR: Sexual expression of mentally retarded people: educational and legal implications, *Am J Ment Retard* 93(3): 328-334, 1988.

Ames TR and Samowitz P: Inclusionary standard for determining sexual consent for individuals with developmental disabilities, *Ment Retard*: 264-268, 1995.

Callanan, CR: Sexuality and sex education. In *Since Owen: a parent-to-parent guide for care of the disabled child*, Baltimore, 1990, Johns Hopkins University Press.

Champagne M and Walker-Hirsch L: *Circles I: intimacy and relationships*, Santa Barbara, Cal, 1989, James Stanfield.

Champagne M and Walker-Hirsch L: *Circles II: stop abuse*, Santa Barbara, Cal, 1989, James Stanfield.

Couwenhoven T: *Beginnings: a parent/child sexuality program for families with children who have developmental disabilities*, ed 2, Wisconsin, 1992, Wisconsin Council on Developmental Disabilities.

Crocker AC, Cohen HJ, and Kastner TA, *HIV infection and developmental disabilities: a resource for service providers*, Baltimore, 1992, Paul H. Brookes.

Friedrich WN et al: Normative sexual behavior in children, *Pediatrics* 88(3): 456-464, 1991.

Furey EM: Sexual abuse of adults with mental retardation: who and where, *Ment Retard* 32(3):173-180, 1994.

Haseltine FP, Cole SS, and Gray DB, editors: *Reproductive issues for persons with physical disabilities*, Baltimore, 1993, Paul H Brookes Publishing Co.

Heighway S and Webster SK: *STARS 2 for children: a guidebook for teaching positive sexuality and the prevention of sexual abuse for children with developmental disabilities*, Wisconsin, 1993, Wisconsin Council on Developmental Disabilities.

Huntley CF and Benner SM: Reducing barriers to sex education for adults with mental retardation, *Ment Retard* 31(4):215-220, 1993.

Klein E and Kroll K: *Enabling romance: A guide to love, sex, and relationships for disabled people (and the people who care about them)*, New York, 1992, Crown.

Lindemann J: *SAFE: an HIV/AIDS curriculum for individuals with MR/DD*, Portland, 1990, Oregon Health Sciences University.

Lutfiyya ZM: *Personal relationships and social networks: facilitating the participation of individuals with disabilities in community life*, Syracuse, NY, 1991, The Center on Human Policy.

Meeropol E: One of the gang: sexual development of adolescents with physical disabilities, *J Pediatr Nurs* 6(4):243-250, 1991.

Monat-Haller RK: *Understanding and expressing sexuality: responsible choices for individuals with developmental disabilities*, Baltimore, 1992, Paul H Brookes Publishing Co.

Morse JS and Roth SP: Sexuality in the nurses role. In Roth SP and Morse JS, editors: *A life-span approach to nursing care for individuals with developmental disabilities*, Baltimore, 1994, Paul H. Brookes Publishing Co.

NICHY 1(3):2-23, 1992.

Niederbuhl JM and Morris CD: Sexual knowledge and the capability of persons with dual diagnoses to consent to sexual contact, *Sexuality and disability* 11(4):295-307, 1993.

People Building Institute: *Human sexuality for the disabled: a manual designed to assist human service professionals*, Sheldon, Iowa, 1991, the Institute.

Schwier KM: *Couples with intellectual disabilities talk about living and loving*, Rockville, Md, 1994, Woodbine House.

Selekman J and McIlvain-Simpson G: Sex and sexuality for the adolescent with a chronic condition, *Pediatric Nursing* 17(6):535-538, 1991.

Sexuality education for persons with severe developmental disabilities, Santa Barbara, Cal, 1991, James Stanfield.

Smith M: Pediatric sexuality: promoting normal sexual development in children, *Nurse Practitioner* 18(8):37-44, 1993.

Sundram CJ and Stavis PF: Sexuality and mental retardation: unmet challenges, *Mental Retardation* 32(4):255-264, 1994.

Valenti-Hein D and Mueser KT: *The dating skills program: teaching social-sexual skills to adults with mental retardation*, Worthington, Ohio, 1991, International Diagnostic Services, Inc.

CHAPTER 15

Systems of Care for Children and Adolescents with Chronic Illness

JAMES M. PERRIN

A GENERIC VIEW OF CHRONIC ILLNESS IN CHILDHOOD

Many children and adolescents have chronic health impairments although the majority of these conditions are relatively minor and have little if any effect on usual daily activities. Estimates of the rates of chronic illness among children and adolescents vary greatly with about 10% to 35% having some chronic health condition.[2,6,7] Estimates of the rates of severe conditions—ones that are likely to interfere on a regular daily basis with the child's activities—vary from approximately 2% to 4% of all U.S. children.[3]

Patterns of chronic illness among children differ markedly from those among adults. Adults face a relatively small number of common chronic illnesses such as diabetes, high blood pressure, heart disease, or arthritis. However, children face a large variety of generally uncommon chronic health conditions such as thalassemia, congenital immunodeficiency disorders, bone cancers, or leukodystrophies. Among the severe health conditions affecting children, only asthma occurs commonly although it too, in its more severe forms, affects fewer than 1 child in 100. Other conditions vary in frequency from relatively rare (for example, diabetes—about 1 in 1000 children under age 16) to extremely rare conditions that may exist in only 20 or 30 individuals worldwide.[1]

Although each health condition has its own pathophysiology, course, complications, and treatment, many of the service requirements of families with a chronically ill child are the same regardless of the specific health condition. These children and their families typically need access to primary and specialty medical care; to other associated therapies such as nutrition, speech and hearing, respiratory, physical, and occupational; to preventive mental health service; to specialized social services; and to educational planning to limit the interference of the conditions with the child's educational progress. Although specialty medical services must generally focus on the specific health condition that the child has, the other services needed by the family better reflect the problem of chronic illness in general than the specific condition.

Families discuss several common issues when describing the tasks involved in raising a child or adolescent with severe chronic illness. These issues include the high costs of care (much of which is not covered by insurance), the burden of daily caretaking for the child (such as in-home physical therapy, special diets, or physical care of the mobility-impaired child), pain and discomfort faced by the child, increased psychologic problems, multiple health providers (often providing conflicting recommendations), and a sense of isolation. This last issue reflects both the decreased time and opportunities for families to maintain activities outside the home and the isolation that comes from having a child with a rare health condition (often previously unknown to the family). Despite the common experiences these families face, services until recently have generally been organized based on the specific condition, taking a relatively narrow view of the needs of the child and family. Recognition in the past several years of the more generic issues that families face has led to the organization of services based more broadly on family needs.

CATEGORIC SERVICES FOR LOW-INCIDENCE CONDITIONS: MEETING LIMITED NEEDS

Organizing services around single or closely related conditions (such as muscular dystrophy or hemophilia) allows the development of a group of specialists sophisticated in variations in prognosis, complications, therapies, and advances in medical care for specific rare conditions. Yet emphasis on specialty medical and surgical care has led to relative neglect of the many other services needed by families. Furthermore, the tendency has been to develop condition-specific specialized therapy such that the multiple associated therapists become increasingly focused on issues affecting the child with, for example, myelodysplasia. This emphasis on specialization requires that most services be highly centralized insofar as the relatively low frequency of each individual condition means that satisfactory numbers of children with the condition can be found only when brought together over a large geographic or population area. This categoric or condition-based approach, although providing some important benefits for children and families, requires that many families travel long distances, face significant disruption of daily lives, and miss school or work to receive most needed services.

Another problem associated with categoric programs has been that children become eligible for services only if they meet specific diagnostic criteria. Thus among two children with similar functional impairment, one child may be ineligible for a program that serves the other child simply because of differing diagnostic criteria. Consequently, a child with a bleeding disorder other than hemophilia may be unable to receive services in a hemophilia center. Many state maternal and child health programs for children with special health care needs have relied on diagnostic listings to determine eligibility for these Title V services.[4] Here too, children may be excluded because of a diagnostic incompatibility even though their functional impairment is comparable to that of children who do receive services. This issue was addressed in a recent Supreme Court decision (*Sullivan v. Zebley*)[13] that required the Social Security Administration to develop new, functionally oriented eligibility criteria for determining children's access to Supplemental Security Income (SSI) benefits.[10] Until this decision children and adolescents qualifying for SSI disability benefits needed to have a condition listed among a group of diagnoses (although some children became eligible by having a condition that was deemed equal to a listed condition). The Supreme Court directed the Social Security administration to develop a means of assessing children's functioning along with consideration of the severity of their specific diagnoses, recognizing that disability is not condition-specific but rather reflects how any health condition may affect the child's ability to function. This court decision, coupled with a legislative mandate for the Title V program to coordinate with the Social Security Administration for children and adolescents with disability, has led to the development of more generic approaches to defining eligibility for a number of public programs.

CHARACTERISTICS AND BENEFITS
OF A NONCATEGORIC SERVICE SYSTEM

Optimal noncategoric or generic service systems complement high-quality, specialized medical and surgical services with community-based services that meet many of the other needs of children and families.[8] When effectively regionalized, such programs ensure that children gain access to specialized medical and surgical care, usually in centralized facilities, but provide the majority of services in or near the child's home community. Thus care such as nursing or respiratory therapy for very young children can be provided in the home community; other associated therapies, such as physical or occupational therapy, can also be provided in the home, through the school, or in a community hospital rather than requiring frequent travel to a distant, more centralized facility.[9] These programs recognize that a wide variety of diverse medical conditions can interfere with the normal functioning of children and adolescents and that much of the effort must be directed toward improving functioning and limiting the interference of the condition with the child's growth and development.

The development of community-based services reflects other key developments as well. First, changing medical technology and access to services in the past 2 decades have markedly improved the long-term survival of children with most severe health conditions. Current estimates are that at least 90% of children, even with severe health conditions, survive to young adulthood.[2] Furthermore, most evidence suggests that the majority of these children and adolescents can become functional young adults who can complete education and become employed and generally be responsible for their own care. Whereas the emphasis a quarter of a century ago was on preventing premature death or otherwise enhancing survival rates, the current high survival rates have intensified attention on improving the quality of life of the children who survive. This attention supports the integration of children and families into community life so that they can benefit from the wide variety of both specialized and general community services.

A second phenomenon that has supported the development of generic, community-based services has been the tremendous growth of programs that empower families to take responsibility for the care of their child with chronic illness. Much of this growth has been directed by parents themselves through local, regional, and national parent groups and by parents experienced in the care of such a child helping families with a newly diagnosed child advocate for appropriate services and learn ways to take responsibility. Many Title V and other public programs have added parents as key members of their staff, in policy making and program-development roles, and as direct service providers.

The growth of community-based programs has been coupled with greater evidence that children grow and develop better and that families can meet their own needs more effectively than through earlier models that emphasized medical and surgical care only.

MODEL PROGRAMS AND FUTURE DIRECTIONS

Community care for children and adolescents with chronic illness will depend heavily on other changes in the organization and financing of health care in general. The current support for programs comes from a patchwork of financing from Medicaid, Title V programs for children with special health care needs, special education, private health insurance, and specific project grants.[9] Developing national agendas for universal access to health care and appropriate long-term care programs may significantly improve these community services. Reviewing effective programs identifies certain basic principles that should characterize appropriate systems of care for children with chronic illness. Some states have developed regional programs that link access to specialty care with a broader base of services at regional and community levels.

For example, Iowa's regional clinics, in collaboration with medicine and special education often coupled with nursing, help assess children's medical and other needs, link them with specialty services in a centralized program when necessary, and help to ensure the local delivery of most services throughout the state.[5] Iowa's program has also pioneered in its collaboration with parent groups and through employment of parents as key staff members of the state program.

In Florida an initial demonstration program in several rural counties (Project REACH) has now been implemented statewide.[11] This program provides coordinating care for children with special health care needs, mainly through specialized community nursing services that help to diminish the reliance of children and families on distant specialized services and improve their access to needed services at home and locally.

Examples at more local levels include the Pediatric Home Care Program at Albert Einstein College of Medicine in the Bronx (New York), where teams of pediatricians and nurse practitioners help families coordinate services when their children have a chronic health condition.[12] In Maryland the Coordinating Center for Children with Special Health Care Needs focuses on families whose children depend on significant technologies, helping them and their families coordinate care from a variety of providers and integrating the children as much as possible into their home and community settings.

All of these programs are characterized by their regional nature, integrating parents actively into program and plan development, and providing an array of services. Programs are regional but decentralized in that they emphasize providing services as close to home as possible, still ensuring that children receive needed specialty care. Recognizing that parents provide the majority of care themselves, these programs have emphasized strengthening parents' abilities to do just that and make appropriate decisions for them and their children. Finally, most programs recognize that, to ensure the best functional outcomes for children and families over time, they must provide an array of services well beyond medical, surgical, nursing, and hospital care.

Changing patterns of financing health care and supporting families will likely continue as important trends in systems of care for children with chronic illness. Universal health care should provide for most traditional medical and surgical services through an insurance mechanism without requiring other funds (such as those from public maternal and child health programs) to support similar services for uninsured people. Public health resources likely will go increasingly to supporting the infrastructure of appropriate regionalized programs and services that cannot be paid for under either direct insurance or long-term care benefits, and experimenting with new models of care. These developments, along with the changes in the SSI program for children, all point toward a move away from diagnostic determinations of eligibility to more functional definitions of children's abilities and disabilities. It is likely that states increasingly will use functional definitions to determine eligibility for programs for children with special health care needs, and that income supplements such as those from SSI will similarly be based increasingly on determinations of functional abilities rather than on specific diagnostic labels.

REFERENCES

1. Gortmaker SL: Demography of chronic childhood diseases. In Hobbs N, Perrin JM, editors: *Issues in the care of children with chronic illnesses*, San Francisco, 1985, Jossey-Bass.
2. Gortmaker S, Sappenfield W: Chronic childhood disorders: prevalence and impact, *Pediatr Clin North Am* 31:3-18, 1984.
3. Hobbs N, Perrin JM, Ireys HT: *Chronically ill children and their families*, San Francisco, 1985, Jossey-Bass.
4. Ireys HT, Hauck RJP, Perrin JM: Variability among state Crippled Children's Service programs: pluralism thrives, *Am J Public Health* 75:375-381, 1985.
5. MacQueen J: *Iowa's mobile and regional clinics*, mimeograph, Iowa City, 1986, Pediatrics, University of Iowa Hospitals and Clinics.
6. Newacheck PW, Budetti PP, McManus P: Trends in childhood disability, *Am J Public Health* 74:232-236, 1984.
7. Newacheck PW, Taylor WR: Childhood chronic illness: prevalence, severity, and impact, *Am J Public Health* 82:364-371, 1992.
8. Perrin JM, MacLean WE: Children with chronic illness: the prevention of dysfunction, *Pediatr Clin North Am* 35:1325-1327, 1988.
9. Perrin JM, Shayne MW, Bloom SR: *Home and community care for chronically ill children*, New York, 1993, Oxford University Press.
10. Perrin JM, Stein REK: Reinterpreting disability: changes in SSI for children, *Pediatrics* 88:1047-1051, 1991.
11. Pierce PM, Freedman SA: The REACH program: an innovative delivery model for medically dependent children, *Children's Health Care* 12(2):86-89, 1983.
12. Stein REK: A home care program for children with chronic illness, *Children's Health Care* 12:90-92, 1983.
13. Sullivan v Zebley, 110S C+ 885, 1990.

CHAPTER 16

Public Policy Advocacy

BEVERLY SCHENKMAN ROBERTS
BRENDA G. CONSIDINE

Parents of children with disabilities or chronic illness travel a difficult road. Sometimes that road seems endless with one obstacle after another—difficulty getting proper diagnosis of their child's condition, difficulty finding a doctor with experience treating the child's condition who is willing to see them, difficulty with the school in developing the child's individualized education plan (IEP), and so on.

Although there is much that the family of a child with a disabling condition needs to learn, there is a wealth of resources available to assist them. In providing individual advocacy the role of the professional is in part to facilitate the family's knowledge of and access to the services and resources that might be of assistance.

Medical and other professionals who provide treatment and support to families may find an emerging role as advocate. This chapter discusses the roles of families and professionals in public policy advocacy and identifies the components of successful advocacy services.

Families often need an advocate to learn how to negotiate the system on behalf of their son or daughter. In this context anyone who has knowledge of the system can be an asset to the family. The advocate may be a social worker at the early intervention program who advises the parents, or may be a case manager who advises low-income parents on the necessary steps to apply for Supplemental Security Income (SSI) for their child. The advocate may be a physician who advises and assists the family in their efforts to access social support services or quality educational services, or the advocate may be a staff person trained to work in that capacity, such as an employee of a non-profit social service organization like the Arc, formerly The Association for Retarded Citizens. Health care professionals, educators, and others not specifically trained in advocacy and case management may step in because the family needs assistance that they can provide.

Webster defines an advocate as "one who pleads the cause of another and one that defends or maintains a cause or proposal." Advocacy on behalf of a child with a disability or a chronic illness can be best examined from two perspectives: (1) individual advocacy and (2) systems advocacy.

In the disability field the goal of advocacy, whether carried out by individuals on behalf of family members or by organizations, is to improve the quality of life of individuals with disabilities or chronic illness or to gain access to a particular program or service.

A pediatrician, for example, may advocate to convince a school system that it is indeed possible to handle a child's medical needs at school. If a school insists that home instruction is required because the school cannot accommodate a child with a gastrostomy tube, the pediatrician can play a pivotal role in easing the fears of the school administrators and instructing the school nurse as to the necessary procedures. Although this type of involvement by the doctor is not taught in medical school, it is as important to achieving a good quality of life for a child with a disability as is the medical care that is provided in the doctor's office. (See the Resources section for a guidebook.)

In the area of developmental disabilities a clinical diagnosis may offer little in terms of treatment. For example, a developmental pediatrician, upon making a diagnosis of autism may recognize that there is little more the medical profession can offer to the patient in terms of treatment for the disability. The treatment in such a case is highly structured, educational programming. Attempting to secure appropriate treatment for a patient can take the physician into the area of special-education advocacy.

Usually, however, individual child advocacy is done by the child's parent or other members of the family. Parents need up-to-date, accurate information about their child's condition, appropriate treatment for that condition, information on available educational and social support services, and information on accessing those services to which their child is entitled. The combined role of parent and advocate is made more challenging by the perception on the part of some professionals that parents are irrational or have failed to accept the extent of their child's disability.

All advocacy begins locally. Until one's own service needs have been met, it can be difficult to engage in advocacy on a systems level. However, millions of families and professionals do get involved in the next stage of advocacy, systems advocacy. Systems advocacy involves an individual or a group of individuals coming together around a common goal or problem to influence public policy. The effort can be on the part of one person or millions of people.

A typical career path for systems advocates begins with personal experience. Many of the leaders in disability policy reform are themselves consumers of services, either directly or secondarily through their own children.

The efforts of Julie Beckett on behalf of her daughter, Katie, provide a good example of how individual advocacy evolves into systems advocacy. In 1978 Julie Beckett, an Iowa mother of a three-and-a-half-year-old child with viral encephalitis, learned that Medicaid would not pay for her daughter's home-based care. Medicaid would, however, pay tens-of-thousands of dollars to keep Katie in a hospital, even though it would be cheaper to let her live at home on a portable respirator. Beckett wrote lawmakers urging that this expensive and unsound rule be eliminated. In 1981 President Ronald Reagan granted what has come to be known as the "Katie Beckett Waiver," allowing Katie and 300,000 others to leave hospital rooms and return to their homes for Medicaid-funded care.

The ability to influence decision makers is a key element of systems advocacy. Powerful lobby groups provide an example for influencing decision makers. These groups provide political donations, information, and, most importantly, voters. While the disability community generally cannot provide large contributions to political parties, it can provide quality information and voters.

HISTORY OF PUBLIC POLICY ADVOCACY

Advocacy pertaining to disability and chronic illness has taken a high profile in the last 3 decades. Prior to the Kennedy era most disability policy centered around the needs of veterans, with the goal of rehabilitating soldiers who had been wounded or maimed in the course of service.

Few formal services or supports for children with disabilities were available from the government, other than institutional, custodial care. During the past 30 years, however, community services have developed as the result of family advocacy.

Parent advocacy networks have been gaining strength since the late 1940s, when the organization now known as The Arc originated. In 1950 the first convention of the National Association of Parents and Friends of Mentally Retarded Children was held in Minnesota. By 1955 the association had more than 400 local chapters with a national membership nearing 30,000. The early members became involved in public policy advocacy, urging Congress to expand teaching and research in the education of children with mental retardation. The members supported expanding Social Security coverage to adults disabled in childhood, funding for medical facilities for people with mental retardation, and increased appropriations for vocational rehabilitation programs. From 1956 to 1961 federal funding for mental retardation services and research increased from $14 million to $94 million. The families involved with the association were successful in moving the federal government to pass landmark legislation such as the Education for All Handicapped Children Act and its amendments, and the Americans with Disabilities Act.

Today, families continue to unite for the purpose of public policy advocacy. Julie Beckett has emerged as a national leader in health care reform efforts related to children with disabling conditions. She and thousands of families have formed Family Voices, an alliance aimed at lobbying Congress on the national debate over health care policy.

ELEMENTS OF AN ADVOCACY PROGRAM

Service organizations can play an important role in facilitating individual and systems advocacy. The following section discusses the major elements of a successful health care advocacy program for people with developmental disabilities as they are handled through a program called Mainstreaming Medical Care, under the auspices of The Arc of New Jersey.

Individual Advocacy Services

Information and referral. Accurate and thorough information is needed by families and professionals so they can make informed choices about available service options. The Mainstreaming Medical Care Program at The Arc of New Jersey operates a Statewide Clearinghouse on Health Care for People with Developmental Disabilities. The clearinghouse provides information and referral to family members and staff at agencies across the state serving individuals with developmental disabilities. The service is free and confidential.

Typically the requests for information include such topics as education for the prevention of sexual abuse, and problems arising from a lack of health insurance. Callers also frequently ask to be referred to a doctor, dentist, psychologist, or psychiatrist in their county. The clearinghouse has a computerized list of more than 500 health care professionals recommended because of their knowledgeable and caring approach to patient care.

Factual printed materials. The dissemination of printed resource materials is central to any quality advocacy program and must include material developed for a number of target audiences. The Mainstreaming Medical Care Program publishes a newsletter three times a year, *Healthy Times,* which highlights efforts of health care providers who treat people with developmental disabilities. The newsletter provides up-to-date information on health care conferences and resources to help families and staff provide better care to this population. The program also offers fact sheets, brochures, medical record forms, and other printed materials to assist families and health care providers.

Problem-solving assistance. One key element of individual advocacy is to provide families with pertinent information on how to access various services; another is to teach families what to do when the system does not work properly. For example, if the application for SSI has been denied, the family needs to know about the appeals process. If a family believes that an inclusive education is best for their child and the school district refuses to provide it, they need to know what recourse they have. The advocate can help the family get in touch with other families who have experienced similar difficulties.

Problems of access to services in areas such as health care and education can turn a simple individual advocacy case into a more complex systems issue.

Systems Advocacy Services

To bring about systems change an advocacy program needs to engage in a number of coordinated activities.

Professional training and education on best practices. Outdated information and lack of quality education and training are major barriers to systems change. Before a group of advocates can reach consensus, they must share a common base of knowledge. The Mainstreaming Medical Care Program provides physicians with a convenient way to keep up-to-date on aspects of medicine that pertain to developmental disabilities. This takes place through continuing medical education (CME) programs offered as part of a hospital's Grand Rounds schedule (educational sessions offered to physicians by various departments within the hospital), an annual conference, and newsletters on the health care needs of persons with developmental disabilities. An example of a monthly medical newsletter that provides CME credit for physicians is *Exceptional Health Care* (see the Resources section at the end of the chapter).

Outreach to other agencies and organizations. Many policy-making agencies are able to make a significant difference in the quality of life of children with disabling conditions. Therefore an advocacy program must engage in active outreach to these agencies. They include departments of county, state, and federal government (health, education, and human services). Advocacy efforts can range from information-sharing sessions that sensitize staff members to health care concerns of people with developmental disabilities, to the examination of proposed legislation and testifying for or against bills.

Grass-roots organizational structure. The members of successful public policy advocacy programs must organize its members and articulate well-planned, carefully timed advocacy campaigns around specific issues. For example, The Arc of New Jersey has created an advocacy network for this purpose. The names, addresses, and phone numbers of hundreds of parents, consumers, and professionals are kept in a database organized by legislative and congressional district. These advocates are provided with up-to-date information on evolving public policy and suggestions for ways in which they may get involved. The Arc also sends advocates fact sheets that explain who their elected officials are and on which key committees their legislators serve. On a national level a similar structure for advocacy activities links individual members with key members of Congress. Such structures allow for one-to-one direct communication between a knowledgeable voter who is personally affected by a matter of public policy and his or her legislator.

Specific organized activities. Once advocates are organized it is up to the public policy advocacy program to mobilize them in effective ways. Traditional activities such as rallies and demonstrations can be very successful, as can letter writing, postcard, and telegram campaigns. These strategies rely on large numbers of advocates participating at once and are vital in debates that are large in scope and are controversial, such as the health care debate and budget issues. The power of targeted personal communication is also important on state and local levels. For example, in New Jersey a legislative committee was moved to act on a bill because of the well-timed and coordinated efforts of six families. The afternoon before the committee was to act on a bill, a statewide organization contacted one family represented by each of the six legislators on the committee. Each family was asked to place a call to their legislator, and to ask three neighbors (each residing in the same legislative district) to make similar calls. By noon the next day, each member of the committee had heard from four constituents on a relatively obscure bill. Despite opposition from the State Department of Education, the legislation was approved unanimously by the committee without hearing any witnesses. A small legislative effort such as this is not likely to be successful if confronted by a well-funded and highly organized opposition.

Accurate, unbiased, quality information. As is true of individual advocacy, systems advocacy requires accessible and readable printed material. Those participating in systems advocacy need to know how a massive national effort, such as health care reform, is likely to affect a specific sector of the population. Accurate, factual analysis of public policy proposals is needed by advocates who wish to get involved in the debate. Those in public office also need unbiased, factual information. The increasing complexity of disability services and health care systems can make the process of researching accurate information very difficult. Elected officials often rely on staff and lobbyists to provide such information. Advocacy programs organized for systems change on behalf of children with chronic illness and disability can provide a similar service to their elected officials by keeping in regular contact and providing information.

A CALL TO ACTION FOR CONTINUED PUBLIC POLICY ADVOCACY

Systems advocacy is currently taking place as the debate over health care reform continues. Whatever the ultimate outcome, disability advocates across America are putting forth a massive effort urging legislators to adopt an equitable plan for individuals with disabilities and chronic illness. Families of children with disabilities know all too well the inequities of a health care system that permits exclusions for preexisting conditions and that locks a parent into a job because leaving the current job would mean a loss of valuable health care coverage. The expenses associated with some disabilities and chronic illnesses are monumental; even with health insurance, out-of-pocket costs for some families can be astronomical.

The growth of managed health care programs presents yet another area in which greater advocacy for children with disabilities and chronic illness is needed. Parents who once had health insurance through their place of business with a fee-for-service plan, are being switched into managed care as a cost-saving measure by companies that are trying to control the skyrocketing costs of their employee health benefits plans. When this occurs families whose children have had many years of excellent pediatric and specialist care are suddenly forced to choose new doctors from a list provided by the managed care organization. In some cases the list contains pediatricians not experienced in caring for children with disabilities, or pediatricians with experience in this field who are not accepting new patients.

It is essential that health care professionals and families educate managed care providers about the needs of children with disabilities and chronic illness and about the hardship created when families are forced to switch to an unknown health care provider who does not have the level of experience caring for children with disabilities that was previously available.

This chapter emphasizes the importance of family and professional advocacy for children with disabling conditions. Suggestions are provided on ways that individuals and groups can advocate for improvements in services for children with disabilities. There are many advocacy organizations that can be helpful in providing answers to specific questions and in sending brochures, fact sheets, newsletters, and other materials to educate families as well as professionals. These organizations will provide information on membership procedures and the locations of their state and local offices. The resources mentioned in this chapter are listed on below, followed by a list on pp. 170 to 171 of the national offices for the most widely known disability organizations serving the needs of children and youth.

RESOURCES

1. Haynie M, Porter SM, and Palfrey JS: *Children assisted by medical technology in educational settings: guidelines for care*, Boston, 1989, The Children's Hospital. Available from: Children's Hospital/Project School Care, 300 Longwood Ave., Boston, MA 02115; cost is $30.00.

   This guide was prepared to help schools feel more comfortable about including children assisted by medical technology. Developed with a grant from the Robert Wood Johnson Foundation and written in an easy-to-understand style, this how-to guide provides sample recordkeeping forms for schools and contains sections on tube feeding, intravenous lines, ostomy care, catheterization, and respiratory care.

2. *Mainstreaming Medical Care Patient Record Form*: This form has been used successfully by families who show it to the physician at the beginning of the office visit whenever the child is being seen by a new physician (e.g., at the emergency room, in a clinic setting, or when visiting a neurologist or other specialist who does not know the child's history). To request this form, specify whether the form is for children or adults. Forms are available at no charge by sending a stamped, self-addressed envelope to: Mainstreaming Medical Care Program, The Arc of New Jersey, 985 Livingston Ave., North Brunswick, N.J. 08902.

3. *Exceptional Health Care*: Edited by Theodore Kastner, M.D, this monthly medical newsletter provides abstracts and commentary on articles from medical literature regarding treatment of persons with developmental disabilities. The newsletter is approved by the Accreditation Council for Continuing Medical Education (ACCME) to provide 12.0 credit hours in Category 1 of the Physicians' Recognition Award of the American Medical Association. The newsletter is also approved for 12 prescribed hours by the American Academy of Family Physicians. It is available through: Developmental Disabilities Publications (#60), 100 Madison Ave., Morristown, N.J. 07960-9886, 1-800-852-7718.

NATIONAL DISABILITY ORGANIZATIONS

The Arc
P.O. Box 1047
Arlington, TX 76004
1-800-433-5255

Autism Society of America
7910 Woodmont Avenue, Suite 650
Bethesda, MD 20814
1-800-328-8476

Cystic Fibrosis Foundation
6931 Arlington Road
Bethesda, MD 20814
1-800-FIGHTCF

Epilepsy Foundation of America
4351 Garden City Dr.
Landover, MD 20785
1-800-332-1000

Learning Disability Association
4156 Library Rd.
Pittsburgh, PA 15234
412-341-1515

Muscular Dystrophy Association
3300 East Sunrise Drive
Tucson, AZ 85718
602-529-2000

National Center for
Learning Disabilities
99 Park Ave.
New York, NY 10016
212-687-7211

National Council on Disability
800 Independence Ave., S.W.
Suite 814
Washington, D.C. 20591
202-267-3846

National Down Syndrome Congress
1605 Chantilly Drive, Suite 250
Atlanta, GA 30324
1-800-232-6372

National Down Syndrome Society
666 Broadway
New York, NY 10012
1-800-221-4602

National Head Injury Foundation
1776 Massachusetts, Suite 100
Washington, D.C. 20036
1-800-444-NHIF

National Information Center
for Children and Youth
with Disabilities
1-800-999-5599

National Information Center
on Deafness
202-651-5051

National Organization for
Rare Disorders
P.O. Box 8923
New Fairfield, CT 06812
203-746-6518

National Organization on Disability
910 16th St., N.W., Suite 600
Washington, D.C. 20006
202-293-5960

National Pediatric HIV
Resource Center
1-800-362-0071

National Rehabilitation
Information Center
1-800-346-2742

Spina Bifida Association of America
4590 MacArthur Blvd., N.W.,
Suite 250
Washington, D.C. 20007
1-800-621-3141

Sudden Infant Death Syndrome
1-800-221-SIDS

The Association for Persons with
Severe Handicaps (TASH)
7010 Roosevelt Way, N.E.
Seattle, WA 98115
206-361-8870

United Cerebral Palsy Association
1522 K Street, N.W., Suite 1112
Washington, D.C. 20005
1-800-USA-5UCP

CHAPTER **17**

Interorganizational Collaboration

MARGO I. PETER
CALVIN C.J. SIA

Contemporary theories of organizational management emphasize collaborative approaches. Walk into any conference room today and you are certain to
hear the words *coordination* and *collaboration*. To that end we are told that
we must establish links and cooperate with one another. Indeed, we are told
this so often that the words themselves are in danger of losing potency. It
behooves us then to take a moment to reflect on just what we mean when we
talk about linkage and cooperation and why they are so important.

WORKING IN THE "BETWEEN"

The overarching goal of recent changes in service delivery for children with
special needs is the development of an integrated system that will reduce
fragmentation, avoid duplication, and close gaps in services. Much must be
done to accomplish this grand goal, including promoting programmatic and
ideologic changes in the way we treat children and families. Fortunately,
much has been done to restructure programs and revolutionize philosophies
so that services are more available, accessible, and family centered. However,
to create a truly integrated system of services we must attend not only to what
happens within individual programs, but to what happens between programs. Links and cooperation are our tools for working in the "between."

A quick look at the dictionary tells us that to link means to join, unite, or
combine; cooperation refers to participation and harmony. Our goal then is to
combine resources and participate jointly in the process of creating and maintaining harmony between programs and agencies.

Who should be working toward this goal? The deceptively simple answer is anyone involved in the provision of services to children with special needs. The inherent complexity of this statement becomes evident when one realizes that this includes public and private agencies at the federal, state, and community levels and individual providers in any given area.

VERTICAL/HORIZONTAL LINKAGE AND COOPERATION

Two factors are important to assure involvement of all appropriate players: (1) vertical and horizontal linkages, and (2) cooperation between private and public sectors. In order to ensure a seamless system of services, public policies must advance consistency throughout the vertical hierarchy. Mandates and missions at federal and state levels must be complementary with one another and supported by community efforts to ensure implementation. For example, success of recent federal initiatives to expand Social Security Income (SSI) benefits for families depends on mandates within each state for aggressive outreach and community-level follow-through with individual providers.

Once complementariness between federal and state programs has been established, it is essential to develop a coherent statewide system comprised of regional programs. Regional systems must maintain enough autonomy and flexibility so they can address needs unique to individual communities. This is especially important in larger states or in states where rural communities may be diverse and widely scattered. Such regional systems of care can assure vertical cooperation by conforming to state policy and communicating regularly with state-level personnel. In addition, regional systems should maximize resources and promote horizontal links by incorporating existing public and private programs.

Horizontal links between providers of care are essential if we are to meet the needs of the total child. Such links between regional community programs assure consistency of program quality and simplifies transitions when a child moves from one region to another. In addition, links between the private and public sectors with a given community are essential to assure that care is comprehensive and coordinated. This means that hospital-discharge planning teams must coordinate with early intervention programs, special educators must communicate with primary care physicians, state health departments must coordinate with private providers, etc.

Seven Steps to Assuring Linkage and Cooperation

Former Surgeon General Koop[4] outlined seven steps requisite to building comprehensive systems. These steps provide a blueprint that, if followed, will assure that horizontal and vertical links are made throughout a state and that professionals at every point along the continuum will cooperate. The seven steps are the following:

1. Institute a process for system development at the local level.
2. Implement community plans based on needs assessment.
3. Establish and maintain organizational mechanisms at the local level to bring about collaboration among community providers.
4. Establish and maintain organizational mechanisms for community-based case management.
5. Develop and implement a statewide plan based on needs assessment for building collaborative service delivery systems among all relevant state agencies.
6. Establish and maintain collaborative mechanisms by state agencies for the purpose of assisting communities in the process of system development.
7. Enact state legislation mandating and facilitating system development at both state and local levels and providing funding for such system development.

Application

The importance of vertical and horizontal linkage and cooperation becomes clear if we focus on the effect they have on the care of an individual child. Consider the case of Sophie. Sophie was born with spina bifida in a large children's hospital where she received state-of-the-art care and was linked to an early intervention program upon discharge. When she was 18 months old, her parents moved to another state where she enrolled in a state-sponsored infant-development program that conforms to standards set by Federal Public Law 99-457. Thus, she received care that was commensurate with her previous experience. When she was 2 years old, her parents moved again within the same state. The only infant-development program in her new smaller community was a private nonprofit program. There was no mass transit and the only children's hospital equipped to handle Sophie's unique medical needs was a great distance away. Fortunately for Sophie her new infant-development program participated in a larger network of early intervention programs in the state, so she was assured continuous quality care. Her previous care coordinator met with her new care coordinator, her parents, and her new pediatrician. A new Individual Family Support Plan (IFSP) was developed that included previous IFSP goals and incorporated new goals relative to problems unique to life in her new community (e.g., vouchers for transportation to and from the program and assistance with arrangements for travel to an evaluation center when necessary). Vertical links assured that Sophie would obtain quality care in a timely fashion in all three of her homes. Horizontal coordination guaranteed that Sophie's services would be comprehensive and not jeopardized by changes in her geographical location.

COMMUNICATE, COOPERATE, COLLABORATE

Henry Ford reportedly once said, "Coming together is a beginning, talking together is a process and working together is success." His comment is particularly relevant today as we consider building collaborative relationships in the service of children and families. It suggests that there is a stepwise process involved in creating integrated services. At least three successive steps, communication, cooperation, and collaboration, need to be considered.

Cooperative interaction provides a foundation for collaborative integrated systems and communication provides its cornerstone. We must learn to communicate with one another before we can work cooperatively and we must cooperate in order to collaborate.

The first step toward integrated services is coming together. This seems rudimentary but it is often neglected. Meaningful dialogue about coordination begins only when all players are brought to the table and given an opportunity to share concerns and identify a common mission. Developing a mission statement can kindle commitment to work together. Indeed, it can be the first in a series of cooperative ventures. Such cooperative efforts provide the opportunity for individuals to learn about one another and to develop mutual trust and respect. Melaville and Blank[6] suggest that where individuals are not ready for collaborative partnerships, cooperative initiatives offer a reasonable starting point. This process cultivates an increasing willingness to work side by side toward similar goals, laying the groundwork for the next step in the process, collaboration.

Collaboration occurs when each individual involved in the process makes a unique contribution to the whole. Participants are no longer simply working in parallel, but are working as a team toward a shared vision. This, as Henry Ford suggested, is true success and is the substructure for successful integrated services.

It is important to remember that collaboration is not an end point, but rather an ongoing process. For this reason, communication, cooperation, and collaboration must be promoted at formal as well as informal levels. Informal telephone conversations and consultation regarding individual cases further collaboration as much or more than formal committees or interagency agreements.

Benefits

The value of linkage and cooperation can be measured in both quantitative and qualitative terms. Economic pressures dictate that we eliminate duplication of services. We can no longer afford to reinvent the wheel at every stop in the service delivery system a family might make. Links between programs allow sharing of professionals yields a more comprehensive picture of a child's strengths and weaknesses in a shorter amount of time than if each individual were pursuing the same picture alone.

Careful consideration must be given to confidentiality and informed consent from families must remain a guiding mandate. Interagency agreements, outlining clear descriptions of what information is needed and how it will be used, can expedite the process of data gathering. If respect for confidentiality and informed consent drive the system, cooperative information exchange will enhance the efficiency of program implementation as well as the quality of care provided to clients.

Enhanced quality of care is perhaps the most important reason for establishing links and promoting cooperation. The complexity of multilayered fragmented systems of care can be daunting to consumers. Some parents may be tempted to give up rather than persevere in the face of a system that seems impossible to navigate. Linkage and cooperation between organizations increase the likelihood that families will access a range of services because individual providers will be knowledgeable about the gamut of available services and advise families accordingly. In addition, cooperation eliminates unnecessary paperwork, allowing professionals more time for direct service, which translates to more service for consumers.

Barriers

Much has been written about the barriers to linkage and cooperation. McLaughlin and Covert[5] list the following 14 potential barriers to collaboration: competitiveness, lack of compelling mutual interest, parochial interests, lack of skill in coordinating, difficulty in communicating across disciplines, preoccupation with administrative rather than functional structures, concerns about client confidentiality, resistance to change, external pressures, lack of accountability, lack of monitoring and evaluation procedures, inadequate knowledge of other agencies, negative attitudes, and little consideration of political bias.

Unfortunately, the various disciplines and organizations serving children often operate as though they are separate countries who lack diplomatic relations with one another. Most have been in place for many years. Each has developed its own culture, complete with unique language, ideology, and mores. Divergent theoretical frameworks, philosophies of patient care, and goals for treatment make cooperation particularly difficult. Establishing and maintaining linkage and cooperation is akin to establishing diplomatic relations between diverse countries. In this way the paradigm of cultural sensitivity is apt as we attempt to promote linkage and coordination.

Gilkerson[3] states that collaboration is enhanced by understanding unique organizational styles and, in essence, it encourages us to be aware of their relative cultures. We must build into the process an awareness of and respect for differences, while capitalizing on commonalities.

It is critical to remember that many organizations and disciplines have a history of competition for funding and clients. According to Baldwin et al,[1] years of mistrust among individuals may go unacknowledged. Fears about losing clients must be addressed and issues of turf confronted. Change in general can be discomfiting; organizational change often breeds distrust and fears of loss of authority and autonomy. It is important that discussions be grounded in the shared goal of helping children and that an atmosphere of give and take be fostered. Individuals must be provided a forum for airing concerns and these should be addressed openly.

One of the most challenging gaps to bridge is that between public and private sectors. Private providers often operate in isolation, have limited knowledge of the "big picture" of the service delivery system, and have no inherent impetus for collaboration. However, inclusion of the private sector promotes access to services because it increases the likelihood that referrals to community services will be made and contributes to the coordinated nature of service delivery.

Strategies for overcoming barriers. Baumeister[2] developed several excellent recommendations for influencing public policy. These can be translated into useful strategies for overcoming barriers to linkage and coordination. They are outlined as follows:

Develop clear and unambiguous consensus about what must be done, by whom, when, and where. Convene a meeting or series of meetings including all relevant parties to discuss benefits and barriers to coordination. Be sure to include individuals from private and public sectors as well as representatives of the consumer group (i.e., parents).

Identify several well-respected individuals who have the interest, time, and energy to study and to understand in detail the political environment, the major players, and the obstacles to implementation. Enlist the involvement of advocacy groups who share the common cause. These people should be involved from the beginning and a smaller group may work more efficiently. Additional members can be added to the group over time, including individuals who can be influential and authoritative when the time comes to implement recommendations.

Generate a plan of action that calls for continuous efforts, coordination among the various professional organizations and disciplines, and constant updating of information. Begin the process by engendering group identity and cohesion. Formulating a name and mission statement for the group is a good way to do this.

Identify legislators and agency officials who, by reason of personal circumstances, can be expected to be sympathetic to your interests and agenda. This is important because at some point it will be necessary to influence the powers that be to institutionalize recommended changes.

Work together politically, rather than competitively, with other organizations also interested in affecting public policy, such as groups and associations serving or advocating for individuals with special needs. This is a good way to facilitate trust building and to assail negative attitudes related to past competition.

Speak English, not jargon—ordinary language advances opportunities for discussion. This should be one of the early explicit ground rules. Group members should be encouraged to ask questions when jargon gets in the way. Individuals are often so comfortable with their own language that they may be unaware that they are using jargon unique to their discipline or agency.

Present information linked to the context of the lives of children. Avoid characterizing them as sets of data and thus nameless faces associated with numbers. This will help keep people cognizant of the human value to your efforts. Having parents involved will help ensure that this happens.

Set realistic annual targets that represent an incremental approach to the ultimate goal. This is important to assure that the group stays on task and feels a sense of success along the way. The sense of accomplishment will fuel continued commitment.

Accept the need for compromise, given that other needs and interests must also be addressed within an already strained system. Everyone will have to give a little, including you.

Establish an ongoing system of information exchange within your own professional groups and those groups with comparable interests, lobbying efforts, and review. Be aware that time constraints make frequent or lengthy meetings difficult to sustain over an extended period of time.

Resist being discouraged—setbacks and tradeoffs are part of the process of public-policy formation in human services. Remember the process is the goal. You may accomplish your goals, but you will never be finished.

CONCLUSION

Interorganizational linkage and cooperation are the foundation of integrated systems of care for children and their families. While many new initiatives have been launched to improve services for children, the last bastion of progress will be addressing problems related to what occurs (or does not occur) between programs, disciplines, and agencies. The integration of service delivery systems will depend upon our efforts to communicate, coordinate, and collaborate. There are many barriers to this and the challenge is great. Fragmentation, duplication, and gaps can be eliminated, however, if we work proactively to assure that linkage is institutionalized in developing systems and that strategies are implemented to overcome existing barriers to coordination. For years many professionals operated as if they could not afford to take the time for linkage and coordination. Today, we cannot afford not to.

REFERENCES

1. Baldwin DS et al: Collaborative systems design for part H of IDEA, *Journal of Infants and Young Children*: 12-22, 1992.
2. Baumeister AA: Policy formulation: a real world view. In Bess FH and Hall JW III, editors: *Screening children for auditory function*, Nashville, Tenn, 1992, Bill Wilkerson Center Press.
3. Gilkerson L: Understanding institutional functioning style: a resource for hospital and early intervention collaboration, *Journal of Infants and Young Children*, 2(3):22-30, 1990.
4. Koop CE: The health education symposium, Surgeon General's Report, Division of Maternal and Child Health, US Department of Health and Human Services, 1987.
5. McLaughlin JA: *Evaluating interagency collaboration*, Chapel Hill, NC, 1986, University of North Carolina at Chapel Hill TADS.
6. Melaville I and Blank M: *What it takes: structuring interagency partnerships to connect children and families with comprehensive services*, Washington, DC, 1991, The Education and Human Service Consortium.

CHAPTER 18

Community-Based Needs Assessment

COLLEEN MONAHAN

Community-based needs asessment (CBNA) is a vital element of the process of achieving a comprehensive, coordinated, community-based system of care for children with disabilities and their families. At the core of a community-based assessment is the recognition that each community has unique characteristics that contribute to the health status of children and families and that can best be reflected by the involvement of community members in the assessment's design and implementation. A CBNA is an empowering process that allows communities to assess and monitor their own system of services and set priorities that have meaning to their own populations.

THE ELEMENTS OF CBNA

An assessment can be conducted for any one or combination of the following reasons: to identify existing needs (i.e., evaluate current adequacy); to monitor progress toward solving one or more identified problems (i.e., after an intervention has been implemented); and/or to provide a basis for planning. To be most effective as an instrument of change, needs assessment should be a part of a planning and monitoring effort that includes the following elements: a defined community, selection of participants, and determination of need.

A Defined Community

A community may be defined geographically (as a neighborhood, township, city, metropolitan area, etc.) or functionally. Functionally, a community is defined as a group of individuals living in proximity to one another, sharing common values or cultural identity, or coming together to address common issues or problems.

Because the definition of community can vary so significantly, the geographic or functional boundaries of a CBNA should be clarified before any assessment is begun. Inappropriate conclusions may be drawn when community boundaries are loosely defined or the community's distinct characteristics are misunderstood or not examined.

Selection of Participants

The collection of information from which to assess or make conclusions about the needs of a specific community requires the involvement of appropriate types and adequate numbers of community participants. This may seem obvious but many needs assessments have been conducted and conclusions attributed to communities with little consideration for community involvement or representative sampling. A valid assessment of needs must reflect the cultural and economic diversity of the population and the unique resources that exist in the community. To ensure that this happens requires that some basic knowledge exists about the community before the assessment is designed. For example, if a community of 100,000 people includes a group of 1000 non–English-speaking migrant workers, their unique issues are likely to be missed by sampling techniques that depend upon random sampling or English-language recruitment of focus groups. However, recognition of the existence of this group and their language barrier prior to selection of participants for the needs assessment can ensure that they are represented and that appropriate resources are available to reach them, such as hiring interpreters or creating surveys in their language.

Determination of Need

Determination of need requires value judgement. The identification of needs is a process of describing and prioritizing the problems of a target population and recognizing potential solutions to those problems.[4] There are four general categories of need: normative, perceived, expressed, and relative. Integrating needs from all of these categories strengthens the validity of the assessment.

Normative need. Normative need is derived from expert opinions about what constitutes appropriate levels of service or health status. These are often promulgated as standards (i.e., Year 2000 Objectives, American Academy of Pediatrics Guidelines, etc.) and used to compare with what is found in a community. If the service level or health status of a group falls below the standard, then the group is defined as in need.

Perceived need. Perceived need is derived from the expectations of the population, such as parents' expectations about the amount or quality of the services that their child should receive. This type of need is important to ascertain because when there is no perceived need for a service, the population will usually not support measures to provide for it, nor will they use those measures once provided.

Expressed need. Expressed need is defined through the utilization of services. Unfortunately, failure of a population to use a service does not necessarily mean it is not needed. Access barriers may exist for some groups in the community. When barriers do exist, comparing expressed need with perceived need may help to identify the particular group having the problem with access.

Relative need. Relative or comparative need is derived from examining the distribution equity of services across populations. For example, if 90% of children with private health insurance receive dental services and only 40% of the children on Medicaid receive dental services, then children on Medicaid can be said to have a greater comparative need for dental services.

PLANNING THE PROCESS OF CBNA

The steps in the community-based needs assessment include the following:
1. Identification of the target population (the community and participants)
2. Organization of the planning group
3. Identification of the needs (the problems and potential solutions)
4. Assessment of the relative importance of the needs to the community
5. Summary and communication of the results

Identification of the Target Population

The target population is the group or groups of individuals about which the information for the needs assessment is desired or for which interventions will be planned and applied. The size and characteristics of the community affect the cost and complexity of the assessment and ultimately the cost of implementing new services.

If comparisons are to be made between subgroups within the target population, it is important to plan for a sufficient number of participants in each subgroup for the analysis. Therefore it is important to identify which comparisons will be made, if any, prior to selection of the target population. For example, if one wishes to compare the views of parents of children with disabilities by their source of funding support, then the samples should include sufficient numbers of those covered by private insurance, Medicaid recipients, and uninsured respondents.

Organization of the Planning Group

Involvement of both service providers and service users is critical to the success of a CBNA. The involvement of these two groups can best be accomplished through the organization of a community team or planning group.

This group can define the purpose of the assessment, identify the target and subgroup populations, assign responsibility for specific tasks, and provide quality control to the assessment process. At a minimum, membership of a community team for needs assessment for children with disabilities should include parents, young adults with disabilities, and representatives from all elements of the community service system.

State-level agencies and organizations that develop policies or offer services that affect systems of care at the community level should work with the community team to facilitate local assessment, to support planning, and to promote local partnerships. These organizations should provide technical assistance, develop joint data bases, and assist communities to obtain the financial support needed to define and achieve planning goals. Organizations that may be able to provide such assistance to communities include the state's Title V Maternal and Child Health Program and Program for Children with Special Health Care Needs, the state's Council on Developmental Disabilities, university-affiliated programs for developmental disabilities, the state's Interagency Coordinating Council for Early Intervention, the state vocational rehabilitation program, the state medical society, and the state chapter of the American Academy of Pediatrics.

Identification of Needs

The data needed to satisfy the assessment of the health care system for children with disabilities and their families should reflect all the dimensions of child and family health. Simple indexes (i.e., infant mortality) or composite measures of child health (i.e., mortality as a function of poverty) are insufficient. Demographic data should be considered that covers all the major domains of health including biologic (disease, longevity, functional capacity), psychological (satisfaction, comfort), and social (ability and achievement).[10]

Because child and family health are also related to the health of the community and the adequacy of its service system, data should be examined about the community's resources and existing services. The type of community-specific data pertinent to a needs assessment related to a system of services for children with disabilities and their families includes population demographics, socioeconomic status, vital statistics (birth and death), hospitalization data, availability of health care providers and programs, and the adequacy of educational, social, and recreation services. These data can be collected from a variety of sources (Table 18-1).

Secondary data. Existing (secondary) data from other sources (census, vital statistics, annual reports, etc.) is relatively easy to obtain, inexpensive, and serves as the usual starting point for a CBNA. Data gathered from such sources contributes to an understanding of the characteristics of a communi-

TABLE 18-1. Inventory of Needs Assessment Data Sources

Secondary Data Analysis	Primary Data Capture	Community Input Processes
Description of health status, services, resources, utilization, etc.	Surveys, questionnaires	Local planning group
	Key informant interviews	Advisory councils
Ranking of indicator data by uni-dimensional, additive, standardized, weighted, multivariate modeling	Focus groups	Town meetings, hearings
	Expert panels	
Risk indices: poverty, socioeconomic status (SES), health	Delphi groups	
Service system matrices		
Old primary data		

Modified from Peck, M: *Putting needs assessment to good use*, Paper presented at the Children with Special Health Care Needs Continuing Education Institute, Columbus, Ohio, November 1993.

ty and should be examined by the planning group before it decides upon issues to address in primary data collection. These data can be used to develop indexes to rank areas by risk. The box on p. 185 lists some common sources of secondary data.

Demographic data describe the numbers of individuals in the community by age, race, ethnicity, or ancestry. *Socioeconomic data*, which describe the income and employment status of the population, are critical in understanding the size of the population at risk for receiving inadequate levels of medical services or care financing. *Perinatal data*, which include infant mortality/morbidity rates and levels of maternal care, help to define the adequacy of prenatal care and identify poor birth outcomes. The numbers and causes of *deaths in childhood* are important for identifying risks by category (i.e., accidents) or by age groups (i.e., infants, adolescents). *Pediatric hospitalization data* describe the reasons for hospitalization and the hospital locations and sources of payment. General *child health data* include the results of hearing, vision, lead, and scoliosis screening programs. *Education data* include the number and location of schools, the total enrollment by program, the number in special education, early intervention, and Headstart, dropout rates, and the number of students with disabilities with documented plans for transition. This data can also be used to examine the issue of children receiving special education in segregated settings. *Financing data* include information about sources of health care funding and the number of children who

---

Sources of Secondary Data

American Hospital Association
   (Number/type of hospitals)
American Medical Association
   (Number/type of physicians)
Department of Employment Security
   (Unemployment)
Department of Health and Human Services Administration for Children
   (Headstart)
Department of Special Education
   (Number of children by disability)
National Center for Health Statistics (NCHS)
   (National Health Interview Survey)
Social Security Administration
   (Number of children receiving SSI)
State Administrator of Medicaid
   (Number served)
State Board (Department) of Education
   (Number of students/schools)
   (Number of early intervention programs)
State Department of Professional Regulation
   (Number of licensed health personnel)
State Department of Public Health
   (Vital statistics)
State Program for Children with Special Health Care Needs
   (Number served/characteristics of)
State Vocational Rehabilitation Agency
   (Number served/characteristics of)
U.S. Bureau of the Census
   (Decennial census and current population survey)

---

are uninsured, receiving Medicaid and/or early periodic screening, diagnosis, and treatment (EPSDT) services, Supplemental Security Income (SSI), and served by a state's children with special health care needs program. Identifying the number of *health care providers* available to a community is important and would include those licensed as physicians, pediatricians, family practitioners, occupational/physical therapists, audiologists, certified school health nurses, and nutritionists/dietiticians. Existing suggested standards for the ratio of many of these provider types to the population may be used to assess the health manpower status of a community. In addition to income and employment, *family data* include the size and composition of families, the number of female-headed households with children, the average number of persons residing in a household, occupational status, primary language, and educational level of the wage earner.

Synthetic estimates can be made using secondary data from population-based surveys and applying the percent with the characteristic of interest to estimate the number of persons with that characteristic in the community. These estimates can be refined further if other factors affecting the characteristic are known (such as age, race, income status). For example, the number of children in a community with activity limitations because of a chronic illness can be estimated by applying the national rate for activity limitation from the most recent National Health Interview Survey.[8] This estimate can be improved by stratifying the community population by income level and applying income-adjusted rates from the same survey.

Although secondary data is usually the least costly to obtain it has some disadvantages. It is important to remember that classic epidemiologic rates are only estimates and that the quality of each estimate varies with the number of cases on which the rate is based. Therefore rates from communities generating small numbers of cases annually (generally those with populations under 50,000 persons) tend to have wide confidence intervals, making it difficult to compare them from year to year. When numbers are small, communities may combine their annual numbers over years or with other communities, but this reduces the applicability of the new rate to a single community.

Primary data. There are a variety of methods used to collect primary data, each with its own unique characteristics of complexity, cost, time requirement, and validity (see the box on p. 187). All should be considered before deciding on the method or methods that will be used in the CBNA.

The approach most commonly used in a CBNA is the survey in which information is gathered through direct interveiws or questionnaires mailed to a sample of the target population. Advantages of properly conducted surveys include high reliability and validity, flexibility, and versatility.

Key informant interviews, unlike surveys, are conducted with specifically identified individuals within the community who are considered experts in the topic area. Key informants can be health care providers, school personnel, parents of children with disabilities, etc. Key informant interviews are easy to conduct, relatively inexpensive, and useful when studying issues beyond common knowledge. They are also useful in involving people of authority in the assessment process. Disadvantages stem from the skewed selection of participants and possible misrepresentation or bias.

Focus groups are comprised of individuals from the community who have first-hand experience with the issues but are not necessarily experts. Use of a focus group follows a structured process and discussion format. The data obtained are qualitative and reflect the diversity in the group's dis-

Examples of Primary Data

Access measures

Affordability
Insurance (private, public, self-pay)
Supply of health professionals
Regular source of medical care
Acceptability
Client-provider relationship
Knowledge and awareness of services
Early intervention
WIC, mental health/counseling
Public health, emergency care
Hot lines/crisis intervention
Title V (CSHCN)
Healthy kids (EPSDT)
Housing, recreation
Transportation/travel time
Perceived barriers to care
Culturally competent providers
Waiting time
Availability of child care/respite

Coordination of service data

The existence of care coordination
  services
Presence of interagency agreements
Presence of coalitions representing
  persons with disabilities
Information and referral
Other indicators of coordination
  and cooperation between primary,
  secondary and tertiary care providers
Other indicators of coordination and
  cooperation between state and local
  agencies providing services to
  CSHCN

Use of services data

Professionals seen in the past year
(e.g., physicians, mental health,
  therapists, etc.)
Services/programs (seen ever/seen
  during past year)
Immunizations

**Family knowledge of and
involvement in local system of care data**

Family knowledge and awareness of
  system of care and applicable laws
Role in coordination of care
Involvement of families in:
  system planning and design
  quality assurance
  standards development
  advisory/planning boards

Community family characteristics data

Marital status of parents of CSHCN
Family functioning and need for support
Sibling coping
Parental adaptation

Availability of local family support data

Parent-to-parent groups
Parent education provided
Respite/day care
Home nursing services
Financial planning and assistance

cussion around each issue. Focus groups can be held at the beginning of a CBNA to discover the perceived needs of the community, or near the end of the assessment to determine priorities. Focus groups have high face validity and are inexpensive to conduct. Because responses are provided in a group setting, however, they can be influenced by a partial moderator or skewed by group dynamics.

If previous data collection efforts have shown uncertain or conflicting results, Delphi (or expert) panels can provide an alternative approach to assessment.[4] In this method a group of anonymous experts are brought together to express their individual opinions about the problem or needs. The panel then completes a questionnaire about the issues and their importance, and the results are distributed back to the panel members. The process continues until group consensus is reached. The advantages and disadvantages of these panels are similar to that of key informant interviews with the addition that this method permits experts with the most strongly held views to influence the other panelists.

Community input processes. General community input is also very important to a CBNA. This can be obtained from the community planning group or an advisory council created for the purpose. Each can help shape and balance the data gathered and its interpretation. Other ways to obtain community input might include town meetings or public community forums.

Assessment of the Relative Importance of the Needs

Analysis of needs assessment data should occur at many stages in a community-based assessment. The community planning group's early comparison of secondary data with national norms or standards and local health objectives begins the process. The community planning group makes its collective values known during the process of selecting areas to address through primary data collection and later when that data is analyzed. When multiple issues are addressed and multiple methods are used to assess them, the needs discovered can be difficult to prioritize. Health professionals and parents of children with disabilities, for example, often identify different needs or see the same issue in different ways; there is no easy answer to decide which should take precedence. However, it should be the role of the community planning group to perform the ultimate analysis and establish priorities.

Software tools designed to assist in this process include EPI-INFO and EPI-MAP for survey development, data management, and analysis,[1] WONDER/PC for secondary data acquisition, telecommunications, and graphical presentations,[2] and MCH-INFO, an analytical software tool specifically for assessment needs.[6]

Summarize and Communicate the Results

Developing a plan to respond to the CBNA is difficult, especially when high-priority needs have been identified, resources are limited, and the distance between need and service is great. First, all of the problem areas identified should be prioritized in the order of perceived importance to the participants in the assessment (i.e., respondents to surveys / focus groups, key informant interviews, etc.). The planning group should then identify short- and long-term goals to address each issue and the interventions required to achieve them. The group must then review each intervention to estimate costs and other resources required for its implementation. At this point the results of this process should be shared with the community through town meetings, newspaper articles, special forums, etc., to provide opportunity for additional feedback and reordering of priorities. Once finalized, the plan should be communicated to all who will be affected by it and all who have a role in its implementation.

Clear communication of the results of the assessment is critical to affecting change. Data should be presented in easy-to-understand narrative and tables with only the most important data items listed. Always allow everyone the opportunity to see all the data if they request it but keep the amount of detail presented in the public report to a minimum. The purpose of the public report is to persuade and educate; the more complex the report and the harder it is for lay persons to understand the data, the more likely that it will be ignored.

MODELS OF COMMUNITY-BASED NEEDS ASSESSMENT AND PLANNING

Two national models of CBNA have been developed that facilitate collaborative assessment and planning: the Assessment Protocol for Excellence in Public Health (APEX/PH),[7] and the Planned Approach to Community Health (PATCH). These models focus on the examination of all health issues affecting a target population, rather than on limited categories of health problems, and promote community involvement in the form of community planning groups. They focus on the entire community population and use classical epidemiologic data (birth, death, and disease) for their secondary data.

The APEX/PH model guides local health departments to assess and improve their own organizational capacity and work with their local community to assess and improve the health status of the citizens. The model provides a structured approach to setting priorities for solving local problems and for developing a local health plan.

The PATCH model also helps communities plan but focuses on the conduct and evaluation of health promotion and health-education programs. PATCH does not focus on the local health department but on a working team comprising representatives from the state and local health departments, the community, and the Centers for Disease Control (CDC). PATCH provides much assistance in the process of community planning (organizing/facilitating groups, presenting data, etc.).

To use these models in planning for children with disabilities ages 0-21, a separate planning process would need to be organized and appropriate secondary data identified to reflect their issues. The FOCUS for Children[5] model is an example of this approach in which secondary data described previously in this chapter was obtained specific to children and children with special health care needs.

CONCLUSION

At the core of a community-based assessment is the recognition that each community has unique characteristics that contribute to the health status of children and families and that can best be reflected by the involvement of community members in the assessment's design and implementation. The CBNA should empower the community to assess and monitor its own system of services and set priorities that have meaning to its own populations.

REFERENCES

1. Dean AG et al: *Epi Info, Version 5*, Incorporated, Stone Mountain, Ga, 1990, USD.
2. Centers for Disease Control and Prevention: *Wonder/PC*, Atlanta, Ga, 1993, Centers for Disease Control.
3. Kreuter MW et al: *Planned approach to community health*, Atlanta, Ga, 1985, Centers for Disease Control.
4. McKillip J: *Needs analysis: tools for the human services and education*, Newbury Park, Calif, 1988, Sage Publications.
5. Monahan C and Craik D: *Facilitating organized community systems for children with special health care needs (FOCUS for children)*, Rockville, Md, 1993, Maternal and Child Health Bureau, Health Resources Administration, U.S. Public Health Service, Department of Health and Human Services.
6. Monahan C and Strassberg M: *MCH-INFO analytical software tool for needs assessment*, Chicago, 1995, University of Chicago Division of Specialized Care for Children.
7. National Association of County Health Officials: *Assessment protocol for excellence in public health*, 1991, Washington, DC.
8. National Center for Health Statistics: *1991 National Health Interview Survey*, CD-ROM Series 10 No 5, 1993, Hyattsville, Md.
9. Peck M: *Putting needs assessment to good use*, Paper presented at the Children with Special Health Care Needs Continuing Education Institute, Columbus, Ohio, November 1993.
10. Walker DK and Richmond JB: *Monitoring child health in the United States: selected issues and policies*, Cambridge, Mass, 1984, Harvard University Press.

CHAPTER 19

Defining Goals and Shared Expectations: The Use of Model Standards to Enhance the Quality of Care

SUSAN G. EPSTEIN
ANN B. TAYLOR

APPROACHES FOR QUALITY ASSURANCE

Health care systems that provide services for children with special health care needs are currently in transition. These changes are based on the broadly accepted belief that such systems must include family-centered, community-based, coordinated, and culturally competent care if they are to provide high-quality services and respond effectively to children and their families.

This chapter describes how it is possible for public or private programs that deliver health care services to assess their system's performance in providing the anticipated high-quality care. This is accomplished by using a process for quality improvement that measures how well the values and principles of family-centered, community-based, coordinated, and culturally competent care have been integrated into that health program.

Human Services Research Institute (HSRI) defines quality assurance as "ensuring that health care service providers, facilities, and agencies have the capability and resources necessary to deliver an acceptable level of service consistent with established beliefs regarding good practice."[2] Central to this definition is the assumption that there are shared and acknowledged standards for acceptable levels of service. Such standards, when established and broadly endorsed, can provide the yardstick by which participants in the health care system can measure quality of care. In the current transition toward family-centered, coordinated, community-based, and culturally competent care, such standards are evolving and not yet institutionalized. Arguably, each community may wish to contribute to a definition of quality care, and articulate standards that reflect the diversity of its own needs and values.

To assist providers and family participants in the difficult task of building a quality-improvement process, this chapter offers as a resource the experience of the New England SERVE Regional Task Force on Quality Assurance* and the 68 standards it produced. Both the methodology developed by New England SERVE and the set of standards, published as *Enhancing Quality: Standards and Indicators of Quality Care for Children with Special Health Care Needs*,[1] can serve as models for any community effort to improve the quality of care. New England SERVE sought to develop a set of generic standards and indicators, or examples of how each standard might be achieved, that expressed mutually agreed-upon "best practices." Such standards and indicators could then be used by families, providers, policymakers, and advocates to assess the progress their programs have made toward delivering a shared vision of what constitutes quality care for children with special health care needs.

DEVELOPING STANDARDS: A SHARED RESPONSIBILITY

Setting standards for quality care entails the complex movement from identifying abstract values that include goals and expectations, to the formulation of concrete statements that express the measurable qualities of these values. To facilitate understanding of this process it is helpful to review the methods used by New England SERVE in guiding its Task Force in developing a set of standards.

The Task Force, a 25-member, multidisciplinary group that included physicians, nurses, social workers, educators, allied health providers, state policy makers, and families, began by defining and elaborating upon shared values. Those values, once adopted by the members, provided the "established beliefs regarding good practice"[1] that form the core of any quality-assurance effort. The Task Force selected values that focused on the process of

*New England SERVE is a planning and technical assistance network working on behalf of children with special health care needs and their families. Administered by the Massachusetts Health Research Institute, Inc., in Boston, Mass., New England SERVE has been supported in part by Grant # MCJ-253878 and Grant # MCJ-255043 from the Maternal and Child Health Bureau, Health Resources and Services Administration, U.S. Department of Health and Human Services.

health care delivery rather than health outcomes or specific clinical treatment methodologies. These values include the following:

- the rights of families to be involved as partners in the delivery of care and to be recognized as central care givers and decision makers for the child
- the recognition that children with disabilities or chronic health conditions need a continuum of primary and specialty care and access to a broad range of community-based medical, nonmedical, and family-support services
- ˏa belief that these services must be provided regardless of financial status, racial and ethnic identity, medical condition, or geographic location

New England SERVE endorsed the idea that all participating groups in the health care system must share the responsibility for developing operational definitions for quality care. Each group has a valuable perspective regarding critical elements that contribute to quality care, and each perspective is essential to any system-based quality-improvement effort. The membership of the Task Force established by New England SERVE reflected this view by including families, health care providers representing a wide range of disciplines and various levels of the care delivery system, and representatives of the six state health agencies in New England. Together this diverse group of stakeholders hammered out issues of what constitutes quality care and were able to reach consensus on the specific language of the 68 standards contained in *Enhancing Quality*.[1] *Enhancing Quality* has received the endorsement of six state health departments and a broad range of consumer and family advocacy groups.

Representation by families on the Task Force contributed significantly to the final content and format of *Enhancing Quality*. Family members, through their experience as consumers of health care on behalf of their children, can offer detailed observations about both supports and barriers to care. In a system such as health care that has been traditionally dominated by professionals, the family or consumer perspective is not commonly sought or incorporated in the development of standards for quality care. As heavy users of the health care system, families of children with chronic illness or disability often have extensive and long-term experience accessing and coordinating care for their child. Opportunities that solicit feedback or confidential criticism from families are a necessary component in assessing family needs and priorities. Professionals working alone are unable to reflect this perspective in the development of systems that define and measure quality.

The participation of health care providers and policy makers representing various disciplines, from community-based and tertiary care settings, ensured that the diverse skills and perspectives of professionals were also included in the standards. In this way, potential users of the standards guided their development and shared the responsibility for assuring the future relevance of the document.

UNDERSTANDING THE SERVICE DELIVERY SYSTEM: WHERE DO RESPONSIBILITIES FOR QUALITY CARE RESIDE?

The Task Force conceptualized the health care delivery system as being organized at five different levels. This framework was then used to determine where specific contributions to building quality care could be made. One way to visualize these levels is to use concentric circles. At the center of these circles is the child and family and their interaction with the health care system. At the second level is the team of health care providers who contribute to a child's care. The third level focuses on the organization or health care agency that supports the team of professional providers who deliver care to children and families. The fourth level of the service delivery system is the state health agency, which the Task Force identified as contributing a critical role in the delivery of care to children with specialized needs. The fifth and broadest circle in this framework of the health care delivery system is the larger community or society in which the health care system operates.

Using this framework, the Task Force identified the concerns, responsibilities and best practices for each participating group regarding quality of care. The sections of *Enhancing Quality* are organized along the five levels of the health care system described above. Each section lists standards that identify key elements contributing to quality health care at each level of the system. Following each standard statement are several indicators, which are examples of how a standard may be implemented.

For example, Section I, *Individualized Services*, focuses on services received by the individual child and family and contains standards based on the recognition that "The child is a member of a family whose partnership and collaboration with health care professionals are essential to the delivery of quality health care."[1] The standards in this section seek to assess how family members participate in decision making, interact with providers to plan and coordinate care, and access services from multiple providers. The first standard in this section is:

1.0 The child has representation through family membership on the health care team.

Listed below this statement are the following indicators that exemplify how this representation might occur:

1.1 Family members participate in team decision making regarding health care services and the development of the health care plan.

1.2 Expectations and roles of all team members are defined.

1.3 The family provides information regarding the child's strengths, needs, and culture, and feedback regarding the services received.

1.4 Interpreter services are available.

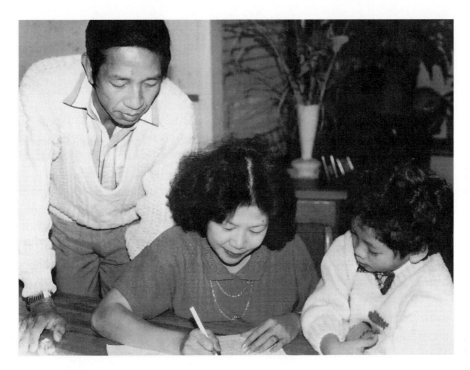

From Danielson et al: *Families, Health & Illness*, ed 1, St Louis, 1993, Mosby–Year Book.

Enhancing Quality[1] follows this format throughout its next four sections. Section II, *Health Care Professional and Team Characteristics*, addresses the activities and responsibilities of health providers in coordinated, community-based, and family-centered care. What are the skills and training necessary for providers to deliver such care?

The standards in Section II propose that, in addition to their specialized technical knowledge, health care professionals must possess well-developed communication skills for effective collaboration in order to provide a continuum of quality care. They must also receive continuous, high-level training in a variety of settings to keep up with technologic developments. Equally as important, they must be responsive to the needs of the child and family. The standards in this section are grouped into three areas that address the health care professionals' needs for continuing training, their effectiveness in coordinating services, and their responsiveness to families.

Section III, *Health Care Agency or Facility Responsibilities*, focuses on the organization that supports the team of professional providers who deliver care to children and families. The agency level includes the facility, organizational structures, operating policies, and financial mechanisms that influence care delivery. What are the health care agency's responsibilities for supporting and organizing services? How does the agency enable the team of providers to deliver quality health care to children with special health care needs? What does it offer to providers to support their ability to meet the needs of children and families?

The standards and indicators of this section address performance at the agency level that most directly affects the delivery of family-centered, coordinated, and accessible care. They evaluate how the agency responds to the needs of children and families, how it supports, trains, and develops staff, and how efficient its administrative procedures and policies are for families.

Section IV, *State Health Department Responsibilities*, addresses the role of the state public health agency in building systems of care and establishing and supporting interagency collaboration. Effective and creative leadership at the public policy level is essential in guiding systems change on behalf of children. Leadership is needed to support and develop family-centered policies and to anticipate and plan for emerging needs statewide. The standards and indicators in this section, therefore, assess the role of the state health department in enhancing the quality of the health care delivery system. The major areas of concern include planning and resource allocation at the state level, promoting health and preventing disability and disease, collaborating with other agencies on health-related issues, and ensuring quality.

Finally, Section V, *Guidelines for Community and Societal Supports*, expands the standards to include the role of the community. Communities influence many spheres in the lives of children and their families, including education, recreation, housing, and employment. These and other community characteristics affect health status, the integration of children with special needs into community life, and the delivery of health care. Section V identifies three major areas of community activity crucial to supporting a quality health care system: (1) public awareness and family support, (2) community-program planning, and (3) the potential contribution of advocacy groups. Because the scope of these activities requires a community effort, this section does not list standards but instead provides guidelines for groups and individual community members.

CONDUCTING A SELF-ASSESSMENT: ARE FAMILY-CENTERED, COMMUNITY-BASED SYSTEMS IMPLEMENTING AGREED UPON STANDARDS OF QUALITY CARE?

The "best practice" standards and indicators in *Enhancing Quality*[1] are presented in a checklist format, which enables groups to use the document as a workbook to guide a self-assessment process. Programs serving children with special health needs can develop surveys or other data collection tools to obtain both family and provider perceptions regarding a mutually-agreed upon set of standards of quality care. By applying these tools, families and health professionals participate in a process that is designed to support their collaboration toward improving quality care.

An assessment based upon the standards in *Enhancing Quality* can be used to:

- Sensitize families and providers to the values of family-centered, coordinated, community-based, culturally competent care
- Determine to what extent these values are reflected in the delivery of care in a particular setting or system of care
- Identify areas of strength and weakness in the service delivery setting or service system
- Assist in setting goals for improved services and guiding resource allocation
- Strengthen the team process in the service setting
- Provide acknowledgment and legitimacy to family participation
- Provide an opportunity for effective family-professional collaboration
- Provide an opportunity to demonstrate a commitment to quality health care

The assessment process should begin with a representative group of families and providers reviewing the 68 standards to ensure that any special concerns they may have are addressed. Such planning groups may choose which of the five sections are most applicable for their settings. New standards and indicators may be added. Vocabulary can also be adapted to more accurately reflect labels or descriptors that are familiar in a given setting.

To provide a larger view of the system's efficacy, the standards can be used to gather information about perceived quality of service delivery. Assuming the existence of an agency, committee, or other entity that has the resources to conduct data collection and analysis, such as an office in the Department of Health, data collection tools based on the standards can be developed. Such survey tools can ask families and providers to rate parallel standards and indicator statements along a Lickert scale. Written questionnaires can elicit both quantitative and qualitative data. Basic demographic information should also be collected from both family and provider respondents to allow comparison of the sample with the overall population served. Focus groups, key informant interviews, and program data can be used to augment the core data collection from families and providers.

Data from families and providers can be analyzed using a database such as EpiInfo[3] developed by the Epidemiology Program Office at the U.S. Center for Disease Control. Frequencies for each level of response for both providers and families can be computed, allowing for comparisons between the two groups. Areas of strength as well as weakness can be identified using this quantitative analysis.

In addition, written comments and answers to open-ended questions can be compiled and edited to protect confidentiality. These direct quotations can be used to illustrate quantitative findings (both positive and negative) and add a qualitative dimension to the assessment. Once data are analyzed and summarized, providers, administrators, and families can review the findings.

An underlying principle for successful implementation of family-centered policies, programs, and practices is that the responsibility for their development is shared by all participants. Families, health care providers, and administrators each have critical roles to play in building and improving the delivery of family-centered care. All three groups must have the opportunity to review findings, seek out examples of best practices both within and outside their program setting, and identify new goals and actions that can improve quality care.

An assessment based upon *Enhancing Quality*[1] is not a complete program evaluation. It does not include discipline-specific professional standards or credentials. It will not provide an assessment of administrative areas such as financial management or personnel operations. It does not measure technical aspects of the medical care delivered, and it does not measure individual child outcomes. It can, however, be used in conjunction with these other types of standards and measurement strategies as part of a complete quality assurance program.

CONCLUSION

As health care policy makers, providers, and families continue the process of revising health care systems to better serve children with special health care needs, methods for reviewing these systems and monitoring the quality of care must also be developed and implemented. As evidenced from the methodology used by New England SERVE, the process of developing standards and designing a quality-improvement process should reflect a set of shared values endorsed by a full range of participants. The approach to creating *Enhancing Quality* began with the Task Force members defining shared values, goals, and expectations and compiling a set of mutually agreed upon "best practices." This resulted in a set of standards that is anchored in the salient concerns of families and a commitment to building effective partnerships to improve the quality of care. Public and private programs that provide health services for children with special health care needs can use the set of standards contained in *Enhancing Quality* as a reference source on family-centered care and as a framework for building quality-assurance systems.

As health care systems and practices continue to evolve in the next decade, families and providers will need to continue to collaborate to refine their definitions of quality. Similarly, standards of care must be dynamic and reflect such changes in expectations to remain responsive to the specialized needs of children and families. By sharing the responsibility to define and refine standards, communities can ensure the full participation of all parties who have a stake in the quality of care and support a more responsive and effective health care system.

REFERENCES

1. Epstein SG et al: *Enhancing quality: standards and indicators of quality care for children with special health care needs*, Boston, Mass, 1989, New England SERVE.
2. Human Services Research Institute: Assessing and enhancing the quality of human services: a guide for the human services field, *Executive summary*, Cambridge, Mass, 1984, The Institute.
3. U.S. Center for Disease Control, Epidemiology Program Office: *EpiInfo*, Atlanta, Ga, 1992.

PART FOUR

SOLUTIONS

Too often we hear only of problems. Yet over the years a considerable store of knowledge about how to address these problems has accumulated.

There are exciting new developments in the prevention and health promotion field. An increasing number of genetic diseases can be detected early and prevented. Successful public health strategies to prevent preterm labor and birth are available. Innovative campaigns to get children to wear helmets when riding bicycles have dramatically reduced the incidence and severity of traumatic brain injury in several communities.

This section on solutions offers a compact summary of the service delivery components of care for children and youth with disabilities and chronic illness. Departing from the traditional focus on health aspects of care, such chapters as those on mental health, education, assistive technology, and vocational preparation are included.

Rather than describing the details of hands-on care, the chapters provide an orientation to the potential contributions to comprehensive care that each professional field or specialized-services cluster can make, provided that a systems viewpoint is maintained.

Integration and coordination of this amazing constellation of sophisticated services remains our biggest challenge. The chapters on service coordination and team function furnish insights on how this might be accomplished successfully.

CHAPTER 20

Evolving Concepts in the Prevention of Developmental Disabilities

JOSEPH G. HOLLOWELL, JR.
MYRON J. ADAMS, JR.

We are entering a second era of prevention in pediatrics. In the past, those concerned with prevention focused primarily on infectious diseases; safe water and food and the promotion of immunizations ensured that the incidence of many such diseases was greatly reduced. Advances in the understanding of disease processes and in medical technologies have further reduced disease-related mortality. However, in some instances the success of mortality prevention has increased the prevalence of disabilities caused by chronic diseases.

The spectrum of approaches for preventing developmental disabilities and other childhood disabilities extends from improving the capacity and coordination of existing public health and medical services to developing targeted methods of prevention. The challenge now is to use epidemiologic research to understand the etiologic relationships involved in the disability process and to evaluate prevention effectiveness.

In this chapter we discuss conventional concepts of prevention and disability in the context of prevention planning, we describe work being done to improve developmental disabilities prevention, and we evaluate the effectiveness of that work. We also summarize other opportunities for preventing developmental disabilities, including proposed models for coordinated prevention.

Because the complex concepts surrounding disability are made even more difficult by different systems of nomenclature, a Department of Health and Human Services task force was established to develop a standardized definition of disability. Various disability and chronic disease models were proposed by the World Health Organization International Classification of Impairment, Disability, and Handicap (WHO ICIDH),[24] the Institute of Medicine Report,[15] and others (Table 20-1).[17] Federal statutes contain as many as 40 operational definitions of disability, usually describing eligibility for services. However, the task force recognized that a common conceptual framework underlay the different definitions of disability and, rather than attempt to redefine terms, the group chose to outline this common conceptual framework and to describe four levels in the disability process: (1) cause, (2) organ function, (3) person function, and (4) interaction with environment.[16] Fig. 20-1 illustrates the levels in this process.

For prevention to be effective it must be directed at the appropriate level in the disability process. The disability process begins at the cause level, *A*, when an etiologic agent interacts with the biologic system of an individual thus producing an impairment at the organ level, *B*. For example, congenital rubella (cause) may seriously impair neural or cochlear functioning (organ). One or more of these impairments may produce a limitation in function at the person level, *C*. To continue with our example, impairment in hearing may interfere with a person's normal age-specific activities such as learning or communication. Such a limitation may in turn limit that person's ability to function at school or work (loss at the interaction-with-environment level, *D*. At the interaction-with-environment level the limitation may be the result of a person-level deficit or an inhospitable physical or social environment. A hearing impairment (organ level) can interfere with a person's ability to communicate (person level).

TABLE 20-1. Comparative Terminology in Disability Classification

Classification Source (PHS Proposed)	Conceptual Framework			
	Underlying Cause	Organ Level	Person Level	Interaction with Environment
WHO ICIDH[24]	Disease	Impairment	Disability	Handicap
Disability in America Model (IOM)[15]	Pathology	Impairment	Functional limitation	Disability
Stein et al[17]		Physiologic severity	Functional severity	

Modified from PHS Taskforce on Improving Medical Criteria for Disability Determination.

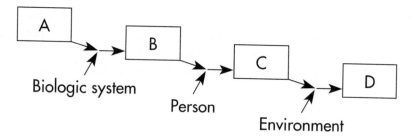

A = Cause level

B = Organ level

C = Person level

D = Interaction-with-environment level

FIGURE 20-1. Common conceptual framework of the disease and disability process.

Unemployment (interaction-with-environment level) can result from either the person-level disability or from the stigma associated with the hearing loss.

Before 1980 developmental disabilities were categorized by specific condition (e.g., mental retardation, cerebral palsy, autism, or epilepsy). Such categorization reflected cause and organ-function levels. After 1980 developmental disabilities were defined in broader, more complex terms that reflected functional loss at the person and environmental-interaction levels.

Using the WHO ICIDH classification, Veen et al[23] documented disability at each level among children with a history of very low birthweight. Such an approach to describing the full array of disability will lead to a better understanding of the disability process and to improved methods of prevention.

THE INSTITUTE OF MEDICINE (IOM) REPORT ON DISABILITY

The IOM report, *Disability in America: Toward a National Agenda for Prevention*,[15] made several important contributions to the understanding of disability. In addition to discussing definitions and models of disability, it introduced the concept of risk factors, a concept that provides a basis for disability-prevention programs. In the report three types of risk factors were identified: (1) biologic, (2) environmental, and (3) behavioral. The disability nomenclature in the IOM report differed from that in the WHO ICIDH.[24] The IOM report used pathology to describe the cause level, impairment to describe the organ level, functional limitation to describe the person level, and disability to describe the interaction-with-environment level (see Table 20-1). The report points out that disabilities at all four levels of measurement can be prevented by reducing risk factors. Organ-level, person-level, and interaction-with-environment–level disabilities may themselves be risks that could contribute to further disability.[14]

The report emphasizes the importance of quality of life in any examination of the outcome of disabling process. Our understanding of the effect of disability on the quality of life is evolving and ways of measuring it are being developed. This concept is clearly important when evaluating the endpoints associated with an intervention's success.

DEVELOPMENTAL DISABILITY PREVENTION

Prevention means averting a health problem before it begins rather than treating or curing the problem once it is established. Traditionally, prevention has been divided into three categories.[2]

1. *Primary prevention* includes measures designed to preclude the development of disease in potentially susceptible populations. The goal of primary prevention is to avoid disorders before they begin. Primary prevention activities are the backbone of many public health programs. For some diseases, such as fetal alcohol syndrome, the etiology is known, but the effectiveness of primary prevention methods is uncertain. For some infectious diseases, however, specific prevention methods have been effective in lowering the incidence. For other problems, such as low birthweight and child abuse, programs are offered because contemporary wisdom leads people to believe that such programs provide preventive benefits, although strong scientific evidence of either the etiology of the condition or the effectiveness of the programs is sparse.

2. *Secondary prevention* involves the early diagnosis and prompt treatment of existing disease to shorten the duration of the disease, reduce discomfort, minimize contagion, and limit sequelae. The goal of secondary prevention is to recognize the beginnings (precursors) of disease and then to limit the progress of the disease. Examples of public health programs that address secondary prevention include programs for screening and early diagnosis. Intensive care neonatal units are used to limit the sequelae of premature birth.

3. *Tertiary prevention* involves methods designed to promote maximum personal and social functioning among patients with diseases that have gone beyond the point of full reversibility; health workers intervene to minimize the disability after it occurs. Examples of tertiary prevention include many of the interventions used in rehabilitation, retraining, and improving the affected person's social access.

CHANGING CONCEPTS OF PREVENTION

As the field of developmental disabilities prevention has developed, the terms primary and secondary have been used to describe disabling conditions as well as types of prevention. The term *secondary conditions* emerged to denote separate conditions that accompany chronic disease or other disabling conditions.[11,14,17] Two major types of secondary conditions can be distinguished. One, a comorbidity secondary condition, is manifest at the same time as the chronic disease of interest. For example, mental retardation may be a comorbidity secondary condition associated with cerebral palsy or visual impairment. The other type of secondary condition occurs as a result of an initial (primary) disabling condition. For example, persons with spinal cord injuries are at high risk for developing decubitus ulcers or urinary tract infections. It is this second group of conditions that may be susceptible to prevention.

Thus the disability prevention field has two sets of meaning for the terms *primary* and *secondary*; one involves a type of prevention, the other, a type of disabling condition. Given this ambiguous background, the term *prospective intervention* may be less confusing than prevention. A specific prospective intervention can be developed to reduce a specific risk that can be anticipated in a person with developmental disabilities. Retrospective intervention, or intervention after the fact, may be much less effective. For example, to prevent decubitus ulcers one cannot wait for the early detection of the decubiti. To be effective, prevention of this secondary condition must be primary prevention. The need for prospective, or primary, prevention is particularly critical when an individual's chronic disease or disability is deemed a risk for additional disabling or secondary conditions.

Surveillance and Epidemiologic Research

Recent developments in developmental disabilities prevention have been driven by epidemiologic research. The results of randomized clinical trials using specific, intensive early intervention for low-birthweight infants[9] and infants with other risks[12] showed that more than half of the mental retardation could be prevented among susceptible children at age 3. The results of other studies demonstrated that folic acid supplementation can reduce the recurrence[13] and occurrence[5] of spina bifida by 70%. These studies were instrumental in the formulation of Centers for Disease Control and Prevention (CDC) recommendations that women of childbearing age should take folic acid supplements.[3]

Developmental disability prevention must encompass more than prevention at the cause level. We must seize opportunities for prevention at all stages of disability causation. Further epidemiologic research is needed, however, if we are to describe the interaction of risk factors at various steps in the disability causal chain and thus provide the basis for new preventive measures.

When collecting surveillance data on chronic diseases and impairments, one must pay special attention to the definitions used and to the age of the patient at the onset of a developmental disability and at the time of surveillance. The latency period between exposure to a causal factor and the manifestation of an outcome presents a special challenge in determining the cause of various types of developmental disabilities. For example, a child's mental retardation may not be manifested until he or she is in school. Because of the great variation in the etiologic relationships associated with developmental disabilities, the type of developmental disabilities being examined must be described precisely.

MODELS FOR PREVENTION

The present public health and medical-care systems offer opportunities for preventing developmental disabilities and other childhood disabilities. Good health care often results in primary and secondary prevention. Improved health care, family-life education, and pregnancy planning can all contribute to the primary prevention of disabilities. In addition, we can decrease behavioral risks by paying more attention to the causes of child abuse and neglect and by assuring that infants and young children learn to meet the challenges of the environment that they will later encounter. Secondary prevention can be accomplished through the promotion of early case finding, such as screening newborns for inborn errors of metabolism, screening women for high-risk pregnancies and following up with infants who may be at high risk for developmental disabilities and intervening early and appropriately. Tertiary prevention, which is most appropriate in the field of disability and chronic disease, involves interdisciplinary team care, case management, and intervention with broad systems of health, education, and social services (Table 20-2).

Failures in prevention occur mainly because health care systems are inaccessible to many individuals with disabilities or chronic diseases and because clinical services often focus on specific organ systems rather than on the whole person or on that person's interaction with the environment.[18]

Crocker[4] has described a system for evaluating the effectiveness of prevention methods in specific and general community systems by assessing the services and risks in the prenatal, perinatal, and childhood periods. In his paper he lists 43 proposals to quantify and evaluate the quality of broad public-health services designed to prevent mental retardation and associated developmental disabilities and to support the good health of all children.

Prospective interventions can be organized according to the period in a child's development that such opportunities occur (e.g., in the preconception, pregnancy, newborn, or early childhood periods). They can be organized according to specific service and educational opportunities, such as health

TABLE 20-2. Strategies for Preventing Childhood Disabilities, by Level of Prevention

Primary Prevention	Secondary Prevention	Tertiary Prevention

Environmental control
  Hazardous or toxic
    substances (lead)
  Injuries
  Alcohol, tobacco, drugs
	Early case finding or care
	  Screening for:
	    Inborn errors of
	      metabolism
	    Hypothyroidism
	    Sensory impairment
	    High-risk factors
		Environmental factors
		  Social supports and
		    awareness
		  Access to all services

Health care
  Preconceptional,
    prenatal, intrapartum
  High-risk infants
  Genetic information,
    testing, counseling
  Family planning
  Immunization
  Nutrition (e.g., folic acid to
    prevent neural tube defects)
	Early diagnosis
	  Treatment for:
	    Infections
	    Injuries
	    Behavioral and
	      social factors
		Comprehensive evaluation
		  and care planning
		  Interdisciplinary or
		    interagency teams
		  Case management—
		    follow-up
		  Coordinated care

Educational or behavioral
  risk reduction
    Teenage pregnancy
    Safety, injury prevention,
      special equipment
    Vehicle-operating behaviors
    Child abuse, neglect, and
      family stress
		Educational enhancements
		  Training and retraining
		  Skill development

education, environmental control, prenatal care, perinatal services, infant care, infant developmental services, and school. Although all of these interventions offer prevention opportunities, the outcome, cost effectiveness, and specificity of many of them is unknown.

Another component is needed to ensure the effectiveness of disability prevention programs; in developing prevention strategies, health officials must identify the specific level in the disability process where the cause or limitation or impairment occurs and then design and target the interventions appropriately. Examples of these approaches were assembled in response to the Year 2000 objectives for *Healthy People 2000*[22] and can be grouped into four major categories: (1) medical interventions, (2) interventions involving assistive technology, (3) interventions based on personal skills and lifestyle choices, and (4) interventions through public policy (Table 20-3).

TABLE 20-3. Targeted Disability Prevention Strategy for Hearing Impairment, by Category of Intervention

| Targeted Level | Prevention Strategy | | | |
	Medical	Assistive Technology	Personal Skills/ Lifestyle Choices	Public Policy
Cause Level	Rubella immunization Meningitis Prematurity/low birthweight Provider education Ototoxicity Patient education Genetic counseling		Public education Noise hazard Ear protection	Regulations Noise abatement Workplace
Organ Level	Neural prostheses Gene therapy			
Person Level	Early detection and treatment Cochlear implants	Hearing aids	Speechreading Signing	
Interaction-with-Environment Level				Supports and services Interpreters Sensory substitution (captioning) Communications access in schools and public buildings Genetic disability programs

We need to conduct further systematic surveillance, preventive epidemiologic studies, and effectiveness research in order to further our understanding of developmental disabilities and chronic disease.[21] Examples of developmental-disabilities surveillance systems include birth-defects surveillance programs based primarily on hospital discharge data[7] and developmental-disabilities surveillance based primarily on public education data.[25] In both instances the information comes from existing records that, although collected for other purposes, are extremely useful in learning about certain developmental disabilities and chronic diseases. Surveys and special studies provide further data on developmental disabilities.

Community Models for Prevention

Since 1987 when the President's Committee on Mental Retardation held a conference on state planning for the prevention of mental retardation and related developmental disabilities, more than a third of all states have developed their own developmental disabilities prevention plans. In 1986 the National Council on Disabilities identified community-based disability prevention as a priority and was instrumental in establishing the Disabilities Prevention Program at the CDC.

Twenty-eight states now have disability-prevention programs that are coordinated by a state office of disability prevention, which is usually housed in the state health department. Each office develops a plan for disability prevention, develops surveillance of developmental disabilities, and stimulates community interest in and planning for prevention.[1] Studies of chronic disease in childhood have heightened public awareness of broad health issues, and their results have offered suggestions for improvement.[20] Models for more effective service delivery are being developed in the areas of pediatric practice,[8,19] family medicine,[10] and interdisciplinary approaches.[6]

CONCLUSION

Prospective interventions can be designed to prevent medical and functional secondary conditions associated with chronic disease and other disabling conditions. Data from surveillance, epidemiologic studies, and prevention-effectiveness research can be used to develop more effective prevention strategies. In evaluating disability outcomes, public-health researchers must consider quality-of-life issues and risks for secondary conditions. Disability planning is beginning systematically at local, state, and national sites. Models for addressing disability and disability prevention are also being developed.

REFERENCES

1. Adams MJ and Hollowell JG: Community-based projects for the prevention of developmental disabilities, *Mental Retard* 30:331-336, 1992.
2. Behrman RE and Vaughan VC, III (editors): Nelson textbook of pediatrics, ed 13, Philadelphia, 1987, WB Saunders.
3. Centers for Disease Control and Prevention: Recommendations for the use of folic acid to reduce the number of cases of spina bifida and other neural tube defects, *MMWR* 41:1-7, 1992.
4. Crocker AC: Data collection for the evaluation of mental retardation prevention activities: the fateful forty-three, *Mental Retard* 30:303-317, 1992.
5. Czeizel AE and Dudas I: Prevention of the first occurrence of neural-tube defects by periconceptional vitamin supplementation, *NEJM* 327:1832-1835, 1992.
6. Dumars KW et al: Prevention of developmental disabilities: a model for organizing clinical activities, *Res Dev Disabil* 8:507-520, 1987.

7. Edmonds LD et al: Congenital malformations surveillance: two American systems, *Int J Epidemiol* 10:247-252, 1981.

8. Harper DC: Paradigms for investigating rehabilitation and adaptation to childhood disability and chronic illness, *J Pediatr Psychol* 16:533-542, 1991.

9. Infant Health and Development Program: Enhancing the outcomes of low-birth-weight, premature infants: a multisite, randomized trial, *JAMA* 263:3035-42, 1990.

10. Knottnerus JA et al: Chronic illness in the community and the concept of "social prevalence," *Fam Pract* 9:15-21, 1992.

11. Marge M: Health promotion for people with disabilities: moving beyond rehabilitation, *Am J Health Promotion* 2:29-44, 1988.

12. Martin SL, Ramey CT, and Ramey S: The prevention of intellectual impairment in children of impoverished families: findings of a randomized trial of educational day care, *Am J of Public Health* 80:844-847, 1990.

13. MRC Vitamin Study Research Group: Prevention of neural tube defects: results of the Medical Research Council Vitamin Study, *Lancet* 338:131-137, 1991.

14. Pope AM: Preventing secondary condition, *Mental Retard* 30:347-354, 1992.

15. Pope AM and Tarlov AR: Disability in America: toward a national agenda for prevention, Washington, DC, 1990, National Academy Press.

16. Seltser R: Unpublished finding of the Public Health Service (PHS) task force on improving medical criteria for disability determination, Washington, DC, 1992.

17. Stein REK et al: Severity of illness: concepts and measurements, *Lancet* 2:1506-1509, 1987.

18. Stein REK and Jessop DJ: What diagnosis does not tell: the case for a noncategorical approach to chronic illness in childhood, *Soc Sci Med* 29:769-778, 1982.

19. Stein REK and Jessop DJ: Functional status II(R): a measure of child health status, *Medical Care* 28:1041-1055, 1990.

20. Stein REK, Jessop DJ, and Riessman CK: Health care services received by children with chronic illness, *Am J Dis Child* 137:225-230, 1983.

21. Teutsch SM: A framework for assessing the effectiveness of disease and injury prevention, *MMWR, Recommendations and Reports* 41:1-13, 1992.

22. U.S. Public Health Service: Healthy people 2000: national health promotion and disease prevention objectives, Washington, DC, 1990, U.S. Government Printing Office.

23. Veen S et al: Impairments, disabilities, and handicaps of very preterm and very-low-birthweight infants at five years of age, *Lancet* 338:33-36, 1991.

24. WHO: International classification of impairments, disabilities, and handicaps, Geneva, 1980, World Health Organization.

25. Yeargin-Alsopp M et al: A multiple-source method for studying the prevalence of developmental disabilities in children: the metropolitan Atlanta developmental disabilities study, *Pediatrics* 89:624-630, 1992.

CHAPTER **21**

Planning Health Education Programs for Self-Management of Pediatric Chronic Disease and Disability

L. KAY BARTHOLOMEW
GUY S. PARCEL
DANITA I. CZYZEWSKI

Self-management is the first priority of health promotion programs for children with chronic disease or disability and their families. Clark et al[10] define self-management of chronic illness as behaviors that minimize the severity of disease symptoms, slow progression, and promote optimum participation in normal activities of daily living. To lessen the effect of the illness family members need to obtain ongoing medical care, perform home treatment regimens, and use a variety of coping and problem-solving strategies.

Self-management has been related to better quality of life (a combination of psychologic, health status, and social factors) in several chronic illnesses. Notably, programs to teach self-management of childhood asthma have enhanced school performance and increased attendance and have decreased acute episodes of reactive airways and medical costs.[1,11,13,17,23] Also, a self-management program for adolescents with juvenile diabetes resulted in decreased family conflict.[22] Integrating and maximizing the diverse goals and behaviors of self-management of chronic health problems may be especially important to enable children to develop normally in spite of their medical conditions.

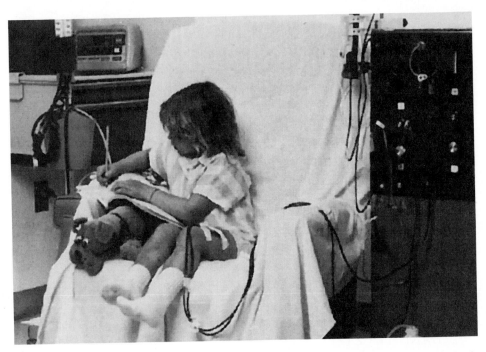

From Whaley LF, Wong DL: *Nursing care of infants and children*, ed 4, St Louis, 1991, Mosby-Year Book.

Self-management is different from strict compliance to medical regimens in that it includes the complex cognitive-behavioral skills of self-regulation, problem solving, and communication.[9,12] What this implies for practice is that health education about chronic disease must emphasize these processes in addition to the disease and its treatment. Enhancing self-management skills through health-education programs that increase self-efficacy and provide feedback on success may be critical to the performance of many self-management behaviors because they are not automatically reinforced by noticeable improvement of physical symptoms or health status.[3,39]

FOCUS ON BEHAVIOR

Planning programs to teach self-management skills requires careful specification of the behaviors required of both child and family.[4] Cystic fibrosis (CF), juvenile rheumatoid arthritis (JRA), and asthma are examples of diseases that, despite improved prognoses and recent medical advances in etiology and treatment, entail significant demands for management by children and parents. Families often have difficulty meeting both medical and psychosocial

demands, as exhibited in the low rates of compliance with medical regimens,*
deficits in psychosocial adjustment,[14,35,45,47,48] and school absenteeism.[18,19,32,44]
The demands and the associated difficulties are interrelated. For example,
inability to manage the pain and stiffness of JRA may keep a child from
attending school, which may in turn negatively influence psychosocial development and adjustment.

There is a need for health promotion interventions that comprehensively
address the behavioral capability of patients and parents to meet the complex
demands of managing a chronic illness. We have used the Predisposing, Reinforcing, and Enabling Constructs in Educational Diagnosis and Evaluation
(PRECEDE) model[20,21] to organize needs-assessment data in order to define
self-management behaviors and to plan educational interventions for patients
with chronic conditions and their families. This problem-focused planning
framework enables the planner to target appropriate problems, behaviors,
and educational factors in health education interventions.[1,5,6,34,43]

PRECEDE AND THE NEEDS-ASSESSMENT PROCESS

The PRECEDE models helps the program planner organize information from
a needs assessment in order to address the following questions:

What are the implications for quality-of-life and health of problems that
emerged from the needs assessment (phases 1 and 2 of PRECEDE)?

What are the behavioral (patient and family) and environmental (health care
site, home, and school) factors that contribute to these problems (phase 3)?

What educational factors (e.g., knowledge and skills) might be important for
families to adopt and maintain new behaviors to manage disease, disability, and related problems (phase 4)? For example, performance of specific
medical regimens may lead to better health outcomes, but what are the
actual behaviors to be performed, and what are the factors related to and
supportive of the performance of these behaviors?

To perform self-management behaviors, families need skills (educational
and behavioral factors), but they also may need the health care system to provide reinforcement (environmental factors). As a specific example, attendance
and participation at school may maximize and appropriate child development,
but what are the factors that support and maintain a child's participation in
school? A child may have to manage the pain and morning stiffness associated
with JRA or the chest physiotherapy regiment required in CF to get to school
and may need classes on the ground floor or may need extra time to climb stairs.

---

*References 7, 15, 16, 25, 27-29, 40, 42.

The careful specification of educational factors in the PRECEDE model is important because they are the variables that become the immediate targets of health education interventions. Predisposing factors within the target population facilitate the adoption of the relevant health behavior, enabling factors determine whether or not the target population can perform the behavior, and reinforcing factors include the elements of the environment that reward the patient for performing the behavior.

For any one health behavior there are many educational or psychosocial variables that influence the performance of the behavior. The integration of any number of psychologic or learning theories into the educational diagnosis phase of the PRECEDE model enables the planner to choose and categorize factors that are the most important contributors to the behaviors and that are most likely to be influenced by an educational intervention.

Case Reports Using PRECEDE

We present two case examples in which PRECEDE was used in population-based program planning for CF and JRA and one example of educational diagnosis for individuals in a clinical setting.

Cystic fibrosis. CF is the most common, lethal, genetic disease among Caucasians. It is primarily manifested by lung infections that lead to lung damage and death. It also affects ducts from the pancreas and causes poor digestion of food, which often results in malnutrition. Although progress has recently been made in understanding the molecular genetics and cellular physiology of CF, the only therapy continues to be the treatment of symptoms and complications.[33] Orenstein and Wachnowsky[37] cite the following four regimens that may influence outcomes in CF: (1) chest physiotherapy and postural drainage, (2) antibiotic and enzyme medication, (3) diet, and (4) exercise.

A needs assessment was done at the Cystic Fibrosis Center of Baylor College of Medicine and Texas Children's Hospital in Houston, that provided care for 256 patients at the time of the study.[5] Structured interviews with 106 mothers, 27 fathers, and 53 adolescent and adult (over age 12) patients were completed. In addition, six group interviews were conducted (13 adolescents and young adults in two groups; 47 parents in four groups). The individual and group interviews addressed issues of diagnosis, hospitalization, knowledge of disease and treatment regimens, confidence in performing treatment regimens, coping, need for information, and death and dying.

The CF planning model is presented in Fig. 21-1. Based on the needs-assessment study, behavioral factors were not limited to the medical self-management behaviors that might have been predominant if the analysis had relied primarily upon clinical impression (e.g., treatment of malabsorp-

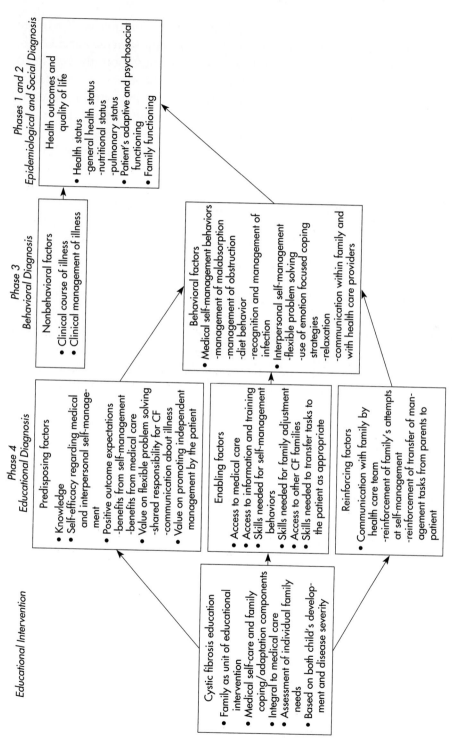

FIG. 21-1. PRECEDE applied to cystic fibrosis.

Modified from Bartholomew LK et al: Planning patient education for cystic fibrosis: application of a diagnostic framework, *Patient Education and Counseling* 13:57, 1988.

tion, management of obstruction, diet behavior, recognition and management of infection), but also included coping and adjustment. Parents who participated in the needs assessment expressed feelings about the burden of home care activities, isolation from other parents, the stress of hospitalizations, and the degenerative nature of the disease. The interviews presented little evidence that psychosocial resources were used effectively in response to the stress of the illness, thus alerting the planners to the need to focus on coping behavior as a potential contributor to improved quality of life and perhaps health status. Because the needs assessment did not provide specific information about coping strategies or needs of the families, the adjustment and coping behaviors in the model were defined by the theoretical and empirical literature on coping and stress[26] as the flexible use of problem-solving and emotion-focused coping strategies and well-developed communication skills to facilitate negotiation within the family, community, and health care system.

Social cognitive theory[2] provided the framework for delineating the educational factors, self-efficacy, knowledge and skills, value expectancies, and outcome expectations related to both interpersonal and medical self-management. Although all predisposing and enabling factors in the model could contribute to the behaviors, they were not all equally important in the educational diagnosis. For example, knowledge and skills regarding medical self-care may be more important in some areas than in others. Based on reports of compliance with medical regimens,[7,15,16,25,40] we proposed that knowledge, skills, and attitudes necessary for adherence to antibiotic regimens already exist in the population to a higher degree than those necessary for diet modification or exercise. Further, attitudes and skills related to coping may need emphasis because they apparently were not recognized by the CF families as being a part of the management.

Juvenile rheumatoid arthritis. The rheumatic diseases of childhood comprise some 50 diverse illnesses, all with the common denominator of inflammation of the connective tissues. JRA is the most common of the pediatric rheumatic diseases with a prevalence of approximately 1.1/1000 school-age American children and a peak age of onset between 1 and 3 years.[8,24,41,46]

Manifestations of JRA may include chronic arthritis, fever, rash, and systemic involvement such as cardiac abnormalities and iritis. The medical regimen required for children with JRA and their families typically includes taking medications, performing range of motion and strengthening exercises, wearing wrist splints, soaking in warm baths to combat morning stiffness, and making routine visits to the physician and other members of a multidisciplinary health care team.

A needs assessment for JRA was performed by the Rheumatology Service of Texas Children's Hospital in Houston and included an analysis of data from several sources: (1) a literature review, (2) a survey of 61 primary caretakers of children with JRA, (3) a group interview of parents of seven children with JRA, (4) results of school liaison pilot programs using a special educator, and (5) clinical experience of an interdisciplinary pediatric rheumatology team.[6] The PRECEDE model for JRA is presented in Figs. 21-2 and 21-3.

The needs assessment suggested that JRA affects several aspects of quality of life, including the child's school attendance and participation and the family's adjustment, specifically the family's ability to participate in recreational and other activities of daily living. JRA also contributes to psychologic distress of the child and other family members. The health of the child, including experiences of acute and chronic pain and disability related to joint function, may mediate some of the quality-of-life effect of JRA.

For JRA two sets of interrelated behavioral and environmental factors were identified throughout the needs-assessment process: (1) those related to managing the school environment to facilitate optimal participation and to minimize school-related disability, and (2) those related to treating pain and stiffness, intervening in the disease process, and preserving joint function. Because of the complexity of these two sets of factors we have depicted them in two figures (see Figs. 21-2 and 21-3) even though we propose their relation to the same set of outcome variables.

Predisposing and enabling factors in our analysis included knowledge, skills, and self-efficacy of the parent and the child regarding medical self-care, pain management, and communication with school personnel and the health care team. Self-efficacy[2] has a demonstrated relation to the self-management of chronic disease, including arthritis.[3,30,31] Because one of the desired outcomes was development of autonomy in the children, the enabling factors of knowledge of child development and expectations for independent behavior, including medical self-care and pain-management behavior, were also included in our planning model.

Reinforcing factors in the school-oriented model (Fig. 21-2) include school personnel's knowledge of JRA related to school functioning of the child and their skills and self-efficacy in communicating with the health-care team. Conversely, the health care team must be knowledgeable of school services and have skills and self-efficacy for evaluating the child's school needs and communicating those needs to the school personnel. One goal is for both the school and the health care teams to encourage the families' attempts to obtain appropriate school services for the child and to support those attempts with information and action.

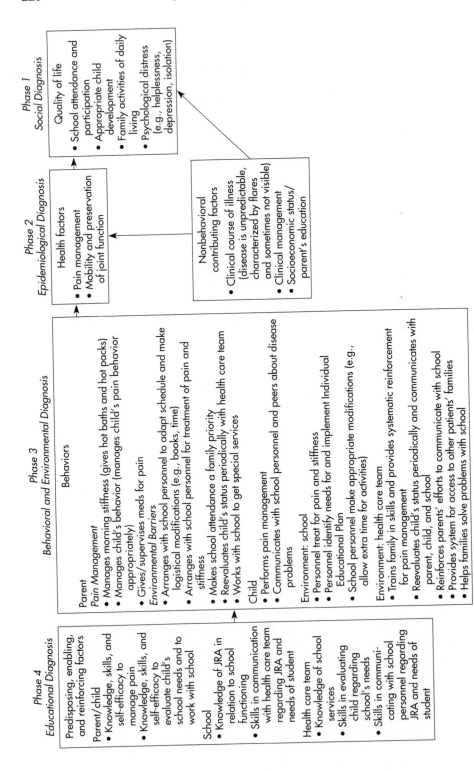

FIG. 21-2. PRECEDE model for JRA factors related to school.

From Bartholomew et al: An educational needs assessment of children with juvenile rheumatoid arthritis, *Arthritis Care and Research* 38:1307-1315, 1994.

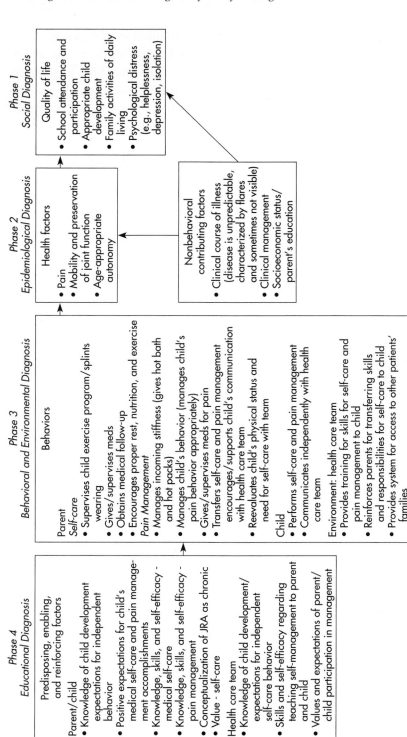

FIG. 21-3. PRECEDE model for JRA factors related to medical self-care.

From Bartholomew et al: An educational needs assessment of children with juvenile rheumatoid arthritis, *Arthritis Care and Research* 38:1307-1315, 1994.

Reinforcing factors in the medical self-care–oriented model (see Fig. 21-3) include the health care team's knowledge of child development and appropriate expectations for self-care behavior by the parent and child. Further, the provider must have skills and self-efficacy regarding teaching self-management to the parent and the child, as well as positive values regarding parent and child participation in the management of JRA. These are then translated into the behavioral goals of providing systematic self-management training for the parent and reinforcing the parents for performing the medical routines and for transferring the skills and responsibility for self-care to the child as the child becomes able to perform them.

Educational diagnosis of individual needs. The PRECEDE framework can also be applied in individual health care or social-service encounters.[38] The diagnostic approach in patient-education encounters is essentially the same as presented in the two previous population-based examples. One begins by defining health and quality-of-life outcomes for a patient and family and then moves to specifying the behaviors that will lead to those outcomes. For example, in the general case of asthma management there are many important potential health and quality-of-life outcomes that can be expected from good management, including the following: decreased acute care and emergency room visits, decreased cost of care, increased social and school participation, decreased sleep disturbance, and increased exercise tolerance.[36] However, self-management for each individual child and family may have a narrower focus. In the case of an eleven-year-old girl whose asthma is fairly well managed with a continuous medication regimen and contingency medications for exacerbations but who refuses physical education (PE) participation, increased exercise tolerance might be the desired outcome. Related to this outcome will be a set of related parent and child behaviors and possibly environmental factors, such as talking to the PE teacher about the child's capabilities, planning a gradual introduction of strenuous PE activities, and increasing exercise activities at home.

Once the desired behaviors and modifications in the environment have been identified, the next step is to assess knowledge, attitudes, and skill that may be determinants of the behaviors. This assessment is usually done by asking open-ended questions. Examples might include the following: What can you tell me about your participation in PE? Tell me how you would go about talking to your teacher about what you can do in PE. Would you tell me about what might happen when you try to get more exercise at home like bike riding, roller skating, or swimming? Do you want to participate in PE?

Once the data on knowledge, attitudes, and skills have been collected, the health care provider is in a good position to identify educational needs. In the example of the patient with asthma, the knowledge that the parent and child may need is the relation between the child's airway reactivity and asthma. The needed attitude change may be enhanced confidence in the child's ability to remain symptom-free during exercise and to manage any symptoms that do occur. They also may need additional confidence in their ability to communicate with the school personnel regarding these issues. The child and family may need skills in managing medication around exercise and in communicating with the school about health issues.

Often educational needs cannot all be met in a single visit or with simple educational techniques and setting priorities becomes necessary. Priority can be assigned according to the importance of a need based on how likely it is to influence behavior and its changeability through available educational techniques.

CONCLUSION

Using the PRECEDE model for planning educational interventions for pediatric chronic illness and disability allows us to consider the complexity of the issues based on information from multiple data sources and multidisciplinary perspectives. It allows us to analyze the determinants of patient and family health outcomes and quality of life so that interventions can be targeted to appropriate problems and behavioral and educational determinants so that potential for impact is maximized. In our example of a JRA population this analysis leads to consideration of both medical self-management and management of the school environment and of the role both of these issues play in child development. Use of the planning model in our example of a CF population facilitates the recognition that both the medical and the psychosocial aspects of self-management should be targets of the educational intervention. The focus on behavior required to promote self-management and that is engendered by the model also facilitates an efficient, effective educational encounter in the clinical setting.

REFERENCES

1. Bailey WC et al: Promoting self-management in adults with asthma: an overview of the UAB program, *Health Educ Q* 14:345, 1987.
2. Bandura A: *Social foundations of thought and action: a social cognitive theory*, Englewood Cliffs, NJ, 1986, Prentice-Hall.
3. Bartholomew LK et al: Measuring self-efficacy expectations for the self-management of cystic fibrosis, *Chest* 103:1524-1530, 1993.
4. Bartholomew LK et al: Performance objectives for the self-management of cystic fibrosis, *Patient Eduction and Counseling* 22:15-25, 1993.
5. Bartholomew LK et al: Planning patient education for cystic fibrosis: application of a diagnostic framework, *Patient Education and Counseling* 13:57, 1988.
6. Bartholomew LK et al: An educational need assessment of children with juvenile rheumatoid arthritis. *Arthritis Care and Research* 38:1307-1315, 1994.
7. Bellisari A: Beating CF: compliance with chest physiotherapy in a group of cystic fibrosis patients, *Proceedings of the 6th Annual Scientific Session of the Society of Behavioral Medicine* 41, 1985 (abstract).
8. Cassidy JT: Definition and classification of rheumatic diseases in children. In Cassidy JT, editor: *Textbook of pediatric rheumatology*, New York, 1982, John Wiley and Sons.
9. Clark NM: Asthma self-management education research and implications for clinical practice, *Chest* 95:1110, 1989.
10. Clark NM et al: Developing education for children with asthma through study of self-management behavior, *Health Educ Q* 7:278, 1980.
11. Clark NM et al: Changes in children's school performance as a result of education for family management of asthma, *J Sch Health* 54:143, 1984.
12. Creer TL: Living with asthma: replications and extensions, *Health Educ Q* 14:319, 1987.
13. Creer T and Winder J: Asthma. In Holroyd K and Creer T, editors: *Self-management of chronic disease: handbook of clinical interventions and research*, New York, 1986, Academic Press.
14. Drotar D et al: Psychosocial functioning of children with cystic fibrosis, *Pediatrics* 67:338, 1981.
15. Finkelstein SM et al: Compliance measures for home monitoring in cystic fibrosis, *Proceedings of 37th Annual Conference on Engineering in Medicine and Biology*, 1984.
16. Finkelstein SM et al: Feasibility and compliance studies of a home measurement monitoring program for cystic fibrosis, *J Chronic Dis* 39:195, 1986.
17. Fireman P et al: Teaching self-management skills to asthmatic children and their parents in an ambulatory care setting, *Pediatrics* 68:341, 1981.
18. Fowler MG, Davenport MG, and Garg R: School functioning of U.S. children with asthma, *Pediatrics* 90:939, 1992.
19. Fowler M, Johnson M, and Atkinson S: School achievement and absence in children with chronic health conditions, *J Pediatr* 106:683, 1985.
20. Green LW et al: *Health education planning: a diagnostic approach*, Mountain View, Calif, 1980, Mayfield Publishing.
21. Green LW and Kreuter MW: Health promotion planning: an educational and environmental approach, ed 2, Mountain View, Cal, 1991, Mayfield Publishing.
22. Gross AM, Magalnick LJ and Richardson P: Self-management training with families of insulin-dependent diabetic children: a controlled long-term investigation, *Child and Family Behavior Therapy* 7:35, 1985.
23. Hindi-Alexander MC and Cropp GJA: Community and family programs for children with asthma, *Ann Allergy* 46:143, 1981.
24. Hochberg MC: The epidemiology of juvenile rheumatoid arthritis: a review

of current status and approaches for future research. In Lawrence RC and Stillman LE, editors: *Epidemiology of the rheumatic diseases*, New York, 1984, Gower Medical.

25. Hubbard V and Mangrum P: Energy intake and nutritional counseling in cystic fibrosis, *J Am Diet Assoc* 80:127, 1982.
26. Lazarus R and Folkman S: *Stress, appraisal and coping*, New York, 1984, Springer.
27. Lemanek K: Adherence issues in the medical management of asthma, *J Pediatr Psychol* 15:437, 1990.
28. Litt I and Cuskey W: Compliance with salicylate therapy in adolescents with juvenile rheumatoid arthritis, *Am J Dis Child* 135:434, 1981.
29. Litt I, Cuskey W and Rosenberg A: Role of self-esteem and autonomy in determining medication compliance among adolescents with juvenile rheumatoid arthritis, *Pediatrics* 69:15, 1982.
30. Lorig K et al: The beneficial outcomes of the arthritis self-management course are not adequately explained by behavior change, *Arthritis Rheum* 32:91, 1989
31. Lorig K et al: Development and evaluation of a scale to measure perceived self-efficacy in people with arthritis, *Arthritis Rheum* 32:37, 1989.
32. Lovell DJ et al: School attendance and patterns, special services and special needs in pediatric rheumatic diseases, *Arthritis Care and Research* 3:196, 1990.
33. MacLusky I and Levison H: Cystic fibrosis. In Chernick V and Kendig EL, editors: *Disorders of the respiratory tract in children*, ed 5, Philadelphia, 1990, W.B. Saunders.
34. Maiman L, Green LW, and Gibson G: Education for self-treatment by adult asthmatics, *JAMA* 241:1919, 1979.
35. McAnarney ER et al: Psychological problems of children with chronic juvenile arthritis, *Pediatrics* 53:523, 1974.
36. National Asthma Education Program Expert Panel: *Executive summary: guidelines for the diagnosis and management of asthma*, Bethesda, Md, 1991, U.S. Department of Health and Human Services.

37. Orenstein D and Wachnowsky D: Behavioral aspects of cystic fibrosis, *Ann Behav Med* 7:17, 1985.
38. Parcel GS: Educating the patient and family. In Daeschner CWJ, editor: *Pediatrics: an approach to independent living*, New York, 1983, John Wiley and Sons.
39. Parcel GS et al: Self-management of cystic fibrosis: a structural model for the relationship of educational and behavioral variables, *Soc Sci Med* 38:1307-1315, 1994.
40. Passero MA, Remor B and Salomon J: Patient reported compliance with cystic fibrosis therapy, *Clin Pediatr* 264, 1981.
41. Petty RE: Epidemiology and genetics of the rheumatic diseases of childhood. In Cassidy JT, editor: *Textbook of pediatric rheumatology*, New York, 1982, John Wiley and Sons.
42. Rapoff MA, Purviance MR and Lindsley CB: Educational and behavioral strategies for improving medication compliance in juvenile rheumatoid arthritis, *Arch Phys Med Rehabil* 69:439, 1988.
43. Roter DL: Patient participation in the patient-provider interaction: the effects of patient question-asking on the quality of interaction, satisfaction, and compliance, *Health Education Monographs* 5:281, 1977.
44. Taylor WR and Newacheck PW: Impact of childhood asthma on health, *Pediatrics* 90:657, 1992.
45. Taylor J, Passo M, and Champion V: School problems and teacher responsibilities in juvenile rheumatoid arthritis, *J Sch Health* 57:186, 1987
46. Towner SR, Michet CJ, Jr., and O'Fallon WM: The epidemiology of juvenile rheumatoid arthritis in Rochester, Minnesota 1960-1979, *Arthritis Rheum* 26:1208, 1983.
47. Townsend M et al: Evaluation of the burden of illness for pediatric asthmatic patients and their parents, *Ann Allergy* 67:403, 1991.
48. Zeltzer L et al: Psychological effects of illness in adolescents: impact of illness in adolescents: crucial issue and coping styles, *J Pediatr* 97:132, 1980.

CHAPTER 22

Case Finding

ANITA M. FAREL

The effect of many chronic and disabling conditions on later development can be minimized if children who either suffer from or are at risk for these conditions are identified and offered appropriate services in a prompt and timely manner.* In lieu of expanding categorical priorities, service delivery systems are being developed to ensure that all children who need services are identified, appropriately referred, and followed. The complex and challenging task of finding eligible children and their families is being approached on diverse fronts, including outreach and public awareness, screening and assessment, surveillance, registries, and tracking.

OUTREACH AND PUBLIC AWARENESS

Several recent legislative initiatives to extend and improve services for children have explicitly recognized the crucial role of public awareness and outreach and include specific guidelines in law and regulations. These legislative initiatives, by increasing public awareness about available services, enlist the community in finding those children who could benefit from referral to health service providers.

- *Head Start.* Head Start programs are expected to increase the visibility of their mainstreaming initiatives and to promote early identification of eligible youngsters with disabilities by including child-service providers on Head Start community-based advisory boards, making presentations at local, regional, and national meetings, and participating in interagency planning activities.[4]

*Case finding refers to all activities related to finding and identifying children with special needs.

226

- *Supplemental Security Income (SSI).* The 1989 Omnibus Budget Reconciliation Act (OBRA) directed the Secretary of Health and Human Services "to establish and conduct an ongoing program of outreach to children who are potentially eligible for SSI benefits,"* focusing specifically on populations for whom such efforts would be most effective. In *Sullivan v. Zebley*[17] the U.S. Supreme Court enlarged the potential pool of new SSI recipients and required that children previously classified as ineligible be identified and contacted. Many of the initiatives for identifying eligible children and their families are based on the premise that eligible families do not know about SSI or that they lack correct information about the application and appeals process. Mailings, presentations, training, informational meetings, and advertisements are directed specifically toward nurses, social workers, doctors, early intervention specialists, educators, parent programs, disability advocates, legal services programs, community activists, and human service providers to inform them about revised eligibility rules for SSI and to engage them in finding eligible children and their families.
- *Individuals with Disabilities Education Act (IDEA).* Through a variety of mechanisms, this IDEA legislation heightened community awareness about and identification of children with developmental disabilities. Under IDEA the child-find system requires each state to ensure that all children, birth through age 21, with disabilities or suspected of having disabilities are located, identified, and evaluated.† This requirement serves both to alert the community to the availability and rationale for early-childhood intervention programs and to stimulate the circumstances or behaviors that might encourage a parent or professional to seek further services. In addition to publicity about available services, the law requires that information be developed and directed specifically toward primary referral sources. Primary referral sources include physicians and hospitals, day care programs, local education agencies, public health facilities, social service agencies, and other health care providers. While health care and child care professionals, teachers, and social workers are usually the first people outside the child's family to suspect that a child's development may be delayed or impaired, such professionals might not otherwise be aware of the range or benefits of public programs that are available in the community.

---

*Omnibus Budget Reconciliation Act 1989 (Public Law No. 101-239).
†Individuals with Disabilities Education Act, 1991 (Public Law No. 102-119).

SCREENING AND ASSESSMENT

Screening activities provide a *coarse* sift of the population to indicate those children for whom diagnostic assessment is a reasonable next step. Screening tests, because they are administered to many children, must be brief, simple, and multifaceted. Assessment, however, is a *fine* sift to yield those children for whom further services and procedures are appropriate. It also serves to delineate as precisely as possible the nature and range of the child's problems, the cause of the problems, and possible strategies for treatment or remediation. Screening should be by means of an inexpensive, easily administered instrument or test, while assessment usually requires a more elaborate set of procedures to determine the extent to which the child is at risk for disability in any of several developmental domains (e.g., cognitive, emotional, sensory, motor).[9]

While screening and assessment procedures are readily described for medical problems such as sickle cell disease, screening and assessing children whose risk status derives from environmental (e.g., poverty) or family-related conditions (e.g., parental substance abuse) is less straightforward in that the relevant data cannot always be obtained solely from examination of the child. Parents provide a necessary and valuable source of assessment data. Depending on the nature of the problem, parents may also be the focus of efforts designed to remediate problems discovered by assessment. Information from screening and assessment contributes to the referral process and yields information useful for surveillance, registries, and tracking activities.

Surveillance

Surveillance includes the ongoing, systematic collection, analysis, and interpretation of data. Although the initial purpose of surveillance activities was to identify communicable diseases, applications of surveillance concepts have become more diverse to include a more complex range of health data, such as risk factors, disability, and health practices.[18] Surveillance also includes the dissemination of results to professionals involved in planning, implementing, and evaluating public health practice. The Centers for Disease Control and Prevention (CDC) are rebuilding established programs in birth defects to include other developmental disabilities such as mental retardation and cerebral palsy.[11] When surveillance systems are active, they are more like registries or tracking systems, and in fact these terms are often used interchangeably.

Registries

Registries are designed with the principal objective of organizing data collected over time, which may be used in treating or preventing diverse conditions, follow-up care, and evaluating and planning services. Successful registers are those that collect accurate, focused data, and meet a need that cannot be satisfied any other way.[20] Such registries also serve to improve the quantity and quality of data about the incidence and prevalence of certain conditions. Registries that evolved as tools for local service delivery may lack the data necessary to answer questions related to etiology or demography.

One of the best-studied registries was that instituted by Great Britain in the early 1960s to monitor infants at risk for handicapping conditions. Lindon[7] argued that by identifying and tracking 20% of the infants most at risk, 70% of the children who eventually develop handicapping conditions would be identified early. On the whole the results of these efforts were disappointing. In one district 41% of all live births were classified as at risk; however, this registry included only 65% of children whose handicaps were determined within the first year of birth. The goal of 70% identification could be reached only if the at-risk population were increased to include at least 50% of live births.[6,14] However, such a large rate of risk designation defeats the purpose of screening procedures and does little to help focus interventions on those who need them most. As a result risk registries were discontinued out of concern that less attention would be paid to children at risk for disability but not identified or that registries may stigmatize those children who were identified but did not develop handicaps. Greater success was obtained in a registry where families of hospitalized children with evidence of abuse, neglect, or high risk for maltreatment were thoroughly investigated and were provided appropriate intervention when necessary.[12]

Tracking

The assumption behind tracking systems is that the enrolled child's growth and development is monitored and assessed by a qualified specialist. Several purposes of tracking systems identified by Blackman include ensuring that children with disabilities and chronic illness are:

- identified as early as possible
- referred to an appropriate service agency or treatment facility
- not lost to the service system

Tracking systems are also useful for:

- determining future personnel needs
- understanding developmental outcomes of children with risk factors
- understanding developmental outcomes of children who were differently managed in different care systems
- identifying personnel training needs
- collecting accurate data for program reporting, planning, and evaluation activities

ISSUES IN DEVELOPING A SYSTEM THAT ENSURES IDENTIFICATION OF ALL CHILDREN WITH SPECIAL NEEDS

Recent amendments to Title V legislation addressed elements of system reform and modified the uneven pattern of eligibility and benefits that have characterized Title V implementation in each state.* The amendments emphasized the leadership role of state Title V programs in organizing services—that is, while not abandoning specialty or categorical care, focusing on the development of service delivery systems to reinforce comprehensiveness and coordination at the community level.

A system ensuring comprehensive child identification processes would (1) encompass the changes envisioned by these amendments and other legislation mandating services for children with special needs, (2) be based on clearly articulated goals, and (3) include a common understanding of eligibility and entitlement. A community-based service system must consider several critical features to ensure that all children eligible for services are identified appropriately and expediently.

Issue #1

The system must ensure that the most appropriate intervention is provided for each child identified and that identifying the special needs of children is a continuous and active process from birth through early adulthood.

It is not enough just to identify children with special needs. Initiatives related to finding the target population must be linked to resources and interventions. In addition to enlisting community programs in outreach and child-find efforts, programs must also be engaged in supporting the growth, development, and integration of this population of children in all aspects of community life.

A service delivery system must recognize and address both similarities and differences in life experiences among children who suffer from chronic illness and disabilities. For example, although children of all ages with sickle cell disease, and their families, have unique concerns in common, considerations of other aspects of chronic illness, such as the effect on families, the child's participation in school, and social development, must continue to affect the organization of services for this population.[16]

Issue #2

The system must attend especially to recalcitrant issues in identification, particularly those involving infants and toddlers at risk for disability and adolescents with chronic illnesses or disabilities.

*Omnibus Budget Reconciliation Act 1989 (Public Law No. 101-239).

Infants and toddlers at risk for disability. Under Part H of IDEA states accepting funds to develop comprehensive, coordinated, multidisciplinary, interagency early intervention programs must provide services to infants and toddlers who are experiencing developmental delays related to cognitive development, physical development, language and speech development, psychosocial development, or self-help skills and to those who have a diagnosed mental or physical condition that has a high probability of resulting in developmental delay.* States have the option also of including children between birth and age three who are at risk for substantial developmental delay if early intervention services are not provided. States that have chosen to serve children at risk for developmental delay are committing more resources to services, interagency processes, and data collection. These activities inevitably generate important deliberation about risk factors associated with developmental delay and outcomes from interventions.[15]

*Individuals with Disabilities Education Act, 1991 (Public Law No. 102-119).

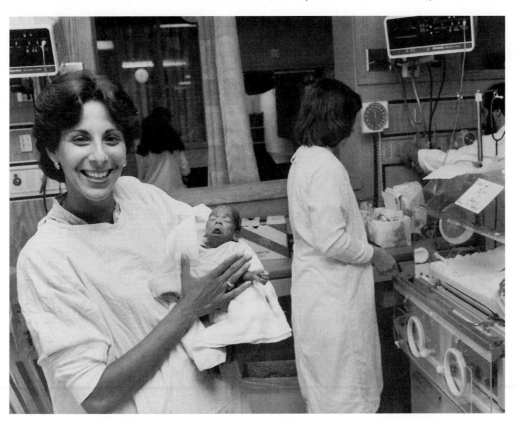

Definitions of risk must of necessity precede the development of services for infants and toddlers. The following three-part classification of risk by Tjossem[19] has traditionally been widely used as a framework for describing the population of children who are at risk for developmental problems: (1) *established risk* factors refer to genetic or congenital conditions, such as Down syndrome, and neurologic disorders; (2) *biological risk* factors include conditions associated with perinatal distress such as prematurity and respiratory disease; (3) *environmental risk* applies to children who are born into extreme poverty or whose families are dysfunctional. Although useful as a general framework, this classification may be misleading in giving the impression that these risk factors are independent and mutually exclusive.[8] The classification does not give explicit recognition to the prevalent view that developmental progress is influenced by the number and interaction of risk factors.[2,5,13] In considering how to make risk classifications operational for children served by Part H, one study has recommended that the traditional classification of established risk be broadened to include child abuse, infectious disease, and parental substance abuse in addition to the traditional conceptualization.[2]

Meisels and Provence[9] identified a number of factors that influence the greater probability that risk will be identified in school-age children than in infants or toddlers. First, signs of delayed or impaired development or conditions that affect development are more likely to be detected in a structured classroom setting where a teacher has the rest of the class as a basis for comparison. Second, developmental rate can vary widely in early years but still be within normal limits. Third, risk among school-age children is often identified on the basis of widely accepted tests and measures that are not appropriate for children served in early intervention programs. Further, because historically there have not been services organized around children between birth to age 3, the incentives to identify children for early intervention have been modest. Discussion about risk conditions must remain current and documented so that conclusions about how infants and toddlers at risk for delayed development should be identified and served are reflected in policy and program implementation.

Adolescents with chronic illnesses and disabilities. A substantial number of adolescents between ages 10 and 17 are affected by chronic conditions. According to the 1988 National Health Information Survey on Child Health, almost one third (31.5%) of adolescents had one or more chronic conditions of whom 16% were reported to be limited in their activities.[3] Adolescents with a wide range of chronic illnesses miss more school than healthy students. School absence attributable to chronic illness influences students' success in school. However, a significant number of teachers are not aware that children with chronic illnesses are in their classrooms. In 1983 an amendment to PL 94-142* included a mandate for services to assist students in the transition from school to work. However, youth with chronic illnesses were seldom identified as candidates for vocational education involvement by the school system, they received limited, if any, prevocational or transitional guidance, and they obtained few of the federal or state vocational rehabilitation services available for adults with chronic illnesses.[21] Also, fewer than 5% of students with chronic illnesses in special education received vocational guidance and only 21% of students who leave special education each year obtain jobs.[21] Problems related to identifying adolescents in need of appropriate preparation for transition from school are compounded when they come from disadvantaged home environments; adolescents with disabilities are much more likely to live in impoverished households than are healthy adolescents.[10]

The unique needs of adolescents, when compounded by chronic illness or disability, require continued special attention and resources. A comprehensive service delivery system must include vigilant outreach and identification of this population. Adolescents with special needs must be integrated into every aspect of community life to be able to take full advantage of the resources available to all youth.

Issue #3

A system must have oversight by all sectors in the community to ensure a comprehensive, coordinated child identification process.

Families, service providers, and members of a community representing private and public sectors must be involved in case finding, outreach, and planning. Successful identification of children with special needs requires the active participation and involvement of agencies associated with recreation, competitive and supportive employment, housing, and transportation in addition to health, education, and social services. The problems faced by children with chronic illness and disabilities and their families are complex and their solutions require involvement of many different institutions. Broad community representation provides the means for overseeing identification policies and processes that are in place and for reviewing and revising identification procedures among all service providers. Information about children being identified, by whom, and the consequences of their identification should influence policy decisions and program evaluation.

*Public Law 94-142, Education for All Handicapped Children Act, 1975.

Issue #4

An ongoing data-collection and needs assessment process must inform the design and implementation of a community-based system.

All agencies serving children with special needs require accurate and timely data as a foundation for policy decisions and program management, and needs assessments are an integral part of an ongoing community-based data collection process. The identification of children with special needs would be enhanced through the development of state and local databases that incorporate information on the population of children in need of services and the number and types of services provided. The database would identify health care providers, school resources, developmental programs, and community agencies providing services to children with disabilities. Such a data system would improve the monitoring of service continuity for children in transition from one program to another, from hospital discharge to community-based services, from school to employment, or from pediatric to adult health services. It would also improve child-finding capacity by enhancing the ability to identify gaps in services and sharpen estimates of the target population.

Data that cross program and service boundaries make it possible to monitor program changes. State-level data must inform community-based planners just as community-based data systems must be used for state program administration and evaluation. Information generated by the data system should be disseminated to and evaluated by both state and community agencies.

CONCLUSION

The past 2 decades represent a watershed for improving and implementing interventions for children with chronic illnesses, developmental disabilities, or who are at risk for poor health and development. Advances in medical technology and their widespread application have enhanced survival rates for premature and low-birthweight infants and improved treatment for children with chronic illnesses. Activism on the part of concerned parents has facilitated the passage of legislation that has greatly improved and expanded available services. At the same time, both research and practice have affirmed the importance of intervening as early in a child's life as possible to maximize developmental potential, and to improve the child's ability to benefit from school and lead a productive, independent life as an adult. These advances have fostered a new paradigm for services that emphasize the development of coordinated, comprehensive, community-based, and family-centered service delivery systems. The development of these systems is entirely dependent upon the ability to identify target populations. Continued attention to successful mechanisms for finding children with or at risk for disabilities is essential.

REFERENCES

1. Blackman J: *Warning signals: basic criteria for tracking at-risk infants and toddlers*, Washington DC, 1986, National Center for Clinical Infant Programs.
2. Carran DT et al: The relative risk of educational handicaps in two cohorts of normal birthweight disadvantaged children, *Topic in Early Childhood Education 9*:14-31, 1989.
3. Geber G and Okinow NA: Chronic illness and disability. In Hendee WR editor: *The health of adolescents*, San Francisco, 1991, Jossey-Bass.
4. Head Start Programs serving infants, toddlers, and pregnant women. Recruitment and enrollment of children with disabilities: Rules and regulations, *58 Federal Register 12* (21 January 1993) 5504-5505.
5. King EH, Logsdon DA, and Schroeder SR: Risk factors for developmental delay among infants and toddlers, *Child Health Chronicles 21*:39-50, 1991.
6. Knox EG and Mahon DF: Evaluation of infant at risk registries, *Arch Dis Child 45*:634, 1970.
7. Lindon RL: Risk Register. Cerebral Palsy Bulletin, 3:(5),481-487.
8. Meisels SJ: Dimensions of early identification, *Dimensions of Early Intervention* 15(1):26-35, 1991.
9. Meisels SJ and Provence S: Screening and assessment: guidelines for identifying young disabled and developmentally vulnerable children and their families, Arlington, Vir, 1989, National Center for Clinical Infant Programs.
10. Newacheck PW: Adolescents with special health needs: prevalence, severity, and access to health services, *Pediatrics 84*(5):872-881, 1989.
11. Pope AM and Tarlov AR, editors: *Disability in America*, Washington DC, 1991, National Academy Press.
12. Rowe DS et al: A hospital program for the detection and registration of abused and neglected children, *N Engl J Med 282*:950-952, 1970.
13. Schraeder BD: The influence of multiple risk factors on very low birth weight infants, *Nursing Papers* 19(4):59-73, 1987.
14. Scott KG and Masi W: The outcome from and utility of registers of risk. In Field TM, editor: Infants born at risk: behavior and development, Jamaica, NY, 1979, Spectrum Publications.
15. Shonkoff JP and Meisels SJ: Early childhood intervention: the evolution of a concept. In Meisels SJ and Shonkoff JP: editors: *Handbook of early childhood intervention*, Cambridge, England, 1990, Cambridge University Press.
16. Stein REK and Jessop DJ: A noncategorical approach to chronic childhood illness, *Public Health Reports 97*:354-362, 1982.
17. *Sullivan v Zebley*, 110 S Ct 885, 1990.
18. Thacker SB and Berkelman RL: Public health surveillance in the United States, *Epidemiologic Review 10*:164-190, 1988.
19. Tjossem TD, editor: *Intervention strategies for high risk infants and young children*, Baltimore, 1976, University Park Press.
20. Weddell JM: Registers and registries: a review, *Int J Epidemiol 2*(3):221-228, 1973.
21. White PH and Shear ES: Transition/job readiness for adolescents with juvenile arthritis and other chronic illness, *J Rheumatol 19* (Suppl 33):23-27, 1992.

CHAPTER **23**

Developmental Screening / Surveillance

FORREST C. BENNETT
ROBERT E. NICKEL
JANE SQUIRES
BARBARA J. WOODWARD

Within the United States and Western Europe there is general agreement regarding the importance of monitoring children's development during regular child health supervision.[8] Both the American Academy of Pediatrics[1] and the British Joint Working Party on Child Health Surveillance[19] recommend routine monitoring of a child's developmental progress as part of preventive health care. The goal of such monitoring is to identify as early as possible developmental delays and deviations that may portend future disabilities. At least 90% of pediatricians in two surveys indicated their support for the early identification of children with developmental disabilities.[5,35] Yet despite these positive recommendations and physician attitudes, Palfrey et al[32] recently documented in five metropolitan communities the medical system's striking lack of success in identifying many of the children with problems that eventually interfere with their ability to function well in school, and especially in identifying them early enough to allow preventive or ameliorative intervention. Still other reports confirm that although a majority of primary care physicians believe that developmental monitoring, including the use of a developmental screening tool, is an important aspect of preventive care for young children and acknowledge that health care providers are in a unique position to perform this function owing to their natural access to this population, most do not actually provide it on a routine basis.[15,25]

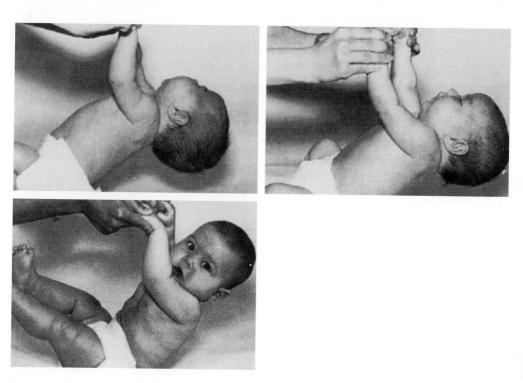

From Wong D: *Whaley & Wong's nursing care of infants and children,* ed 5, St Louis, 1995, Mosby–Year Book.

Why identify early? The stated support for the concept of early developmental identification is based on three principal assumptions: 1) early intervention services are effective in improving child and family functioning, 2) services are available and affordable, and 3) young children with disabilities can be accurately identified. The success of such early intervention programs as the Perry Preschool Project,[3] the Abecedarian Project,[33] and the Infant Health and Development Program[20] has contributed to an increasing emphasis by physicians, educators, psychologists, and parents on the early recognition of developmental problems. Recent federal legislation, Public Law 99-457 (reauthorized as the Individuals with Disabilities Education Act), has established requirements for early intervention services to all eligible children and accordingly promotes the early identification of developmental delay.[7] The accuracy of developmental diagnosis is markedly improved by using repeated measures at several ages.[17] The predictive accuracy of a single developmental screening test or even comprehensive developmental assessment in early childhood is limited. Therefore the success of a developmental monitoring program is dependent on the use of repeated measures at several ages.

CURRENT PRACTICES

Despite the uniformity of international opinion concerning the importance of developmental monitoring, there is currently no consensus as to how such monitoring should best be performed.[8] Pediatricians may use a wide array of eclectic techniques such as relying heavily upon clinical judgment based on history and office observation, reviewing developmental milestones with parents, and performing formal screening with a standardized test. While exemplary developmental history-taking has great intuitive appeal in terms of rapid and efficient monitoring, several authors have suggested that reliance solely upon such subjective data may lead to inaccurate conclusions about the child's developmental status.[25,13]

In fact it was in part these concerns about the highly variable reliability of developmental histories that led Frankenburg and Dodds[14] in 1967 to standardize and publish the Denver Developmental Screening Test (DDST). The goal of the original DDST was to increase the objectivity of developmental monitoring, not to replace the most subjective yet useful information obtained by parent interview. This single screening tool, revised and restandardized in 1990 as the Denver II,[11] has enjoyed worldwide utilization in more than 50 countries and individual standardization in more than 15 nations.

Since the development and dissemination of the DDST, a screening test for global development delay, a myriad of other general and specific screening instruments have been published. In the United States at the present time there are substantial regional and even university-based differences of practice concerning the developmental screening tools of choice. However, the reason most often cited for the lack of use of any formal developmental screening test, even when there is an identified concern, is lack of sufficient time in a busy office practice.

DEFINITIONS AND TERMINOLOGY

It is important to distinguish between developmental screening and developmental surveillance because both terms are in current use in debates about specific mechanisms of developmental monitoring.[8,19]

Development screening is a brief formal evaluation of developmental skills applied to a total, asymptomatic population of children that is intended to identify those children with suspect problems who should receive a complete developmental diagnostic assessment. It typically involves the administration of one or more standard measures at set ages throughout early childhood. Like other screening programs, it does not yield definitive diagnoses or developmental quotients but rather functions as a red flag to indicate which children merit further comprehensive investigation.

Developmental surveillance is a relatively new concept, broader in scope, and encompassing all activities relating to the detection of developmental problems and the promotion of development during primary child health care. In this more informal approach the physician should identify parental concerns and make regular skilled observations of a child's behavior to monitor his or her developmental progress. It is a flexible, continuous process involving input from multiple health professionals, parents, teachers, childcare staff, and others. It may or may not involve the use of developmental screening tests.

Contemporary recommendations for universal developmental monitoring generally imply the process of developmental surveillance. This ideally will include a two-level screening system (basic and focused), a combination of formal screening tests with informal observations, repeated measures at different ages, and the use of multiple sources of information, particularly parental report. Thus developmental screening alone is rarely if ever sufficient to adequately monitor a child's developmental progress but can be a valuable component of quality developmental surveillance.

ADVANTAGES AND DISADVANTAGES
OF DEVELOPMENTAL SCREENING TESTS

Some investigators have cautioned against the routine use of general developmental screening tests.[8,19] Expressed concerns include the following: 1) screening tests are not necessary to identify most children with mental retardation, 2) screening tests will not identify most children with language/learning disabilities, 3) screening tests will not identify most of the developmental dysfunctions experienced by biologically at-risk infants, and 4) screening tests are impractical because they require too much professional time to properly administer. In recent years the DDST has particularly been the subject of intense scrutiny and criticism.[16,29]

Are these concerns and criticisms fair or, as has been suggested, are we "expecting the impossible" of developmental screening?[9,10] There is no single, perfect screening test that combines excellent psychometric properties (e.g., reliability, validity, sensitivity, specificity) with rapidity of administration and that is applicable to multiple developmental domains for children at widely varying levels of developmental risk; nor is there likely to be such an ideal instrument in the near future. However, the limitations of screening tests are outweighed by the well-documented limitation of the average physician's clinical judgment regarding the presence or absence of mild to moderate mental retardation (approximately 90% of all cases of children with mental retardation).[25]

Most general development screening tests, such as the Denver II, were standardized to identify global developmental delay/mental retardation and not specific language/learning disabilities. Focused language screening tools are readily available and may be particularly helpful with children of low socioeconomic status and increased environmental risk. Screening for learning disabilities in the preschool years is notoriously inaccurate and probably contraindicated.[34] Likewise, focused neuromotor, language, and/or adaptive screening tests may frequently be useful adjuncts to basic screening instruments when monitoring the development of low birthweight, premature, and other infants with increased biomedical risk.

Because of the very real practical concerns associated with universal, periodic developmental monitoring, an increasing number of parent-completed screening tools have been developed that involve very little professional time. In fact, parent report measures may save substantial amounts of time by focusing the physician's attention on concerns raised by the parents and by providing relatively complete information about the child's developmental skills. It is clear that parent report instruments offer a cost-effective, valid means of basic-level, general screening if information is obtained by a structured interview or questionnaire.[26] However, these measures may not be appropriate for some parents because of poor reading or communication skills.

SELECTED SCREENING TOOLS

Screening tools may be conveniently divided into two functional groups. First-level or basic screening instruments are intended to provide relatively rapid, cost-effective screening for global developmental delay. They are designed to make the universal developmental monitoring of asymptomatic, low-risk children a feasible component of child health supervision but may also be appropriate for general screening of high-risk populations (e.g., Neonatal Intensive Care Unit [NICU] graduates). They are typically administered by primary care physicians, nurse practitioners, public health nurses, and office nurses but may also be used in special circumstances by childcare staff and preschool teachers. Parents frequently participate directly in this level of screening by means of parent report measures.

Second-level or focused screening instruments are intended to be used with children who have developmental concerns or suspect abnormalities identified by basic screening. They are also appropriate aids in the identification of some of the specific developmental sequelae of at-risk infants and children (e.g., neuromotor problems following prematurity or cognitive/

language problems associated with poverty). They are intermediate tools not intended to replace comprehensive developmental assessment but that allow the health professional to obtain a preliminary functional assessment. They may be particularly valuable in communities with limited access to multidisciplinary diagnostic teams.

The number and variety of available screening tools continue to escalate.[18] Many are aggressively marketed to child health and childcare providers. Because new psychometrically improved, user friendly measures (e.g., FirstSTEP, the Psychological Corporation) may appear even prior to the publication of this book, Table 23-1 briefly outlines several of the best studied and most recommended basic and focused screening instruments. We acknowledge that there are reliable and valid tools that, due to space limitations, are not included in this table. Also not included here are useful screening tools for specific areas such as adaptive behavior, school readiness, and home environment.

Fig. 23-1 presents a simplified algorithm for a model developmental-monitoring program. Level 1 and 2 screening activities may occur in a variety of community settings including private physician's offices, public health clinics, and childcare centers (primarily Level 1). Level 3 assessments generally require a tertiary child development center, a community neurodevelopmental center, or public school district multidisciplinary teams.

WHEN SHOULD SCREENING TESTS BE USED?

Because of the limitations of informal clinical judgment and parent report in unstructured interviews, as well as the need for repeated measures, we recommend that formal developmental screening measures be added to informal observations for all children at certain ages. We recommend slightly different developmental monitoring protocols for low-risk children and for high-risk children.

Low-Risk Infants and Children

- Screen the development of children at 6, 12, 18, 24, 36, 48, and 60 months and whenever a parent expresses a specific concern.
- Use a neuromotor screening for infants with delay in gross motor skills on first-level screening
- Use a language screening for children up to age three with language delay on first-level screening and whenever the parent expresses a concern about language delay.

High-Risk Infants and Children

- Using corrected age (age adjusted for the number of weeks of prematurity), screen the development of children at 4, 8, 12, 18, 24, 36, 48, and 60 months and whenever a parent expresses a specific concern.
- Use a first-level general developmental screening test and a second-level neuromotor screening at 4 months.
- Use a language screening for children up to age 3 with language delay on first-level screening and whenever the parent expresses a concern about language delay.

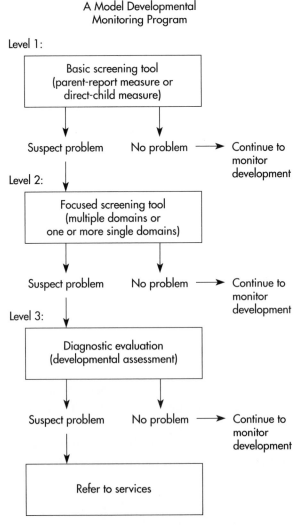

FIG. 23-1. A model development monitoring program.

TABLE 23-1. Selected Screening Tools

FIRST-LEVEL (BASIC) SCREENING TOOLS

Instrument	Age Range	Description	Psychometrics/Utility
Denver II[12]	0-6 years	Revision of DDST. 125 items in personal-social, fine motor-adaptive, language, and gross motor domains; language items added; some items deleted. The paired parent report measure (Denver Prescreening Developmental Questionnaire) is being newly revised to match the Denver II.	Renormed on 2000 children of diverse backgrounds. High reliability. Preliminary validity data: sensitivity = 0.83 specificity = 0.43
Ages and Stages Questionnaires[2]	4-48 months; Questionnaires at ages 4, 8, 12, 16, 20, 24, 30, 36, and 48 months; alternate forms at 6 and 18 months	Each questionnaire contains 30 items in areas of fine motor, gross motor, communication, adaptive, and personal-social. Parent report measure completed in 10-15 minutes; Spanish version available.	Concurrent validity with standardized measures: sensitivity = 0.45-0.94 specificity = 0.83-0.94 reliability = 0.86-0.91
Minnesota Infant Development Inventory[22]	0-15 months	Items taken from the Minnesota Child Development Inventory. A parent report measure with 60-80 items on each inventory asking about child's development, possible problems, and parent concerns.	Concurrent validity with standardized measures: sensitivity = 0.50-0.76 specificity = 0.76
Minnesota Early Child Development Inventory[21]	1-3 years		Revising/renorming underway.
Minnesota Preschool Development Inventory[23]	3-6 years		

Continued

TABLE 23-1. Selected Screening Tools—cont'd

SECOND-LEVEL (FOCUSED) SCREENING TOOLS: MULTIPLE DEVELOPMENTAL DOMAINS

Instrument	Age Range	Description	Psychometrics/Utility
Battelle Developmental Inventory Screening Test[30]	0-8 years	Items derived from Battelle Developmental Inventory. Two items per age level in areas of personal-social, adaptive, gross motor, fine motor, receptive language, expressive language, and cognitive. Battelle has been adopted by several states for PL 99-457 eligibility. Takes 30-35 minutes to administer.	Limited psychometric data on screening instrument. Preliminary validity data: sensitivity = 0.80 specificity = 0.74
Developmental Indicators for the Assessment of Learning-Revised[28]	2½-6 years	Designed to identify problems in domains of gross motor, fine motor, concepts, and communication. Takes about 30 minutes to administer.	Strong psychometric data; norms revised in 1990.
Revised Developmental Screening Inventory[24]	4 weeks-36 months	Selected items from full Gesell; domains of gross motor, fine motor, adaptive, language, and personal-social; takes 15-20 minutes to administer. A paired parent report measure (Parent Developmental Questionnaire) available.	Concurrent validity only with Gesell. Underscreening = 0% (sensitivity = 1.00) Overscreening = 5.1% (specificity = 0.94) No reliability data available.

SECOND-LEVEL (FOCUSED) SCREENING TOOLS: LANGUAGE DEVELOPMENT

Instrument	Age Range	Description	Psychometrics/Utility
Clinical Linguistic and Auditory Milestone Scale[4]	0-3 years	Assesses language milestones through parent interview and child observation. Takes 3-5 minutes to administer. May be combined with items from the Cattell Infant Intelligence Scale as the CAT/CLAMS.	Concurrent validity data with Bayley: sensitivity = 0.66 specificity = 0.74
Early Language Milestone Scale[6]	0-3 years	Domains of visual, auditory receptive, and auditory expressive. Developed for use in medical offices. Three minutes to administer.	Validity data with several groups of at-risk children.

SECOND-LEVEL (FOCUSED) SCREENING TOOLS: LANGUAGE DEVELOPMENT—cont'd.

Instrument	Age Range	Description	Psychometrics/Utility
MacArthur Communicative Development Inventories[27]	Infant: 8-16 months Toddler: 16-30 months	Parent-completed checklists and questions covering expressive and receptive vocabulary, actions and gestures (infant), and sentences and grammar (toddler).	Excellent psychometric studies; inventories are more in depth than most screening tools; short forms are under development.

SECOND-LEVEL (FOCUSED) SCREENING TOOLS: NEUROMOTOR DEVELOPMENT

Instrument	Age Range	Description	Psychometrics/Utility
Infant Motor Screen[31]	4-16 months	Twenty-five items measure muscle tone, primitive reflexes, automatic reactions, and motor asymmetries; items scored on three-point scale.	Predictive validity at 4 months: sensitivity = 0.93 specificity = 0.89 Predictive validity at 8 months: sensitivity = 1.00 specificity = 0.96 Good interobserver reliability data; no normative data reported.
Milani-Comparetti Motor Development Screening Test[37]	0-24 months	Twenty-seven items measure volitional movement, automatic reactions and primitive reflexes; original scoring system is descriptive.	Excellent normative and reliability data; two quantitative scoring systems have been used; very limited predictive validity data.

Modified from Squires, Nickel and Bricker, Use of parent-completed development questionnaires for child-find and screening, *Inf Young Children* 3(2):46-57, 1990.

SUMMARY AND RECOMMENDATIONS

- Developmental monitoring should be a component of regular child health supervision, particularly during the first 5 years of life.
- Developmental monitoring programs should include both structured (developmental screening) and unstructured (developmental surveillance) activities.
- Developmental screening tools vary widely in terms of ease of administration, required professional resources, psychometric properties, and purpose; no single tool meets all needs.
- Parent report measures offer a practical, cost-effective means of basic, first-level screening for large populations. However, education and communication barriers may compromise their use in some settings.
- Focused, second-level screening tools provide the opportunity for preliminary assessment, particularly with at-risk populations and in communities with limited access to formal developmental assessment services.
- Primary care physicians and community nurses/nurse practitioners are uniquely positioned to conduct developmental monitoring with additional input from childcare providers, preschool teachers, and others.

REFERENCES

1. American Academy of Pediatrics, Committee on Practice and Ambulatory Medicine: *Guidelines for Health Supervision*, Evanston, Ill, 1981, American Academy of Pediatrics.
2. Bricker D et al: *Ages and stages questionnaires: a parent-completed, child-monitoring system*, Baltimore, 1995, Paul H Brookes Publishing Co.
3. Bryant DM and Ramey CT: An analysis of the effectiveness of early intervention programs for environmentally at-risk children. In Guralnick MJ and Bennett FC, editors: *The effectiveness of early intervention for at-risk and handicapped children*, Orlando, 1987, Academic Press.
4. Capute AJ et al: The Clinical Linguistic and Auditory Milestone Scale (CLAMS), *AJDC* 140:694, 1986.
5. Carr J and Stephen E: Pediatricians and developmental tests, *Dev Med Child Neurol* 6:614, 1964.
6. Coplan J: *The Early Language Milestone Scale*, Austin, 1987, PRO-ED.
7. Downey WS: Public Law 99-457 and the clinical pediatrician. I. Implication for the pediatrician, *Clin Pediatr* 29(4):223-227, 1990.
8. Dworkin PH: British and American recommendations for developmental monitoring: the role of surveillance, *Pediatrics* 84:1000, 1989.
9. Dworkin PH: Developmental screening: (still) expecting the impossible? *Pediatrics* 89:1253, 1992.
10. Dworkin PH: Developmental screening–expecting the impossible? *Pediatrics* 83:619, 1989.
11. Frankenburg WK et al: The Denver II: a major revision and restandardization of the Denver Developmental Screening Test, *Pediatrics* 89:91, 1992.
12. Frankenburg WK et al: *Denver II Screening Manual*, Denver, 1990, Denver Developmental Materials.
13. Frankenburg WK, Chen J, and Thornton SM: Common pitfalls in the evaluation of developmental screening tests, *J Pediatr* 113:1110, 1988.

14. Frankenburg WK and Dodds J: The Denver Developmental Screening Test, *J Pediatr* 71:181, 1967.

15. Frankenburg WK and Thornton SM: A child development program for a busy office practice, *Contemporary Pediatrics* 6(2):90-106, 1989.

16. Glascoe FP et al: Accuracy of the Denver II in developmental screening, *Pediatrics* 89:1221, 1992.

17. Glascoe FP: Developmental screening: rationale, methods and applications, *Inf Young Children* 4(1):1, 1991.

18. Glascoe FP, Martin ED, and Humphrey S: A comparative review of developmental screening tests, *Pediatrics* 86:547, 1990.

19. Hutchison T and Nicoll A: Developmental screening and surveillance, *Br J Hosp Med* 39:22, 1988.

20. Infant Health and Development Program: Enhancing the outcomes of low birth-weight, premature infants, *JAMA* 263:3035, 1990.

21. Ireton H and Thwing E: *Early Child Development Inventory*, Minneapolis, Minn, 1988, Behavior Science Systems.

22. Ireton H and Thwing E: *Minnesota Infant Development Inventory*, Minneapolis, Minn, 1980, Behavior Science Systems.

23. Ireton H and Thwing E: *Preschool Developmental Inventory*, Minneapolis, Minn, 1980, Behavior Science Systems.

24. Knobloch H, Stevens F, and Malone A: Manual of developmental diagnosis: the administration and interpretation of the revised Gesell and Armatruda Developmental and Neurological Examination, New York, 1980, Harper & Row.

25. Korsch B, Cobb K, and Ashe B: Pediatrician's appraisals of patients' intelligence, *Pediatrics* 27:990, 1961.

26. Lichtenstein R and Ireton H: Preschool screening: identifying young children with developmental and educational problems, New York, 1984, Grune & Stratton.

27. MacArthur Communicative Development Inventory: Infants and Toddlers, San Diego, CA, Center for Research in Language, UCSD, 1989.

28. Mardell-Czudnowski CD and Goldenberg DS: *Developmental indicators for the assessment of learning*, Circle Pines, Minn, 1990, American Guidance Service.

29. Meisels SJ: Can developmental screening test identify children who are developmentally at risk? *Pediatrics* 83:578, 1989.

30. Newborg J, Stock JR, and Wnek L: *Battelle Developmental Inventory Screening Test*, 1984, Allen, Tex, DLM Teaching Resources.

31. Nickel RE: *The manual for the Infant Motor Screen*, Eugene, Ore, 1987, Oregon Health Sciences University.

32. Palfrey JS et al: Early identification of children's special needs: a study in five metropolitan communities, *J Pediatr* 111:651, 1987.

33. Ramey CT and Campbell FA: The Carolina Abecedarian Project: an educational experiment concerning human malleability. In Gallagher JJ and Ramey CT, editors: *The malleability of children*, Baltimore, 1987, Paul H. Brookes.

34. Shapiro BK et al: Detection of young children in need of reading help: evaluation of specific reading disability formulas, *Clin Pediatr* 29:206, 1990.

35. Smith RD: The use of developmental screening tests by primary care pediatricians, *J Pediatr* 93:524, 1978.

36. Squires, Nickel, and Bricker: Use of parent-completed development questionnaires for child-find and screening, *Inf Young Children* 3(2):46-57, 1990.

37. Stuberg WA et al: Milani-Comparetti Motor Development Screening Test: test manual, 1987 edition, Omaha, 1987, Meyer Children's Rehabilitation Institute, University of Nebraska Medical Center.

CHAPTER **24**

Developmental and Behavioral Assessment

THOMAS R. MONTGOMERY

Parents of children with abnormal development and behavior want to know what is wrong with their child, why, how to treat it, and will it happen again. A comprehensive clinical assessment of development and behavior should answer these questions for the parents, and the assessment should then lead to appropriate intervention.

The clinical assessment is a sophisticated approach to developmental and behavioral disorders. It allows the examiner freedom in obtaining the assessment, but with such freedom comes the responsibility of precision. The assessment describes abilities as well as disabilities; it determines the quality of performance, not just the level of performance. The assessment also includes a search for the etiology of abnormal development and behavior—the "why" question that must be answered for parents.

Clinical assessment differs from screening and from formal protocol testing; screening identifies children that may demonstrate development or behavior outside expected norms, and formal evaluations, which require adherence to rigid protocols using standardized test instruments to generate performance levels, were not devised for the evaluation of abnormal children. Often the protocol of administration must be broken to assess an abnormal child; once this occurs the evaluation becomes a clinical assessment.

Behavior assessment belongs within the context of development. Until developmental abilities are known, behavior cannot be interpreted in a sophisticated fashion. Observation of behavior without knowledge of developmental levels leads to inappropriate and inaccurate interpretation. Likewise, abnormal behavior may affect performance. The interrelationship between behavior and development is an important aspect of the clinical assessment.

Clinical assessment is appropriate for any child who has failed screening, either formal or informal. Formal screening with the Denver Developmental Screening Test (DDST), revised as the Denver II,[6] during health maintenance visits continues to be a standard approach to identification of children needing a clinical assessment. Preschool children often are screened with a checklist for school readiness. School children who have failed a grade or who have been identified by a behavioral observation scale to be at high risk for developmental disorders are candidates for a clinical assessment. The screening process often involves an analysis of risk factors for developmental and behavioral disorders (see the box on p. 250).

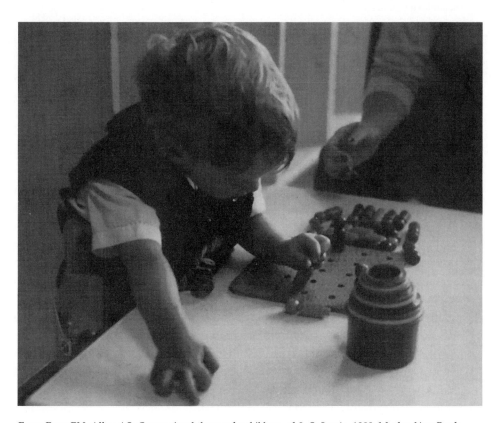

From Pratt PN, Allen AS: *Occupational therapy for children*, ed 2, St Louis, 1989, Mosby–Year Book.

Risk Factors *

Infants

Significant prematurity
Prenatal exposure to drugs/alcohol
Failure to thrive
Neonatal neurologic disorders (seizures)
Congenital anomalies
Failed formal screening

Preschoolers

Infant risk factors
Failed formal screening
Neurologic disorders
Short stature
Failed checklist for school readiness

School-Age Children

Preschool risk factors
Failed grade
Failed behavior checklist screen
Failed formal screening
Neurologic disorders

*A positive risk factor indicates the need for clinical assessment of development and behavior.

STREAMS OF DEVELOPMENT

Development can be divided into different areas or streams. Each stream of development needs to be assessed individually and then reconstructed into a framework of overall functional abilities. Behavior and developmental interrelationships are to be interpreted within this framework. Streams of development flow in a predictable fashion during childhood. Gross motor development, very prominent in infancy and early childhood, tends to reach a functional plateau at a young age. Early visual development evolves into the stream of fine motor development and then into the stream of visual motor problem solving, which then merges into the stream of visual performance. Language begins with visual communication, such as a social smile, and evolves into prelinguistic development and eventually flows into verbal language. With age, the ability to use language in a sophisticated fashion defines the stream of verbal development.

Throughout these streams of development are specific areas referred to as perceptual skills, which are subsets of the major streams of development. For example, visual perceptual development is a portion of the fine motor/visual problem-solving stream, and auditory perception and auditory processing are portions of the language/verbal stream. Whenever an abnormality of the entire stream occurs, these subsets likewise are affected. However, they can present as specific problems dissociated from the stream of development. Combined, language and visual problem-solving developmental streams reflect overall intellectual development—cognition. Personal social development and adaptive development are streams that involve interrelationships between language, visual problem solving, and the social setting. Environmental abnormalities can produce impairments within the personal social and adaptive streams unrelated to cognitive development. However, impaired cognitive development interferes with personal social development even in the best environment.

Certain aspects of behavior flow along as a developmental stream. These aspects include attention, concentration, adaptation, and habituation. Failure to recognize the developmental nature of these aspects of behavior leads to inappropriate interpretations. Once the developmental nature of these aspects of behavior is identified, the social and emotional aspects of behavior can appropriately be assessed.

Milestones

Milestones mark the flow of development within each stream (see the box on p. 252). An isolated milestone may have very little importance; it is the sequential achievement along milestones that provides validity to the clinical assessment. The physician can determine a developmental age for each area of development. A developmental quotient for each stream can be calculated by the following equation:

$$\text{Developmental Quotient (DQ)} = \frac{\text{Developmental Age (DA)}}{\text{Chronological Age (CA)}} \times 100$$

Delay, dissociation and deviancy. Disorders of progression through the milestones of development can be divided into three categories: (1) delay, (2) dissociation, and (3) deviancy (see the box on p. 253). *Developmental delay* is an abnormally slow progression through the milestones of development. The milestones are achieved in the usual order but at a much slower pace than normal. A developmental quotient (DQ) less than 75 represents developmental delay.

Developmental dissociation is a significant discrepancy in the rates of development between two different streams—a significant difference between two DQs. Delay usually is present in at least the slower stream. For example, a child may have normal language development and significantly delayed

Developmental Milestones

Gross Motor

In prone position

Head up	1 mo
Chest up	2 mo
On forearms	3 mo
On wrists	4 mo

Roll over	4 mo
Sit alone	6 mo
Come to sit	8 mo
Crawl	9 mo
Pull to stand	10 mo
Walk alone	12 mo
Walk Up Stairs	18 mo
Walk Down Stairs	24 mo
Pedals	3 y
Skips	5 y
Rides 2 wheeler	6 y

Fine Motor/Adaptive

Visual

Fix	birth
Follow	1 mo
Threat	3 mo
Unfisted	3 mo
Reaches	4 mo
Transfers	5 mo
Hold 2 blocks	7 mo
Scissor grasp	9 mo
Pincer grasp	11 mo
Release	12 mo
Cup/spoon	12 mo
Fork	24 mo
Knife	5 y
Cooperate with dressing	12 mo
Undresses	2 y
Dresses	3 y
Unbuttons	3 y
Buttons	4 y
Ties	5 y

Expressive Language

Social smile	2 mo
Coos	3 mo
Laughs	4 mo
Razzes	5 mo
"Ah-goo"	5 mo
Dada (nonspecific)	8 mo
Mama (nonspecific)	9 mo
Dada (specific)	10 mo
Mama (specific)	10 mo
1st word	11 mo
2nd word	12 mo
Jargons	15 mo
4-6 words	16 mo
2-word phrases	21 mo
2-wd sentences	24 mo
Pronouns	3 y
Plurals	3 y

Receptive Language

Alerts	1 mo
Recognizes mom	2 mo
Orients to voice	4 mo
Orients to bell	5 mo
Understands "no"	9 mo
Gesture games	9 mo
1-step command	
with gesture	12 mo
without gesture	16 mo
Knows 1 body part	18 mo
Points to 1 picture	18 mo
2-step command	24 mo
Points to 7 pictures	24 mo

Modified from Illingworth RS: *The development of the infant and young child, normal and abnormal,* Edinburgh, Scotland, 1985, Churchill Livingstone.

Developmental Milestones—cont'd

Developmental Quotient (DQ)

$$DQ = \frac{\text{Developmental Age (DA)}}{\text{Chronological Age (CA)}} \times 100$$

Developmental Delay-a delay in the rate of development such that it is progressing at less than 75% of normal rate—a DQ of less than 75.

Developmental Dissociation-A significant difference between the developmental quotients of two streams or substreams of development.

Developmental Deviancy-A significant deviation from the normal milestones of development. Deviancy can be a result of out-of-order progression of milestones or abnormal milestones/performance.

---

gross motor development (i.e., language DQ=100 and gross motor DQ=50)—a dissociation between the gross motor and language streams. Another child may have normal verbal development but delays in auditory processing—a dissociation within the language/verbal stream between overall verbal and a specific perceptual substream.

Developmental deviancy refers to an abnormal progression along milestones. Deviancy involves abnormality of function and disorder of milestones. The child with cerebral palsy, for example, who stands before sitting or crawling has deviant development; the milestones are out of order and the performance of walking is abnormal. Deviancy in language development is often referred to as language disorder, distinguishing it from language delay, although delay is usually present whenever deviancy exists. Significantly deviant development is often misinterpreted as emotional disturbance. The clinical assessment should differentiate emotional disturbance from developmental deviancy.

CLINICAL ASSESSMENT

Assessing a child's flow through the milestones of development begins with his or her developmental history. Developmental history reconstructs the pattern of achievements and provides evidence for delay, dissociation, and deviancy. Keepsake baby books may be helpful in providing information about a child's achievements. Generally the greater the delay in development the more accurately the parents recall such attainment. It is helpful to have parents recall behaviors and activities at certain ages such as, what their child was saying on his or her second birthday. Also important dates or events in family life may be reminders for the parents. The discovery of delay, dissociation, and deviancy in the developmental history of a child will guide the assessment of current function.

It is prudent to begin assessing skills below a child's current function level to gain his or her confidence and sense of success during testing. It is unusual for a child to persist at attempts to perform difficult or developmentally impossible tasks. Some children may quietly recognize their inability and act as if they are refusing to perform. Other children may become inattentive or excessively active in avoidance of the task. These behaviors are not refusals but are signs of inability to perform. Indeed such behaviors are excellent measures of peak developmental skills.

Children with significant refusal behavior or other behavior problems display such behaviors for tasks at all developmental levels. Even tasks known by the child to be below his or her historical abilities are refused or generate the abnormal behavioral responses. Such behaviors should be handled by rewards for performance.

Infants and toddlers. Infants and toddlers can be assessed using the CAT/CLAMS,[1,9,14] which divides development into visual problem-solving and language skills, each of which has appropriate items of personal social and adaptive skills. An interpretation of receptive and expressive language can be made within the language scale, and the gross motor milestone scale[3] serves to complete the assessment. DQs for language, visual problem solving, and cognition are derived from the CAT/CLAMS; a DQ in gross motor development is calculated from the gross motor milestone scale.

The Early Learning Accomplishment Profile (E-LAP)[7] also is used for infants and toddlers. It has subtests for gross motor, fine motor, self-help/personal social/emotional, language, and cognitive skills. These multiple subtests overlap in items assessed. The cognitive subtest consists of visual problem solving and language items. Many of the self-help skills involve either problem solving or language. DQs for each subtest can be calculated.

The generation of developmental ages and developmental quotients alone is not sufficient for a clinical assessment. The nature of the items failed is important to determine the overall nature of the disability. Low DQs in language, cognition, and self-help streams may all be due to impaired language. This pattern of development is significantly different from a child that has a low DQ in cognition because both language and visual problem-solving streams are delayed. Careful attention to the quality of performance is crucial. Aberrantly performed tasks are a sign of developmental deviancy.

At the beginning of the assessment it is necessary to find an activity that the child likes, and that activity should be pursued to the point of inability. If blocks are of particular interest to the child, then block play to the point of inability should be pursued. Additionally, the blocks can be used as a reward for attempting other tasks. The child is allowed to return to the blocks to play after attempting tasks with other objects. The examiner needs to be prepared to move quickly and to take advantage of the first sign of sustained interest by the child.

For many infants and toddlers the ideal test setting is in the mother's lap; some may also tolerate the examiner's lap, and a floor mat is another possible arrangement. Children with significant motor coordination impairments may be tested best while in their adaptive seat. The examiner must adapt to the child to find the most appropriate test setting. The setting can change many times during the assessment.

Preschoolers. It is important to have an understanding of the preschooler's abilities from the developmental history. For the impaired preschooler—below 3-year level—the CAT/CLAMS can be used. For the child above the 3-year level, visual problem-solving skills can be assessed with Gesell figures[16] and the Draw-a-Man Test as scored by Goodenough[8]; receptive language skills can be assessed with the Peabody Picture Vocabulary Test.[5] Informal tests of expressive language include the 4-year level ability to tell a story and the 5-year level ability to be fluent in verbal expression. The gross motor milestone scale can be used to generate the gross motor DQ.

The Learning Accomplishment Profile (LAP)[15] is another test that may be used for preschoolers. It has the same subtests as the E-LAP plus a prewriting subtest. It also has the same limitations as the E-LAP with the same overlap of areas assessed.

Preschoolers deemed untestable generally are not tested at low enough levels. The developmental history should help to identify a preschooler that is functioning at very low levels and that requires infant and toddler tests. Preschoolers often tolerate a table and chair if of the appropriate size, however, the floor is another frequently used setting for the preschooler. Others prefer to stand at an appropriately sized table. The low-functioning preschooler requires the same testing environment as an infant or toddler, and like the toddler, the child should determine the appropriate setting.

School-age children. Visual problem-solving skills in school-age children can be assessed with Gesell figures, the Draw-a-Man test, and Bender-Gestalt figures as scored by Koppitz.[12] DQs for each test can be determined and an overall DQ for visual problem solving can be calculated. Auditory memory can be assessed by the age-graded scheme for recall of digits—4 digits at $4\frac{1}{2}$ years, 5 digits at 7 years, 6 digits at 10 years, and 7 digits at adulthood.[13] Developmental-age–graded tests of vocabulary can assess verbal/language development, and graded reading, spelling, and arithmetic tests can assess academic achievement.[11] However, each score needs to be converted to a developmental age with a generated DQ. Otherwise it becomes difficult to compare streams of development. Developmental dissociation, an important aspect of learning disabilities, may not be appreciated if DQs are not generated.

The objective assessment of behavior in school-age children remains controversial because the observed behavior in an assessment setting may not reflect behavior in the classroom or at home. The Conners behavior rating scales[4] and others are widely used by teachers and parents. These rating scales are an important part of the developmental history and must be interpreted as such. The etiology of abnormal behavior in the classroom or at home is not identified by rating scales. The clinical assessment needs to incorporate the reported and the observed behaviors within the context of the whole child to determine etiology. (For a summary of clinical assessment tools see the box on p. 257.)

Diagnostic Formulation

A diagnostic formulation completes the clinical assessment. The degree of delay dissociation and deviancy and the quality of skills performed needs to be determined, and a comprehensive neurologic and neuromotor examination needs to be performed. The pattern of delay, dissociation, and deviancy directs the diagnostic formulation. Observed and reported behaviors need to be incorporated into this formulation, and an assessment of the effect of behavior upon performance needs to be included.

The assessment may identify many specific difficulties in perceptual and processing skills. However a comprehensive diagnosis, such as mental retardation, may appropriately include all of these specific difficulties. Multiple mini diagnoses are confusing and do not accurately reflect the nature of a child's developmental disability.

Assessment and Service Provision

An accurate assessment of a child is necessary before an accurate treatment can be considered. A partial evaluation results in partial and possibly ineffective intervention. Occasionally a child will have severe problems that will require immediate intervention. Such treatment may precede a comprehen-

Clinical Assessment Tools

Infants and Toddlers
CAT/CLAMS
Gross motor milestone scale
Early Learning Accomplishment Profile (E-LAP)

Preschoolers
Draw-a-Man test
Gesell figures
Peabody Picture Vocabulary test
Auditory memory for digits
Informal sample of expressive language
Learning Accomplishment Profile (LAP)

School-Age Children
Gesell figures
Bender-Gestalt figures/Koppitz
Draw-a-Man test
Auditory memory for digits
Vocabulary test
Wide Range Achievement test—revised (WRAT-R)
  Reading
  Math
  Spelling
Conners behavior scales

sive assessment, provided the assessment is eventually completed. Although it is tempting to begin treatment for children with known diagnoses such as Down syndrome, a clinical assessment is necessary to assure that intervention is accurate. Likewise, serial assessments without effective therapy are not beneficial.

CONCLUSION

Accurate clinical developmental and behavioral assessment of children requires a sophisticated and comprehensive approach. The freedom to evaluate development must not be considered less sophisticated; rather it must be respected as the most accurate method of determining the comprehensive nature of an abnormally functioning child. Effective intervention will be the result of accurate clinical assessment.

REFERENCES

1. Capute AJ and Accardo PJ: CAT/CLAMS: A comprehensive language assessment tool. In Capute A and Accardo P, editors: *Developmental disability in infancy and childhood*, Baltimore, 1991, Paul H. Brookes.

2. Capute AJ et al: Clinical linguistic and auditory milestone scale: prediction of cognition in infancy, *Dev Med Child Neurol 28*:762, 1986.

3. Capute AJ and Shapiro BK: The motor quotient: A method for the early detection of motor delay, *Am J Dis Child* 139:940, 1986.

4. Conners CK: A teacher rating scale to use in drug studies with children, *Am J Psychiatry* 126:884, 1969.

5. Dunn LM and Dunn LK: *Peabody Picture Vocabulary Test Form L-M*, Circle Pines Ill, 1981, American Guidance Service.

6. Frankenburg WK et al: The Denver II: a major restandarization of the Denver Developmental Screening Test, *Pediatrics* 89:91, 1992.

7. Glover EM, Preminger JL and Sanford AR: The Early Learning Accomplishment Profile for developmentally young children. Winston-Salem, NC, 1978, Kaplan Press.

8. Goodenough FL: *Measurement of intelligence by drawings*, New York, 1926, Harcort, Brace and World.

9. Hoon AH et al: Clinical adaptive test/clinical linguistic auditory milestone scale in early cognitive assessment, *J Pediatr* 123:51, 1993.

10. Illingworth RS: *The development of the infant and young child, abnormal and normal*, Edinburgh, Scotland, 1985, Churchill Livingstone.

11. Jastek J and Jastek S: *The Wide Range Achievement Test Revised*, Wilmington, Del, 1984, Jastek Associates.

12. Koppitz EM: *The Bender-Gestalt Test for young children*, New York, 1963, Grune and Stratton.

13. Montgomery TR: The neurodevelopmental assessment of the school age child. In Capute A and Accardo P, editors: *Developmental disabilities in infancy and childhood*, Baltimore, 1991, Paul H. Brookes.

14. Rossman MJ et al: Infant assessment: comparison of the CAT/CLAMS and the Bayley MDI, *Dev Med Child Neurol Suppl* 66(34):8, 1992.

15. Sanford AR and Zelman JG: *Learning Accomplishment Profile*, Winston-Salem, NC, 1981, Kaplan Press.

16. Taylor EM: *Psychological appraisal of children with cerebral defects*, Cambridge, Mass, 1961, Harvard University Press.

CHAPTER **25**

Case Management and Service Coordination

ROBERT F. BIEHL

The complexity of our existing service systems for children with chronic illness and disability creates an almost impenetrable obstacle to families seeking to understand and address the problems of their child with special needs. This is particularly true during those times when a family's coping ability and resources are especially taxed, such as: when the child's condition and its implications are first identified and the family must learn new terminology, interface with unfamiliar professionals, and find funds and other supports to manage the new burden; when interventions fail and new and often more expensive or dangerous options are proposed; or during periods of transition when the child moves from one set of expectations to another (i.e., hospital to home, home to school, school to employment, etc.).

During such times for nearly all families, and at almost all times for families with lesser coping reserves, families need a ready source of support, information, guidance, direct assistance, and individual advocacy. This source must be perceived as accessible, concerned, competent, and effective. Case management has been created to address this need.

DEFINITIONS

The terms *case management* and *service coordination* are used by various professions and industries in differing ways. For example, the insurance industry commonly uses the term *case management* to describe benefits management functions, while physicians may use it synonymously with *medical management.* Social service professionals have long used the terms to

259

describe strategies for "promoting coordination of human services, opportunities, or benefits,"[5] and more recently, as an "active process for implementing intervention services that promote and support a family's capacities and competencies to identify, obtain, coordinate, monitor and evaluate resources and services to meet its needs."[4] In the Omnibus Reconciliation Act (OBRA) of 1989, Title V, the legislation responsible for guiding the federal Maternal and Child Health Program, defined care coordination as "services to promote the effective and efficient organization and utilization of resources to assure access to necessary comprehensive services for children with special health care needs and their families."*

As used in this chapter the term *case management* includes the common elements of patient focus, direct and indirect service provision, service coordination across programs and over time, and assurance of achieving planned goals. These services are directed not only at meeting immediate needs but also at building a family's competence and independent capacity to meet future needs. Benefits management, medical management, and system advocacy functions are addressed in other sections of this book.

FACTORS RELATING TO THE NEED FOR CASE MANAGEMENT

The importance of case management and its emergence as a crucial component of the system of services for children with special needs can be related both to changes in the structure and process of the service delivery system and to the increasing numbers of children surviving with chronic impairments who once would have perished at birth or in early childhood.

The system changes include a major shift from center-based, large-institutional care to community-based services, fragmentation of the delivery system through the creation of multiple, parallel, and uncoordinated categorical programs, growing specialization in service provision, increasing technologic sophistication, and proliferation of new funding mechanisms. Relatively simple plans of care that once were managed by a single center-based physician have become highly complex and sophisticated, involving services from several types of providers, operating through many organizations, delivering care at various geographically separated sites, and funded through uncoordinated benefits plans, often with conflicting eligibility criteria.

Interfacing with this complicated new service system is a growing population of children with complex and often expensive service needs that not infrequently exceed the comfort level if not the professional capacity of their

---

*Omnibus Reconciliation Act of 1989, Title V, Section 501, 1989.

community providers. Children with chronic conditions of moderate or greater severity now make up approximately 10% of the childhood population,[6] and their effect on the service delivery system is different and proportionally much greater than that of children who seek care only for acute illnesses and injuries[1] (Table 25-1).

Because effects are cumulative over the duration of a chronic illness or disability, the cost of duplication or misutilization of resources and services can become very significant, exhausting time, energy, and funds that neither the individual nor society can afford to waste. Case management seeks both to avoid duplication and ensure appropriate use of the services provided, thereby reducing cost while maintaining benefit.

Table 25-1. Differentiating Characteristics of Acute and Chronic Illness

Characteristics	Acute Illness	Chronic Illness
Duration	Brief	Prolonged; often lifelong and crossing many developmental periods
Scope	Often limited to a single organ or system; little effect upon self-image or independence	Typically involves multiple functions/systems; strong effect on self-esteem and independence
Presentation and course	Limited variation, course highly predictable; often a tendency for improvement without medical help	Much variation within diagnostic categories; tendency to lose further function without help
Effect	Limited	Coping skills and resources of individual and family stressed over prolonged periods
Management	Commonly managed by single discipline (medicine)	Often involves many disciplines, each with their own terminology
Cost of mismanagement	Often not recognized; unnecessary studies and over-management costs occur over limited duration	Unnecessary costs accumulate over time; drain on limited resources may preclude needed measures

Modified from Wallace HM, Biehl RF, and Oglesby AC: *Handicapped children and youth: a comprehensive community and clinical approach,* New York, 1987, Human Sciences Press, Inc.

GOALS AND PRINCIPLES

From the system's perspective, case management has the dual goals of containing costs and improving the distribution and utilization of limited resources. While avoiding misutilization and ensuring economy are also important to the individual, the principal goals for patients relate more to better service access, improved outcomes of treatment, patient satisfaction, and development of the individual's capacity to act independently in the system.

Case management can facilitate the achievement of these goals through observance of certain basic principles. Case management services should be accessible; they should not be limited by artificial categories of eligibility or restrictive program mandates. Services should be easily accessible to families where they live (decentralized, community based) and when families wish to use them. They should recognize and be responsive to the unique individual and cultural characteristics of the child, family, and community and should respond to the family's own perception of needed services rather than the system's preconception of those needs (family centered, culturally sensitive). Services should be structured to provide coordination across all involved programs and services at each point in time (cross-sectional continuity) and over time (longitudinal continuity). Finally, they should involve the child and family as partners in the process, building the family's competence, comfort, and self-sufficiency and preparing them to assume eventual responsibility for their own service coordination and self-advocacy.

CASE MANAGEMENT ACTIVITIES

Each child and family functions within a support network that includes three major components: (1) a professional component served by physicians, other human service providers, public and private programs, etc.; (2) a mutual care component comprising the informal supports available from other family members, friends and neighbors, church groups, and community service organizations; and (3) a self-care component that includes the sum of the disabled individual's daily living skills, education, physical mobility, interpersonal skills, and capacity for self-advocacy.[5] Case management activities involve interactions affecting all of these components, doing so through a process of individual needs assessment, prioritization and planning, resource discovery, access facilitation, and outcome monitoring. Typical activities might include working with a family and involved professionals to identify a child's self-care strengths and needs; creating a comprehensive and coordinated individual service plan that addresses each identified need in accordance with the family's perception of its importance;

identifying existing options for needed services and funding; helping a family obtain professional services, coordinate appointments, and arrange transportation; and assisting families to develop and use interim, neighborhood, mutual care resources.

In addition to patient-focused activities, case management can also involve certain system-focused activities performed on behalf of the individual child and family. Such activities are intended to influence the system to serve or improve service to the case manager's patient and might include, for example, efforts to have a community program expand eligibility, modify an administrative procedure, or add a specific accommodation needed by the specific patient. Although changes resulting from these activities may also benefit others in the community, the focus here is on meeting the needs of the targeted patient, a difference that distinguishes the advocacy of case management from that practiced by advocacy groups interested in general system expansion or reform.

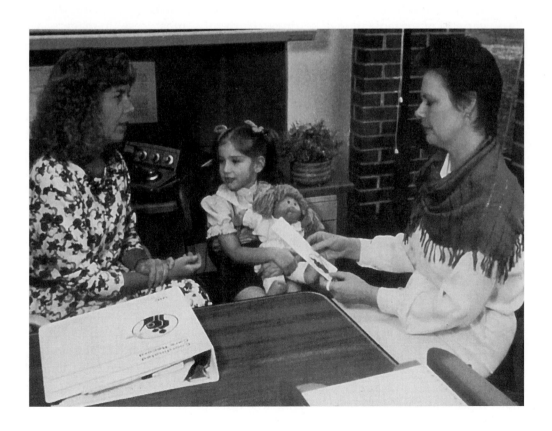

The type and level of activities performed on behalf of, or with the family, also vary according to the capacity of the family to participate in the process. Although a basic objective of case management is the promotion of patient autonomy and independence, most case managers initially exercise a high measure of direct involvement in their patient's service plan. At this initial stage the case manager's activities might include direct referrals, assisting with completing applications for program benefits, or arranging transportation to appointments. As competence and confidence increases, however, families are encouraged to reduce their dependence, and the role of the case manager shifts from direct agency to that of teacher, guide, facilitator, and collaborator. Finally, as the family acquires the competence to exercise full self-direction, the case manager retreats to the role of consultant, responding with information and providing services only when and to the degree requested by the family.[7]

CASE MANAGEMENT SETTINGS

The above activities can be performed by case managers working from a variety of organizational settings. Currently, most case managers are employed in institutional settings such as public and private agencies, hospitals, managed care organizations, etc., where they commonly have the coexisting responsibilities of allocation and conservation of their employer's program benefits. Others work in grant-supported programs where their activities are dictated by the scope and limitations of the grant. It can be argued that a conflict of interest exists between the benefits management functions of an agency-employed case manager and those functions performed primarily in support of an individual child and family. For example, a case manager must constantly ask whether scarce program resources should be allocated to their own patient or conserved for use by others with perhaps greater need.

A logical solution to this conflict would be the creation of independent case management entities, free from the influence of service and funding providers, where a case manager has only one loyalty. Unfortunately, case management as currently practiced is labor intensive and relatively expensive.

Health insurance plans seldom include independent case management as a reimbursable benefit, few families are able to afford case management out of pocket, and the few existing publicly supported independent entities (i.e., those associated with programs like IDEA and Medicaid) tend to be limited by the scope and requirements of their sponsoring programs. Practically then, at least as long as the service system is constituted and funded as it is now, the conflict must be mitigated through strict separation of the benefits management and case manager functions within the responsible agencies. Though an imperfect solution, agencies can be structured to preserve the integrity of both functions and the conflict can be rendered manageable if staffs are regularly reminded of their differing responsibilities.

AUTOMATION IN CASE MANAGEMENT

Many of the more time consuming, labor intensive, and tedious activities associated with case management have the potential to be eased considerably through the use of modern electronic information storage and data processing. The advantages of this new tool can be realized in three general areas: (1) patient records and plan monitoring, (2) resource identification, and (3) program management.

Patient-related information can be stored, retrieved, and corrected electronically far more quickly than with paper-dependent systems. Service plans can be updated to reflect the child and family's latest array of services and can be preprogrammed to issue reminders to the case manager at important plan junctures (scheduled follow-ups, eligibility redetermination dates, etc.). Plan activity can also be monitored to follow service usage, identify missed appointments, and track progress toward plan objectives.

Information about the location, type, benefits, and eligibility criteria of community resources can also be stored, corrected, and kept current in user-friendly electronic directories. Using these databases, case managers can search for and identify appropriate services in a fraction of the time that a paper or phone search would require. In addition, lookup capability can be expanded to any site with a phone link, and with minimal training these data can be made available to patient families for independent use.

Finally, managers of case management agencies can use automated systems to improve agency efficiency and effectiveness. Caseloads can be monitored and balanced, case manager activity and performance can be compared against agency standards, and patient satisfaction with agency services can be routinely and automatically surveyed and assessed.

These potential advantages of automation are only just beginning to be realized in this country. Organizations such as the National Center for Case Management and Automation are actively exploring and promoting automation and can predict with some assurance that future case management systems will employ this very valuable tool in ways not yet imagined.[8] However, even the best of systems will be hampered until certain basic problems are solved.

UNMET NEEDS

As stated at the beginning of this chapter, the existing fragmented, highly categorical, and uncoordinated system of services for children with special health care needs taxes not only the capacity of families seeking care but that of all those attempting to assist them. Until the system is simplified, uniform eligibility criteria developed, gaps in type and distribution of services eliminated, access assured, and funding streams unified, even the most efficient and cost-effective case management program will fail to some degree.

The problem of the inherent conflict between benefits management and patient advocacy discussed earlier also requires a better solution than currently exists. For children with special health care needs (CSHCN), this may occur as Title V CSHCN programs give up their traditional roles as service providers and third party payers and redirect their attention and funding to individual and family service planning, plan coordination, resource promotion, and quality assurance.

To ensure that case management services are available to all those with the potential to benefit from them, the system must also address the issues of professional preparation, qualification, and numbers of case managers. Most current case managers gain their skills through on-the-job experience. Though many possess a foundation in a health or human service discipline, few have received any formal training in such areas as group process, planning, service coordination, resource utilization, or quality assurance. Some colleges of social work are now beginning to offer their students opportunities for cross training in health-related areas, and nursing education has long recognized the importance of social support and patient advocacy in a nurses practice. Unfortunately, there is as yet no formal discipline of case management nor any nationally recognized standard curriculum for the training of independent case managers. Only recently has there been any attempt made to certify practitioners working in the field to ensure that they possess the basic knowledge and experience required. If the health care system is ever to benefit fully from the advantages of case management, it must first produce professionals with a consistent and reliable set of competencies, ensure that they are trained in adequate numbers, credential them appropriately, and then place them in positions with the authority, resources, and tools to do what is needed.[2,3]

CONCLUSION

The growing number of children with chronic disability and illness and the increasingly complex system serving their needs and the needs of their families produce an overriding need for competent case managers working from an independent base and possessing the skills and tools necessary to engage families, access needs, identify appropriate resources, and ensure necessary service delivery. Case management services should be easily accessible, community based, family oriented, culturally sensitive, and coordinated across programs and over time. Although managers commonly exercise a high degree of control over a new patient's service plan, the basic objective of case management is the promotion of patient autonomy and independence.

Because case management is labor intensive it tends to be expensive and managers have difficulty serving large caseloads. Automation can make the process more efficient and offers additional opportunities for improvements in practice management and resource identification.

Unsolved problems in case management include unnecessarily complex health care and funding systems, inherent conflicts between the case management and benefits management activities of organizations that engage in both functions, and the lack of any formally recognized and uniformly prepared discipline with primary responsibility for the activity. Despite these problems, case management has been accepted as an essential component of today's system of services for children with chronic impairments and their families. It offers one of the most effective means of matching recognized needs with available services and ensuring optimal use of existing

REFERENCES

1. Biehl RF: Definitions. In Wallace H et al, editors: *Handicapped children and youth*, New York, 1987, Human Sciences Press.
2. Certification of Insurance Rehabilitation Specialists Commission: Certification for Case Managers, Rolling Meadows, Ill, 1993, The Commission.
3. Dinerman M: Managing the maze: case management and service delivery, *Administration in Social Work*, 16(1), 1992.
4. Jackson B, Finkler D, and Robinson C: A case management system for infants with chronic illness and developmental disabilities, *Children's Health Care 21:4*, 1992.
5. Moxley DP: *The practice of case management*, Newberry Park, Calif, 1989, Sage Publications.
6. Newacheck PW and Taylor WR: Childhood chronic illness: prevalence, severity, and impact, *Am J Public Health* 82:364-371, 1992.
7. Swan WW and Morgan JL: *Collaborating for comprehensive services for young children and their families: coordination of case management*, Baltimore, 1992, Paul H. Brookes.
8. Wainstock L, Director, National Center for Case Management and Automation: unpublished correspondence, 1993.

CHAPTER 26

Team Organization and Function

CORDELIA C. ROBINSON

The concept of teams comprising professionals from a number of disciplines has been a ubiquitous concept in the diagnosis and treatment of persons with disabilities or chronic illness since the inception of the concepts of rehabilitation and habilitation services. Added to this emphasis on the use of interdisciplinary teams for the last 8 to 10 years has been the concept of culturally competent[24] community-based, coordinated, family-centered care[5,20,25] as the value base for the design of services for children with disabilities or chronic illness and their families. In this chapter we examine the progression in concepts of team organization and function over the past 5 decades in the context of the current value base and legislative mandates for services for children with disabilities or chronic illness.

DEFINITION

In this text the focus is on interdisciplinary teams that address the combined health and habilitative, educational, psychologic, and social needs of children with disabilities or chronic illness and their families. In this regard Ducanis and Golin,[6] and Golin and Ducanis[14] define an interdisciplinary team as "a functioning unit, composed of individuals with varied and specialized training, who coordinate their activities to provide services to a client or group of clients."[6] In developing this definition the authors drew upon dictionary definitions of team and teamwork that, in this case, included the essential elements of (1) "a number of persons," (2) "function[ing] as a collaborative unit," (3) "each doing a clearly defined portion," and (4) "subordinating personal prominence to the efficiency of the whole."[6] Each of these elements is important to the underlying rationale for and philosophy regarding the importance of interdisciplinary teams in providing family-centered, community-based, coordinated, culturally competent care for children with disabilities or chronic illness.

In addition to considering the basic definition in their books on interdisciplinary teams in health care[6] and education of exceptional children[14] Golin and Ducanis address team composition, functions, and tasks as characteristics that will help clarify the concept of team approach. These characteristics are summarized in the box on p. 270 and will be addressed in more detail as we consider the issue of how to build well functioning interdisciplinary teams that address the functional outcomes of independence, productivity, inclusion,[34] and participation[29] for the children with whom we are concerned.

Ducanis and Golin[6] cite three major factors as particularly significant in the emergence of the team approach: (1) the concept of the whole patient, (2) the needs of the organization, and (3) mandates from outside the organization.

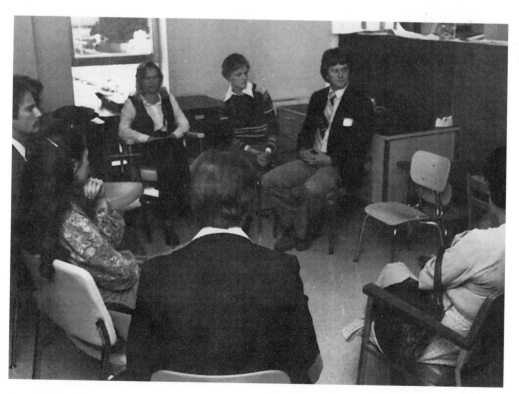

From Stanhope, Lancaster: *Community health nursing,* ed 3, St Louis, 1992, Mosby–Year Book.

Summary of Characteristics of Interdisciplinary Teams[6]

- A team consists of two or more individuals.
- There may be face-to-face or non–face-to-face configurations.
- There is an identifiable leader; however, leadership may shift.
- Teams function both within and between organizational settings.
- Roles of participants are defined.
- Teams collaborate.
- There are specific protocols of operation.
- The team is client centered.
- The team is task oriented.

The whole client. A holistic view of the individual is one of an integrated whole in which problems are interrelated and cannot be adequately treated in isolation and therefore require the expertise of many disciplines working together. A holistic view includes a recognition that development is integrated and organized across domains[32] and therefore health care and habilitative treatment efforts require knowledge and expertise of child development drawn from multiple disciplines.

Needs of the organization. As intervention services for children with disabilities have grown over the past 2 decades, the interaction between health, education, and social service systems has increased considerably, thereby requiring interdisciplinary teams to function both within and across organizations. As more specialized interventions become available the " ...need for clarifying the lines of communication and authority within the agency becomes increasingly acute."[6]

Mandates external to the organization. The last 3 decades have been ones where an interdisciplinary team approach has been supported by federal mandate, particularly federal education mandates.[2,8] The fact that a team approach is mandated is at least in part a function of the consensus in health and education disciplines that such an approach is necessary for quality comprehensive diagnosis, treatment, care, and education for children with developmental disabilities or chronic illness.

DEVELOPMENT OF THE TEAM APPROACH IN DEVELOPMENTAL DISABILITIES OR CHRONIC ILLNESS

The need for a team approach in health and human services has long been noted.[15] In briefly tracing this history Ducanis and Golin[6] noted that during the 1940s the team concept gained importance in the context of rehabilitative needs for veterans and in community-based primary health care teams. During the 1950s, 1960s, and 1970s the interdisciplinary team concept was applied to a range of issues. In the field of mental retardation and related disabilities, considerable impetus was given to the interdisciplinary team approach through the initiation in the middle and late 1960s of University Affiliated Facilities—now University Affiliated Programs (UAPs)—by the Bureau of Maternal and Child Health (MCH).[3,21,24] MCH placed a priority on preparing leadership personnel from a number of disciplines including pediatrics, psychiatry, nursing, nutrition, clinical psychology, and physical, occupational, and speech therapy. Collaboration among these disciplines was considered to be essential for effective diagnosis and treatment for persons with mental retardation and related disabilities. A unique feature of the UAPs was the requirement that this leadership training include training in working on interdisciplinary teams. In the 1970s and 1980s the number of UAPs expanded through funding from an additional federal agency, the Administration on Developmental Disabilities. Thus much of the articulation of the interdisciplinary team concept and a significant extent of the preparation of professionals from many disciplines has occurred within the UAP network.

Types of Teams

In this chapter the term *interdisciplinary team* has been selected as the most inclusive term to describe the collaborative efforts of health and education disciplines involved in diagnosis and treatment of children with developmental disabilities or chronic illness. Other terms that have been used extensively include *multidisciplinary* and *transdisciplinary* and consequently warrant some attention here. The term *multidisciplinary* was used especially in the late 1960s and early 1970s, particularly in the context of UAPs[24]; it was intended simply as a description of the fact that a number of disciplines were included among the team members. The term *interdisciplinary* came to be emphasized with the reasoning that *interdisciplinary* carried more of a connotation of collaboration. Most recently the term *transdisciplinary* has received considerable attention, particularly in the field of early intervention.[28] The concept of a transdisciplinary team was introduced in early intervention work by Haynes[17] in the United Cerebral Palsy early intervention program. The concept of transdisciplinary teamwork includes all of the concepts already discussed but adds the characteristic of identifying a lead person who works directly with the patient incorporating the recommendations and strategies from the other disciplines.

The transdisciplinary approach was originally developed in response to a lack of available personnel to carry out individual early intervention services, particularly from occupational, physical, and speech therapies. By identifying one person as the primary person to work directly with the client, the resources of the team were extended to a greater number of children and families. Early intervention leaders[13,23,28] argue that the transdisciplinary model represents the most refined and laudatory level of teamwork. In my opinion some of the contrasts drawn among the models are artificial and use multidisciplinary and interdisciplinary as foils for a transdisciplinary model.[28] Parent participation, for example, is portrayed in the transdisciplinary model as encompassing the current values of parent empowerment at the expense of the other models. For me, the meaningful distinction between interdisciplinary and transdisciplinary is the use of a primary interventionist in the transdisciplinary model.

The other elements presented by Woodruff and McGonigel[28] are qualitative standards that may serve as guidelines for the functioning of any health and/or educational intervention team. For example, in regard to guiding philosophy, the characterization of transdisciplinary team is the only statement that captures the characteristics previously cited as defining teamwork. Critical features of this statement regarding guiding philosophy include the following: (1) the emphasis on collaboration (i.e., commitment to teach, learn, and work together), and (2) the patient as the focus (i.e., to implement a unified service plan). Thus while much has been made in the early intervention literature of distinctions among the types of teams, these distinctions tend to be more rhetorical than real,[22] and the ultimate test of a team is not how it refers to itself but how it functions.

ESSENTIAL ELEMENTS OF EFFECTIVE TEAMWORK

Literature from various fields, including education, health, and policy, is all convergent in the identification of the importance of teamwork.* In promoting the concept of teams there is also considerable agreement regarding the elements of effective teamwork. An example of an effective program for developing an interdisciplinary team is Project Bridge. Project Bridge,[16,24] conducted by the American Academy of Pediatrics, was a nationwide effort in which states participated by sending interdisciplinary teams to a central location in their state to participate in inservice training as a team. Since this effort a number of programs advocate that training for teams should occur within the context of the team if the training is to be effective.

References 2, 5, 8, 10, 11, 13, 14, 18, 20, 21.

Group development/endorsement of mission. There is unanimity across fields regarding the necessity for group development/endorsement of a mission statement and guiding philosophy if a team is to be effective.[1,11,16,26] A team's mission will be influenced by the context of the team, which may be individual child and family oriented or systems-development oriented such as a community interagency team. To address this mission, "best practice" in relation to team work indicates that the group needs to put the mission into the form of a statement defining the target group or beneficiaries, the goals of the team, and the anticipated outcomes.[16,26]

Principle of interdependence. Members need each other to accomplish their goals. Effective interdisciplinary teams working with children and families need to recognize that "no one area of the child's functioning is the exclusive concern of any one discipline; no one discipline should limit others' participation in the decision-making process, and that each member should be encouraged to share observations and contribute recommendations."[16]

Commitment/consensus. Each individual team member must be committed to accepting the team's mission, goals, and strategies as defined within the group process.

Resources. Teams must have the resources to accomplish their mission and goals. Included among the resources are leadership, access to information, agreements and cooperation, and opportunities to increase knowledge and skills.

Accountability. The context of the team (agency/interagency) will influence its functioning. While ultimate accountability is to children and families, the context and culture of the host agency will influence the team's functioning.

BUILDING A TEAM

Project Bridge offers a process for team building that begins with an individual and team assessment to clarify values. One of the key benefits of a team approach is the value derived from the diversity of team members. With this diversity of disciplines there also will be diversity in points of view. To be effective teams must acknowledge that this diversity exists, and where there are differences in underlying values these differences must be examined and agreements forged that everyone can accept. A sampling of the items included in the Project Bridge assessment tool are presented in the boxes on p. 274 and 275. The basic core of Project Bridge training is a problem-solving process. The five-step decision-making process presented in Project Bridge is a general one that comes from work on problem-oriented record keeping and strategic planning. The steps of the process are outlined in Table 26-1. These same steps are used in Project Bridge to address team building itself.

Self-Assessment

Practice Attitudes

To what extent do you think a child's family should be involved in selecting and implementing a service plan for an at-risk child or a child with disabilities?

1	2	3	4	5

They should be treated as a full member of the team throughout the process

They should be involved only at critical points in the decision process

They should be kept fully informed of decisions so they can cooperate effectively

Decision Making

How satisfied are you with your role in the team's decision making?

1	2	3	4	5

Completely satisfied

My role should be modified (either expanded or reduced)

Not at all satisfied

Team Dynamics and Personal Characteristics

To what extent have you worked to enhance team cohesiveness and mutual understanding?

1	2	3	4	5

A great deal

I try occasionally but could do more

Not at all

Developing the Team Action Plan

The Project Bridge self and team assessments are designed to assist teams in identifying characteristics of its members and aspects of team functioning that may affect the teams' effectiveness. These areas of team functioning include: (1) consistency in values/philosophy among team members, (2) decision-making strategies, and (3) team dynamics and characteristics of leadership. In Project Bridge teams use the same process for addressing their development and refinement that the team is expected to use to address its mission. A point that has become very clear with review of the literature on teams, and from clinical experience, is that development and maintenance of effective interdisciplinary team functioning is difficult, time consuming, and requires constant vigilance.

Team Assessment

Practice Characteristics

	Response 1	Response 2
Attitudes toward people with disabilities	Value of the child as a human being with worth and potential is a major influence on team discussions and decisions.	Team discussions and decisions focus primarily on the difficulties presented by the developmental disabilities.

Characteristics of the Decision-Making Process

	Response 1	Response 2
Implementation	An organized plan for implementation is developed to which all team members are committed.	Plan for implementation and the commitment of members to the plan is not always clear.

Characteristics of Team Dynamics

	Response 1	Response 2
Attitudes	Team members feel a strong commitment to team goals.	Some members pursue individual goals at the expense of team goals.
Cohesion	Team's mission is clear and there is a high level of cooperation in achieving it.	Mission is unclear and team members act like a collection of individuals each with his or her own agenda.
Goals	Our team's overall goals are clear and strongly supported by all team members.	Overall goals are vague, poorly understood, and/or not accepted by all team members.
Conflict	Our team has generally effective methods of resolving inter- and intra-group conflicts quickly and constructively.	Inter- and intra-group conflicts are often allowed to escalate to the point of impeding effective team functioning.

TABLE 26-1. Problem Solving Process

Step	Action
1. Problem Definition/ Information Gathering	Questions and methods of information gathering will vary depending upon the function (assessment, individual plan development, systems development) team is addressing.
2. Generating Alternatives Relative to Exemplary Services	In this step of problem solving the process involves generating a number of alternatives and solutions to the identified problem. It is essential that a number of approaches be identified and at this step no judgment be made as to the worthiness of individual ideas.
3. Selecting Alternatives	In this step the task is to systematically evaluate the benefits of each alternative in light of congruence with program mission/philosophy, quality indicators or optimal standards, family preferences, intended outcomes, and possible unintended effects.
4. Implementation	This step involves the actual testing of the selected alternative. The team should have developed a detailed plan. If for some reason the plan cannot be implemented as developed, then the team needs to meet again to revise the plan.
5. Monitoring	The plan developed in Step 3 should have included statements of desired outcomes. In monitoring, the team evaluates whether those outcomes have been accomplished. If the desired outcomes are not accomplished, explanations are sought. If the results are unacceptable, the team should do the following: • consider the reasons for the lack of success • select another alternative to implement • go through the problem-solving process again

Involvement of the Consumer on the Team

A major and welcome innovation that has occurred in the context of the current values base for the development of teams is that of consumer involvement on the team.[12] However, involving consumers as respected team members is certainly easier in word than in deed.[1] A number of reasons for this difficulty as well as strategies for addressing them are presented in the top box on p. 277.[1] To the extent that teams consist primarily of a group of employed individuals and the consumer, the team will have a structure and a history to which the consumer does not have access. This inherent inequality needs to be articulated, and the team must work with consumers to identify strategies that will address this inequality and accomplish meaningful consumer involvement. Some possible strategies are outlined in the bottom box below.[1]

Emphasis on Functional Outcomes

It was noted earlier in the chapter that part of the rationale for interdisciplinary teamwork is the nature of development and how development in one domain is related to development in other domains.[32] The recognition of the interrelated nature of development across domains, the growing maturity of interdisciplinary teams, and the mandate for including people with disabilities have all led to an emphasis on setting functional goals that are integrated across areas of development and that are not discipline specific. The top box on p. 278 lists five essential components for teams to consider when developing functional integrated goals.[11]

Family Involvement in the Team Meeting and Decision Making[1]

Why is it difficult for families to feel like they are really part of a team?
- Professionals often discount parent perspectives or priorities.
- Professionals often see the child only from their discipline's perspective.
- Parents often enter poorly functioning groups.
- Parents often are not involved in the initial planning stages.
- Parents are not given legitimate/meaningful roles on the team.
- Parents often are not prepared for or supported in their involvement in meetings.
- A group of professionals can be very intimidating, whether it is intentional or not.

Strategies for Facilitating Family Involvement[1]

- Offer choices for involvement from the beginning.
- Focus the assessment process and the team meeting on parents' concerns.
- Involve families in child assessment to the extent they want to be involved.
- Conduct individual preconference meetings with families.
- Ensure good communication skills on the part of all team members.
- Organize meetings in ways to maximize parent involvement.
- Agree on team goals and philosophy.
- Develop a structure or plan for decision making.
- Learn to disagree effectively.
- Support the development of each team member.
- Ensure effective leadership.

Standards of Interdisciplinary Team Functioning

Another recent influence on the functioning of teams is the identification of standards for quality assurance. An interdisciplinary/interagency group known as New England SERVE has identified a number of standards for the practice of professionals and teams and the agencies in which they function that are based on the values of family-centered, community-based, coordinated care. Areas of responsibility for quality assurance practice standards for teams and agencies from this group are presented in the bottom box below.[7]

Guidelines for Functional Goals

- Goals and objectives belong to the learner, not to individual team members.
- All team members are responsible for contributing information and skills to the process of defining goals and objectives.
- Many specialized disciplinary methods and skills, many of which can be taught to other team members.
- Activities that the individual child selects are the logical and necessary focus for the identification and integration of effective intervention.
- Combining methods from a variety of disciplines allows the team to address the needs of the learner more successfully.

Enhancing Quality Standards

The health care professional or team:
- delivers care resulting in health status outcomes consistent with optimal expectations for children with special health care needs
- maintains a high level of education and training
- responds to the needs of families as defined by families
- coordinates care with others delivering services
- derives professional satisfaction and growth in delivering care

The health care agency or facility:
- delivers and/or collaborates in delivering a wide range of services
- facilitates family-centered care through its administrative practices
- supports providers in their delivery of care to children
- delivers care in a cost-effective manner
- ensures safe care within its physical facility

Benefits of Effective Team Functioning

There are a number of benefits to be derived from effective team functioning. These benefits occur for staff and agencies and to children and their families. Interdisciplinary teams provide benefits to children with disabilities or chronic illness and their families by providing services that address all the interrelated needs of the individual: emotional, social, economic, educational, and medical. Best practice draws upon the skills and knowledge of all team members with the needs of the children and their families defining the desired outcomes and strategies for accomplishing those outcomes. Interdisciplinary teams also provide benefits to professional members with opportunities for collaboration with others that enable team members to test their own assumptions and subject them to rigorous review. Effective team decision making ensures that all members have participated in, are satisfied with, and are committed to the decisions made. Such effectiveness in team functioning increases the probability of appropriate services for the child and family and enhanced functioning of the professionals and ultimately the agencies that employ them.

REFERENCES

1. Bailey DB, Jr. et al: *Implementing family-centered services in early intervention: a team-based model for change*, Chapel Hill, NC, 1992, Carolina Institute for Research on Infant Personnel Preparation, Frank Porter Graham Child Development Center, University of North Carolina at Chapel Hill.
2. Brown W: *Early intervention regulation: annotation and analysis of Part H*, Horsham, Penn, 1990, LRP Publications.
3. Crocker AC and Cullinane MM: The use of teams and their limitations. *Developmental-Behavioral Pediatrics*, Philadelphia, 1983, WB Saunders Co.
4. Dokecki PR and Heflinger CA: Strengthening families of young handicapped children with handicapping conditions: mapping backwards from the "street level." In Gallagher JJ, Trohanis PL, and Clifford RM, editors: Policy implementation and PL 99-457: planning for young children with special needs, Baltimore, 1989, Paul H. Brookes.
5. Edelman L: *Recognizing family-centered care: a group exercise*, Baltimore, 1991, The Kennedy Institute.
6. Ducanis AJ and Golin AK: *The interdisciplinary health care team: a handbook*, Germantown, Md, 1979, Aspen Systems Corporation.
7. Epstein SG et al: *Enhancing quality*, Boston, 1989, New England SERVE.
8. Federal Register. Title I, Part H, Early Intervention for Handicapped Infants and Toddlers. Individuals with Disabilities Amendments to the Education of the Handicapped Act of 1975. Federal Register. November 18, 1987; 52:44,352-44,363.
9. Fenichel E: *Promoting health through Part H*, National Early Childhood Technical Assistance System (NEC*TAS) and National Center for Clinical Infant Programs (NCCIP).
10. Fenichel ES and Eggbeer L: Preparing practitioners to work with infants, toddlers, and their families: four essential elements of training, *Infants and Young Children* 4:56-62, 1991.

11. Forbes EJ and Fitzsimons V: Education: The key for holistic interdisciplinary collaboration. In Hoeman SP, editor: *Holistic Nursing Practice*, Vol 7(4):1-10, Aspen Publishers.

12. Gallagher JJ, Trohanis PL and Cliffort RM: Policy implementation & PL 99-457: planning for young children with special needs, Baltimore, 1989, Paul H Brookes Publishing Co.

13. Garland CW and Linder TW: Administrative challenges in early intervention: staffing patterns and team models in infancy programs. In Jordan J et al editors: *Early childhood special education: birth to three*, Reston, Vir, 1989, Council for Exceptional Children.

14. Golin AK and Ducanis AJ: *The interdisciplinary team: a handbook for the education of exceptional children*, Rockville, Md, 1981, Aspen Systems Corporation.

15. Halstead LS: Team care in chronic illness: a critical review of the literature of the past 25 years, *Archives of physical medicine and rehabilitation* 57:507-511, 1976.

16. Handley EE and Spencer P: *Project Bridge: Decision-making for early services: a team approach*, Elk Grove, Ill, 1986, American Academy of Pediatrics.

17. Haynes U: The National Collaborative Infant Project. Tjossem TD editor: *Intervention strategies for high risk infants and young children*, Baltimore, 1976, University Park Press.

18. Hoeman SP: Forward. In Hoeman SP, editor: *Holistic nursing practice* 7(4):vi-vii, July 1993, Aspen Publishers.

19. Jaffe KB and Walsh PA: The development of the specialty rehabilitation home care team: supporting the creative thought process. In Hoeman SP, editor: *Holistic nursing practice* 7(4):36-41, July 1993, Aspen Publishers.

20. Johnson BH, McGonigel MJ and Kaufmann RK: *Guidelines and recommended practices for the Individualized Family Service Plan*, Washington, DC, 1989, Association for the Care of Children's Health.

21. Kilgo JL, Clarke BA and Cox AW, editors: *Interdisciplinary infant and family services training: a professional training model*, Richmond, Vir, 1990, University Affiliated Virginia Institute for Developmental Disabilities, Virginia Commonwealth University.

22. Lynch EW and Hanson MJ: *Developing cross-cultural competence: a guide for working with young children and their families*, Baltimore, 1992, Paul H Brookes Publishing Co.

23. McCollum J and Hughes M: *Staffing patterns and team models in infancy programs*. In Jordan J et al editors: *Early childhood special education: birth to three*, Reston, Vir, 1989, Council for Exceptional Children.

24. O'Neil SM and Newcomer B, editors: Social Systems and UAC Nursing. Proceedings of the sixth national workshop for Nurses in Mental Retardation, Cincinnati, Ohio, March 20-22, 1974, Maternal and Child Health Bureau of Community Health Services, U.S. Department of Health, Education and Welfare and The University Affiliated Cincinnati Center for Developmental Disorders.

25. Shelton T, Jeppson E, and Johnson B: *Family-centered care for children with special health care needs*, Washington, DC, 1987, Association for the Care of Children's Health.

26. Spencer P and Coye R: *Project Bridge: a team approach to decision-making for early services. infants and young children*, Aspen Publishers, 1988.

27. Stein REK: *Topics in early childhood special education: promoting communication between health care providers and educators of chronically ill children*, vol 5, Austin, Tex, 1986, PRO-ED Inc.

28. Woodruff G and McGonigel MJ: Early intervention team approach: the transdisciplinary model. In Gallagher JJ et al, editors: *Early childhood special education: birth to three*, Reston, Vir, 1988, Council for Exceptional Children.

CHAPTER **27**

Health Services

WILLIAM C. COOLEY

The confluence of four developments has illuminated new horizons for children with disabilities and chronic illness. First, the recognition of families as primary caregivers has refocused services on a consumer-driven agenda and has broadened the scope for the evaluation of needs and outcomes. Second, early, family-centered development and education interventions in natural, age-appropriate settings have emerged as fundamental entitlements for children with educational challenges. Schools have become more comfortable with and informed about fully including children with chronic medical conditions and disabilities in all aspects of school life. Third, communities have become more accepting of their citizens with special needs and have been enriched in the process. Finally, children with disabilities and chronic illnesses have benefited from technologic revolutions and attitudinal progress in health care and health services. This chapter addresses the final of these areas of importance while recognizing how the evolution of health services is inextricably related to issues of families, schools, and communities.

Nearly all children with chronic illnesses and most children with developmental disabilities enter the world of exceptionality through a door in the health care system. The diagnosis of chronic illness or major developmental disability is usually established and initially explained by a health care provider. More than 50% of the services provided to very young children with developmental disabilities are health care related.[3] Chronic conditions require ongoing medical monitoring, direct medical and surgical interventions, management of exacerbations and complications, health-related services at home, and individualized health care planning at school. As other chapters in this text describe, children with special health care needs utilize a complicated array of health services with multiple sources of funding, diverse histories, missions, and policies, and frequently, limited coordination and cohesion.

Adopting a community-based perspective, this chapter examines the range of health services important to children with chronic conditions. The discussion focuses on the critical importance of a primary care medical home and its vertical links to other levels of medical care and horizontal links to related services in the community. This chapter presents the concept of chronic illness management (CIM) in the primary care setting as an undeveloped and undersupported activity for primary health care providers, with suggestions for the expansion of this role.

COMMUNITY HEALTH SERVICES

The menu of health services provided in regional and community settings has grown over the past 25 years.[1] Availability of many services, including primary health care and access to financing for services, is still a problem for many socioeconomic levels and geographic regions. Many forces, such as earlier hospital discharge of medically complex children, the struggle of community hospitals to compete and survive, the growth of public and home health agencies, and the incorporation of health-related services into the educational plans of children with special needs, have fostered the expansion of community-based therapeutic and habilitative services.

Ideally, community-based services of importance to children with chronic conditions should revolve around an axis of primary health care services. These services are commonly provided by pediatricians, family physicians, physician assistants, and nurse practitioners in private office and clinic settings. Increasingly, medically underserved urban and rural areas are the sites for federally-supported community health centers if they are not already served by state maternal and child health programs or city/county health departments. Increasing responsibility for care and decision making has shifted toward the primary care level under new policies of community-based care and under new pressures from the economics of managed care.

Work such as that of Sia[10] in Hawaii has developed the concept of a primary care "medical home" for all children. Children with special health care needs are particularly vulnerable to fragmentation of care and to problems of communication and coordination because of their dependence on multiple levels of health care services and multiple agencies and programs for support services. These factors make the establishment of accessible primary care medical homes of particular importance to such children. The readiness and capacity of community primary care settings to assume new responsibilities for a population of children who use more services is a challenge discussed later in this chapter.

Primary care services in community settings often are closely linked to community hospital services through the hospital affiliations of the primary care providers. This link provides locally accessible diagnostic services, such as laboratory and medical imaging, and connections to secondary level specialists (e.g., ophthalmology, otolaryngology, and orthopedics) and to hospital-based nutrition or rehabilitative services (e.g., physical and occupational therapy). Home health or visiting nurse services have traditionally been organized around public health departments or through local, nonprofit, semicharitable organizations. As the demand for these services has grown and, in particular, become better reimbursed by third party payors, providers of home health care services now include large regional and national for-profit corporations. Some children with complex health care needs living at home require the services of several vendors of home-based services for a combination of nursing care and support for technical and mechanical devices (respirators, feeding equipment, and intravenous fluid pumps).

School Health Services

Like most children, children with chronic illness and disabilities who are at least 3 years old spend a substantial portion of their time in school settings. Health services for children with special educational needs, such as intermittent clean catheterization of the bladder in children with spina bifida or management of gastrostomy tube feedings for children unable to consume food orally, have been the subject of intense debate and litigation in the past. It is now widely accepted that such services must be provided as part of a child's individual educational plan to allow participation in public education in the least restrictive environment. Though direct health services at school have been perceived as the domain of the school nurse, many health-related procedures performed at school are organized and undertaken by nonmedical personnel such as teachers or classroom assistants.[7] In some areas the level of supervision of such procedures by school nurses or other qualified professionals is limited.

In addition to direct health services, many children receive therapeutic services including physical or occupational therapy as part of an individual educational plan. Many of these services are carried out at school on an individual or group basis in the context, more or less, of the educational environment (i.e., classroom, physical education program, or therapy room) as

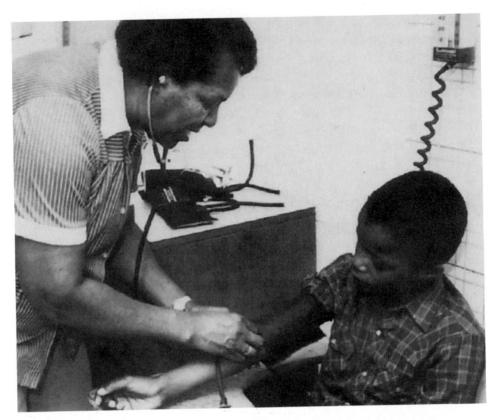

From Case-Smith J, Allen AS, Pratt PN: *Occupational therapy for children*, ed 3, St Louis, 1996, Mosby–Year Book.

opposed to the context of the school nurse or school-based health clinic. Though deemphasizing the medicalness of these therapeutic services is appropriate, the services themselves often require a medical authorization or doctor's order under state licensure and practice regulations for therapists. Primary care physicians are often called upon to sign orders for these services even when they may have been minimally involved in the decision making about what constitutes necessary or appropriate services for a given child.

Communication with a child's primary health care provider can be an even more complex dilemma for a school nurse. In many schools, the school nurse is the only noneducation professional. There are frequently indistinct lines of authority and poor interdisciplinary awareness of professional codes of conduct that place school nurses in stressful and vulnerable circumstances with regard to their responsibility for the health and well-being of children with chronic conditions. School nurses may or may not be involved in the educational plans for children with disabilities, they may or may not be expected to develop individual health care plans for children with complicated health problems, and they may or may not be supported to devote time to their own educational needs in serving such children. Many school nurses are uncertain about when to communicate with a child's primary health care provider, when to communicate with a child's specialists, and under what circumstances issues of confidentiality will affect the communication process. Often school nurses assume that a child's parents will provide the communication link between the school nurse and other health care services while parents may assume that the school nurse and a child's other health providers will communicate directly.

Under the Individuals with Disabilities Education Act (IDEA) individual states have planned and most have implemented an extension of entitlement to early developmental and educational services for young children with established conditions affecting development or with developmental delays. Some states have also chosen to include children at risk for developmental delay based on child- or family-based risk factors. These new entitlements reduce the age of eligibility for services from age 3 to birth. This early intervention component is referred to as Part H of IDEA, and policymakers have made strong efforts to clarify the role of health care providers in these services.[4]

CHALLENGES AND SOLUTIONS FOR HIGH-QUALITY HEALTH SERVICES

Other chapters in this volume emphasize the importance of service coordination and interorganizational collaboration. One of the fundamental prerequisites for successful coordination and collaboration is a clear, mutual understanding of the roles of key participants serving young children with disabilities and chronic medical conditions. Confusion based on implicit assumptions and poorly communicated expectations as well as insufficient attention to the full assessment of family needs has led to well-documented misconceptions about roles and responsibilities.[8,9] Though the solutions to this communication issue involve an array of training and technical support issues, the simple notion of explicitness, particularly in communications to parents and children, could help to clarify consumers' perceptions of professional roles. If primary care physicians, for example, set aside a role-defining and agenda-setting time with parents and children to review needs and to define the primary health care role in meeting those needs, then parents would experience less uncertainty about who will assist them with which specific issues.

The quality of health care services is an important aspect of the current national debate about health care reform. Though expanded access to services and control of health care costs have been the rallying points for most reform plans, the issue of quality services has been raised both as a need and as a variable among the effects of particular plans. Families of children with special health care needs have been particularly concerned about protecting the patchwork of supports and services developed over the past 60 years and with the opportunity to redefine those supports as components of a more generic and universal health care system.

Regardless of the outcome of health care reform at the statutory level, a revolution in the organization and financing of health care is nevertheless underway. The development and expansion of an array of managed care approaches is discussed in Chapter 5 of this book. However, the effect of managed care developments on health services for children with chronic conditions has important implications. Most managed care systems place the responsibility for decision making (sometimes called "gatekeeping") about specialized diagnostic and therapeutic health services in the hands of the primary health care provider. In many managed care plans there is a financial disincentive for primary care physicians to utilize more specialized services, particularly if they must be obtained outside the plan. There is also a financial disincentive for primary care providers to spend extra time with particular children since the monthly capitation payment for each child served by a provider remains the same regardless of how many visits occur or how lengthy the visits may be. Though these phenomena tend to reduce the overall cost of care in the system, they work specifically against the needs of many children with chronic conditions and their families.

Beyond issues of health care funding and reimbursement, primary care physicians have made clear statements about their lack of preparation for the provision of a medical home for children with disabilities and chronic conditions. Multiple studies and surveys over the past 25 years have documented a belief among practicing primary care physicians that they have received insufficient training in such areas as developmental disabilities, organization of community-based services, and the long-term care of children with chronic illnesses.[5,11,12] Most preservice training has involved practice models based in a medical center setting in which the care of children with special health care needs is presented through the eyes of the specialist or, at best, in the context of the multidisciplinary specialty clinic. While this training model may provide useful information about chronic conditions, the importance of care coordination, and interdisciplinary communication, it provides little exposure to community-based services and to the potential co-management role of the primary care provider. In addition, many specialty-based service models still fail to follow guidelines for the provision of family-centered care and therefore fail to model such approaches to trainees.[6]

Clearly the training of health service providers, particularly those planning careers in community-based, primary care settings, remains a crucial element in the enhancement of community care for children with special health care needs. It is important that training involve cross-disciplinary elements not only within the health-related professions, but within education, early intervention, social work, and mental health disciplines as well. Professionals in training need to develop a common, jargon-free language and a sensitivity to the roles, demands, and work ecology experienced by other professionals. Even more important, the voice of consumers, both parents and children, must be heard in medical school and university classrooms, and trainees must have multiple opportunities to experience the day-to-day demands that families face.[2]

Chronic Illness Management

Finally, a new role and set of primary health care activities called chronic illness management in primary care should be added to the traditional health maintenance and acute illness management services of the primary health care provider (see the box below). Providers of adult primary health care have always monitored the status of chronic health conditions through periodic problem-oriented visits; a similar role has not been developed in the primary health care of children. CIM in primary care requires a new mind-set during training, during service provision by specialists and primary care providers, and on the part of reimbursement systems. However, if properly prepared and reimbursed, primary care physicians could play a crucial role in the co-management of chronic conditions, in the coordination of community-based services, in the development of self-care skills in families and children, and as a reliable advocate for families.

Chronic Illness Management in the Primary Care Setting

Chronic illness management in the primary care setting is a specific primary care practice that acknowledges that children with chronic conditions and their families may require more than the usual well-child preventive care and acute illness interventions. Incorporating the elements of family-centered care and founded on a belief in community-based services, CIM involves explicit changes in the roles of the primary health care provider and the office staff. CIM goals include improving access to needed services, improving communication with specialists, schools, and other resources, and improving outcomes for children and families.

Chronic illness management may be initiated if a child's chronic medical condition meets one or more of the following criteria:

- significantly affects daily living and family life
- affects school performance
- affects development
- involves significant, ongoing specialty care
- involves multiple agencies or professionals
- causes a new crisis (because of hospitalization, accelerating office or ER visits, or major family stress)

REFERENCES

1. Brewer EJ et al: Family-centered, community-based, coordinated care for children with special health care needs, *Pediatrics* 83:1055-1060, 1989.

2. Cooley, WC: Pediatric training and family-centered care. In Darling R and Peter M, editors: *Families, physicians, and children with special health care needs: collaborative medical education models*, Southport, Conn, 1994, Greenwood Press.

3. Crocker AC: Partnerships in the delivery of medical care. In Rubin IL and Crocker AC, editors: *Developmental disabilities: delivery of medical care for children and adults*, Philadelphia, 1989, Lea & Febiger.

4. Fenichel E: *Promoting health through Part H*, Arlington, Vir, 1992, National Center for Clinical Infant Programs.

5. Guralnick MJ et al: Training future primary care pediatricians to serve handicapped children and their families, *Topics in early childhood special education* 6(4):1-11, 1987.

6. Johnson BH, Jeppson ES, and Redburn L: *Caring for children and families: guidelines for hospitals*, Washington, DC, 1992, Association for the Care of Children's Health.

7. Johnson MP and Assay M: Who meets the special health care needs of North Carolina school children? *J Sch Health* 63:417-420, 1993.

8. Liptak GS and Revell GM: Community physician's role in the case management of children with chronic illness, *Pediatrics* 84(3):465-471, 1989.

9. O'Sullivan P, Mahoney G, and Robinson C: Perceptions of pediatricians' helpfulness: a national study of mothers of young disabled children, *Dev Med Child Neurol* 34:1064-1071, 1992.

10. Sia CCJ and Peter MI: Physician involvement strategies to promote the medical home, *Pediatrics,* 85:128-130, 1990.

11. Task Force on Pediatric Education: *The future of pediatric education*, Elk Grove Village, Ill, 1978, American Academy of Pediatrics.

12. Wender EH, Bijur PE, and Boyce WT: Pediatric residency training: ten years after the Task Force report, *Pediatrics* 90:876-880, 1992.

CHAPTER 28

Oral Health Services

LYNETTE A. LANCIAL

Normalization and integration of children with disabilities into the community has made them and their families dependent on a community-based health care system for dental care. While integration into the community has been a boon to the social and emotional well-being of many children with special needs and their families, frustrations with disjointed health service provision exist. Before deinstitutionalization many children and young adults in residential facilities received their daily oral care assistance and supervision from institutional care staff and their dental treatment from an institutional dentist or in a tertiary care setting. However, in community settings families have a very difficult time finding accessible, affordable, and appropriate dental services for their children with disabilities and chronic illness.

Further complicating this situation is the fact that children with special health care needs are at greater risk for oral diseases and have greater unmet oral health care needs than other children.[11,14] In fact, dental treatment has been said to be the greatest unmet health need of persons with disabilities. There is general agreement that persons with disabilities experience higher rates of poor oral hygiene and periodontal disease.[15] Although there is less agreement relative to dental caries, recent data suggest children with special needs also experience a higher rate of tooth decay and have more untreated decayed teeth than other children.[22] Currently, dental caries is probably the most common disease found among all children in the United States, affecting more than 84% by age 17.[16] Therefore the even greater need for dental care by children with disabilities and chronic illness is a serious concern.

BARRIERS TO ORAL HEALTH

Why is there such a great unmet oral health need in this population of children who are known to be at risk for dental problems? This question has been discussed and researched by dental service providers with an interest in persons with special needs for more than 3 decades.[15,18] Unfortunately, data collection has often been specific to small regional groups or select disabilities and illnesses and therefore conclusions cannot be generalized.[20] However, there is no doubt that the barriers to acceptable oral health are substantial.

FINANCIAL BARRIERS TO DENTAL CARE

Payment or lack of funds for payment for dental care is the largest single problem for persons with disabilities.[18] Unlike traditional medical services, 97% of payments for oral health services are either out of pocket or through private dental insurance,[12] and more than 150 million Americans have no dental insurance.[4] Furthermore, those persons with the greatest oral health needs are also least likely to have dental insurance or the personal financial resources to purchase care. Families with special health needs incur substantial out of pocket expenses such as noncovered medical expenses and prescription medications, therapy, and special equipment. These extraordinary expenses, in addition to basic needs like housing, food, clothing, and transportation, leave little money for oral health services.

Medicaid (Title XIX of the Social Security Act of 1965) is the safety net provided by the government to fill health care gaps for families with very low incomes or for those experiencing extreme medical hardships. Many children with disabilities and chronic illness use Medicaid to obtain needed health care services.[13] However, even when a child is eligible for Medicaid, which reportedly pays for a minimum level of dental care, there is no guarantee that he or she will receive dental services; four out of five children eligible for Medicaid received no dental care in 1989.[2] In many states the dental benefits available through Medicaid do not even include basic services. Administrative hassles and paperwork associated with prior approvals and low reimbursement rates are dilemmas for dental practitioners who are willing to open their practices to children with Medicaid. In addition to these programmatic obstacles, there are nonfinancial factors that contribute greatly to the lack of use of Medicaid benefits by eligible children and their families.

Nonfinancial Barriers to Oral Health

Simply having financial access to clinical dental services through personal finances, dental insurance, or Medicaid is not synonymous with having oral health. Substantial nonfinancial barriers exist, especially for children with disabilities.[14,17] These barriers to oral health include the following:

- personal attitudes, behaviors, and knowledge of consumers, parents, caretakers, and communities regarding oral health
- environmental and/or physical barriers or lack of equipment
- access to transportation
- knowledge, experiences, attitudes, and behaviors of dental providers and other health care disciplines
- failure to integrate oral health professionals into the health planning team

Children with disabilities and chronic illness may require modifications or special considerations in their preventive and restorative health programs. Undergraduate and graduate dental programs contain varying degrees of coursework in dental care for persons with disabilities. Not all dental practitioners can accommodate children with special needs for reasons of inadequate information, attitude, or willingness.[10]

Some dental providers also seem apathetic about preventive practices. This apathy compounds the potential for dental disease in children whose oral health is already at risk because of circumstances created by their disability. Preventive oral health measures, including the optimal use of both systemic and topical fluorides, dental sealants, oral hygiene measures, decay-limiting dietary

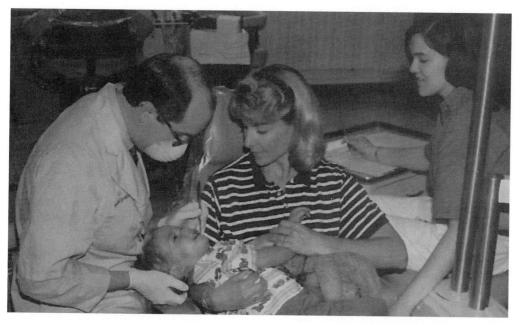

From McDonald, Avery: *Dentistry for the child and adolescent*, ed 6, St Louis, 1994, Mosby–Year Book.

practices, and habits such as wearing mouthguards and abstaining from tobacco use, must be taught, accepted, and integrated into daily lives.[17] Unfortunately, there is great inconsistency among dental health professionals relative to regular application of these preventive measures. While some dentists religiously promote preventive practice, others provide little other than checkups and corrective measures.[5] The superficiality of the current system of provision of dental services is evidenced when extensive restorative services are provided to a child without thoroughly teaching daily home preventive measures.

Furthermore, it can be difficult to convince families of the importance of oral health in overall health care when health professionals also fail to recognize its value. For example, therapists and teachers may use sweets as reinforcements or prescribe diets high in carbohydrates without discussing the need for increased oral care measures with the child's dentist, family, or caretakers. Many physicians do not even conduct a basic examination of a young patient's mouth or provide children or their parents with oral health counseling or referral for dental care.[19] Unfortunately, many dentists also fail to integrate the value of their oral findings or to consider a special patient's other health care needs when providing for the oral health of their patients.

The attitudes, knowledge, willingness, and cultural backgrounds of parents, caretakers, advocacy organizations, and other health care professionals toward oral health also act as great barriers to oral health care for children with special health care needs. Some dentists feed that consumer attitudes toward dentistry in general and the priority that dental care is given in a family's budget are greater barriers to care than financial problems and the availability and willingness of practitioners[10]; it is true that some families do not have social, cultural, or educational backgrounds that promote an understanding of the value of oral health.[17]

Perspectives From the Community

Parents, caretakers, and advocacy organizations have confirmed the existence of both financial and nonfinancial barriers to dental care for children with special health care needs.[3,7,8] In California parents of 500 developmentally disabled children between birth and age 21 were surveyed about obtaining dental care and how they perceived their children's dental health.[8] Fifty percent of 277 respondents reported problems seeking care. The most significant problem was cost; finding a willing dentist in California may actually be more of a financial factor, as many dentists in California do not accept the state Medicaid program, Medi-Cal, because of extremely low reimbursement rates.

A survey of 64 group homes in north central Florida to determine the availability of dental care for developmentally disabled clients indicated that only 33% received comprehensive dental services.[3] Fifty-seven percent of the clients received examination and cleaning only and 10% received emergency treatment only. These figures seem low considering that caretakers reported that 75% of their residents were cooperative dental patients. Dentists were reported to be reluctant to provide services because of financial disincentives or lack of proper equipment. Group home operators commented on the need for more dentists willing to see their clients and indicated their clients would benefit from a mobile dental unit.

National advocacy organizations for persons with disabilities were also surveyed to assess their perceptions of barriers to oral health and needs and knowledge relative to dental resources and oral health information.[7] Thirty-one questionnaires were returned from the 83 organizations surveyed. Responses indicated that the most commonly perceived obstacle to dental care was payment, followed by unfavorable professional attitudes, locating accessible offices, funding transportation, and communicating with dental staff. More than half of the organizations surveyed provided information about dental care resources but only 14% provided financial assistance or counseling regarding financial resources for care.

FINANCIAL SOLUTIONS

The solution to the multifaceted problems of dental access for children with special health care needs is not simple. Providing the financial resources for oral health care does not necessarily make it available, accessible, or acceptable to special-needs children and their families. However, because cost is a principal barrier to oral health, financial access to dental services is a prerequisite to solving other nonfinancial barriers.

Some dental services have been financed through a variety of privately funded programs for persons with special care needs. Most notable is the Donated Dental Services (DDS) program initiated in Colorado in 1985 by the Foundation of Dentistry for the Handicapped.[11] This program matches elderly persons and persons with disabilities with dentists willing to donate their services to a limited number of patients yearly; persons receive up to $900 worth of donated services. Through a Robert Wood Johnson Foundation grant, DDS programs have been developed in 12 states with more than 5000 participating dentists providing $6.5 million of donated care to 12,000 indigent children and adults annually. Unfortunately, programs of this scale are rare and other efforts consist of small local or state efforts or assistance programs specific to certain disabilities or illnesses.

These current financial assistance programs are not sufficient to provide needed dental care to persons with disabilities.[6] To remove financial barriers for children with special needs, oral health services must be recognized as essential health care measures and integrated into the basic health care package.

An Essential Oral Health Benefits Package

On March 30, 1993 the Coalition for the Inclusion of Oral Health in Health Care Reform proposed that a basic oral health care benefit package for all Americans in connection with the Clinton administration's national health care reform effort.[4,21] It was developed on the assumption that the federal government would pay for dental care for Americans without dental insurance who are at or below 200% of the federal poverty level. This proposed package includes:

1. Primary Preventive Services
   - a thorough annual oral examination for those age 2 and above
   - dental sealants for permanent molar teeth in children
   - professionally applied topical fluoride for persons at risk of dental caries
   - oral prophylaxis: an annual dental cleaning
   - fluoride supplements (available to children age 13 and younger whose water supply contains suboptimal levels of fluoride)
2. Acute Emergency Dental Services: treatment to eliminate acute infection, control bleeding, relieve pain, and treat injuries
3. Early Intervention Services
   - dental restorative services; basic dental restorative services to prevent tooth loss
   - periodontal maintenance services: removal of subgingival calculus for those 15 or older
4. Services for Special Needs Patients: includes benefits described above (1-3) and additional services that this group requires for a functional dentition including, when necessary, hospitalization and general anesthesia, orthodontic care for handicapping malocclusions, and prosthodontic care for those with ectodermal dysplasia
5. Dentures: full dentures to restore function to adults using a phased-in approach

The Coalition stressed the importance of retaining the preventative, acute emergency, and early intervention services for all children in any potential phased implementation should the Oral Health Benefit's Package be accepted.[21] It was also recommended that some provision be made for oral rehabilitation of patients with special needs who might otherwise be subject to catastrophic expenses based on dental care treatment needs alone.

Persons ultimately responsible for health care reform in the United States must recognize oral health as essential to total health if oral health benefits are to be included in any public health plan. Unfortunately, even if oral health benefits were to be funded by the government, there are no assurances that the services would be fully utilized or readily accessible to children with special needs in the community unless steps are also taken to reduce the nonfinancial barriers to oral health services.

SOLUTIONS TO NONFINANCIAL BARRIERS

Even if financial barriers are resolved integration of oral health into overall health teaching by all health disciplines will not be accomplished by slogans or dental health week programs or even strong dental office preventive practices.

To reduce nonfinancial barriers two types of measures are necessary: (1) basic, community, oral health measures, and (2) specific advocacy measures taken by an agency charged with coordination of the special health care needs of children. First, all children and their families need to be involved in oral health care planning and intervention on a community level. The fragmented oral health education and research efforts that have taken place in the past have been insufficient. Appropriate standardized data regarding individual community oral needs should be gathered, and needed interventions should be planned and implemented by the public.[9] Strong working relationships between dental and nondental professionals must be cultivated, and oral health education efforts with groups and agencies working with women, infants, and children are necessary.

Second, coordination of oral health services is necessary for the many children with complex oral health needs such as craniofacial anomalies, hemophilia, ectodermal dysplasia, and convulsive disorders. This coordination and the community integration desired by families could be included in the scope of services provided by state Title V programs charged with the development of community-based service networks and care coordination for children with special care needs and their families.[1]

Some Proposals for Care Coordination

A number of programs for persons with special needs employ dental hygienists as coordinators and dental social workers. One such project is the State of Iowa Dental Care for Persons with Disabilities Program.* Through a

*Iowa Department of Public Health, Dental Care for Persons with Disabilities Program, Department of Pediatric Dentistry, University of Iowa College of Dentistry, Iowa City, Iowa.

statewide network of 13 local dental practitioners, this program provides free dental care to persons under age 21 with special health and educational needs. The dental hygienist is the project coordinator and acts as gatekeeper for the program. She consults regularly with families, health care providers, advocates, and educators to refer, finance, and coordinate appropriate dental care for qualified children and young adults.

Another example of a program that employs a dental hygienist as a dental coordinator is a project funded by Maternal and Child Health, the Great Plains Regional Hemophilia Program.* The University of Iowa portion of this program has a dental hygienist who is the dental coordinator of an interdisciplinary health care team that provides coordinated health care to hemophiliacs located throughout rural Iowa and west central Illinois. In addition to the burden of large health care expenses, families dealing with hemophilia must find dental care providers capable of and willing to work with the medical management of potential prolonged bleeding caused by dental treatment and with patients who may have contracted blood-borne viruses from blood or blood products. The dental coordinator removes barriers to dental care by advocating and coordinating needed care horizontally between the family and community health care providers, as well as vertically among the family, community providers, and the tertiary care center. By providing education to families and health professionals regarding dental treatment regimens for persons with hemophilia, the dental coordinator also improves patient access to community dental care providers.

On a larger scale, the National Foundation of Dentistry for Handicapped Campaign of Concern employs hygienists in 11 states in the capacity of dental social workers.[11] The Campaign of Concern has three objectives: (1) to teach participants with disabilities oral hygiene skills, (2) to identify disease early and make referrals to community dentists, and (3) to help disabled patients overcome barriers to needed dental treatment. The dental social workers screen participants and help resolve problems that prevent dental care by working with the family and community personnel.

The common theme in these three programs is that advocacy and care coordination are needed by children with disabilities and chronic illness to make appropriate oral health care services accessible in the community. If statewide programs such as the Iowa Child Health Specialty Clinics—an Iowa Title V care coordination program for children with special health care needs—are

*Maternal and Child Health Great Plains Regional Hemophilia Program, University of Iowa Hospitals and Clinics, Iowa City, Iowa.

already mandated,[1] it seems prudent to complement these well-established networks with oral health components. For example, the joining of the Dental Care for Persons with Disabilities Program and the Child Health Specialty Clinics in Iowa could be an efficient and effective use of resources and community networks. The integration of such services, if successful, could be used as a model for integration of oral health services into community services for children with special health care needs in other similar state Title V programs. In addition to the potential efficiencies gained from the joining of two such programs, a large step would be taken toward the recognition of the importance of oral health and the integration of the special oral health care needs of children with disabilities and chronic illness into their total health care.

REFERENCES

1. Association of Maternal and Child Health Programs: *The coordination of care for children with special health care needs: responsibilities of state Title V programs*, Washington DC, 1988, U.S. Government Printing Office.
2. Bloom B, Gift HC, and Jack SS: *Dental services and oral health: United States, 1989*, Vital Health Stat series 10, No. 183, Washington, DC, 1992, National Center for Health Statistics.
3. Burtner AP: A survey of the availability of dental services to developmentally disabled persons residing in the community, *Spec Care Dent 10*:182-184, 1990.
4. Coalition for Oral Health: Statement of the Coalition for Oral Health submitted by oral testimony to the Subcommittee on Health, Committee on Ways and Means, March 30, 1993, U.S. House of Representatives.
5. Coffee L: Developing a dental program for the handicapped citizen in the community. In Nowak AJ, editor: *Dentistry for the handicapped patient*, St Louis, 1976, Mosby.
6. Coffee L: Executive Director, National Foundation of Dentistry for the Handicapped, Personnel communication, March 1993.
7. Entwistle BA and Casamassimo PA: Advocacy organizations and dentistry: a survey, *Spec Care Dent 6*:114-116, 1986.
8. Finger ST and Jedrychowski JR: Parents' perception of access to dental care for children with handicapping conditions, *Spec Care Dent 9*:195-199, 1989.
9. Frazier PJ and Horowitz AM: Oral health education and promotion in maternal and child health: a position paper, *J Public Health Dent 50*:390-395, 1990.
10. Marinelli RD et al: An undergraduate dental education program providing care for children with disabilities, *Spec Care Dent 11*:110-113.
11. National Foundation of Dentistry for the Handicapped: *Special smiles*, Denver, 1990, The Foundation.
12. National Medical Expenditure Survey: *Annual expenses and sources of payment for health care services*, Rockville, Md, 1992, Center for General Health Services Intramural Research, Agency for Health Care Policy and Research.
13. Newachek PW and McManus MA: Financing health care for disabled children, *Pediatrics 81*:385-394, 1988.

14. Nowak AJ: Dental care for the handicapped patient—past, present, future. In Nowak AJ, editor: *Dentistry for the handicapped patient*, St. Louis, 1976, Mosby.

15. Nowak AJ: Dental disease in handicapped persons, *Spec Care Dent 4*:66-9, 1984.

16. Oral Health of United States Children: *The National Survey of Dental Caries in U.S. School Children: 1986-1987*, Epidemiology and Oral Disease Prevention Program, NIH Pub No 89-2247, Bethesda, Md, 1989.

17. Steffensen JE: Literature and concept review: issues in maternal and child oral health, *J Public Health Dent* 50:358-369, 1990.

18. Strom T: Access: meeting the needs of special patients, *J Amer Dent Assoc 116*:319-327, 1988.

19. U.S. Preventive Services Task Force Guide to Clinical Preventive Services: *An assessment of the effectiveness of 169 interventions*, Baltimore, 1989, Williams and Wilkins.

20. U.S. Public Health Service: *Equity and access for mothers and children*, Washington, DC, 1990, National Center for Education in Maternal and Child Health.

21. U.S. Public Health Service Oral Health Coordinating Committee: *An essential oral health benefit package*, unpublished working draft, Feb 24, 1993.

22. Waldman HB: Oral health status of women and children in the United States, *J Public Health Dent 50*:379-389, 1990.

CHAPTER 29

Nutrition Services for Children with Disabilities and Chronic Illness

MARION TAYLOR BAER

Nutrition services are an essential component of any health delivery system. They are especially important in the prevention of disabilities as well as in the treatment and/or habilitation of children with chronic illness or other disabling conditions.

Primary prevention is not the major focus of this chapter. Research findings suggest, however, that improved prenatal nutrition would greatly lower the incidence of low birth weight,[17,23] which is the single most important risk factor for the subsequent development of disabling conditions in infants.[30] Other studies indicate that micronutrient deficiencies, either dietary or resulting from drug-nutrient interaction, may be responsible for more environmentally caused birth defects,[20,19,29,36] as well as subtle but possibly permanent learning disabilities or cognitive impairments,[12,34,46,47] than has been previously recognized.

Dietary treatment, as a form of secondary prevention, also can attenuate the devastating effects of hereditary metabolic disorders. Phenylketonuria (PKU), for example, which used to result in severe mental retardation if untreated, can now be treated by dietary means. If the treatment is instituted early in life, the child's growth and development are nearly normal.[32] Diet is also the key in the treatment of chronic illnesses such as diabetes and cystic fibrosis.

Nutrition is important as well to tertiary prevention (habilitation), or the minimalization of the potentially debilitating effects of an existing disabling condition. A well-nourished child has a greater chance of remaining healthy and of reaching potential development both physically and cognitively. This is true of all children, but is especially so for the child with a disability. In addition to the nutritional risks facing normal children, those with special health care needs may have risk occasioned by structural anomalies, neuromuscular dysfunction, mental retardation, behavioral abnormalities, or any combination thereof. Also, the medical condition itself, or the drugs required to control it, may alter nutrient needs or interfere with nutrient absorption and utilization.

The recognition of the importance of nutrition services has grown steadily in the last 50 years.[9,27,37] This increased national concern has been reflected in legislation mandating the inclusion of nutrition services, for example, as part of comprehensive services for children with special health care needs (CSHCN) under the various provisions of Title V of the Social Security Act. Nutrition screening and assessment are included in Title IXX-funded Early and Periodic Screening, Diagnosis and Treatment (EPSDT) protocols and, under the Omnibus Budget Reconciliation Act of 1989 (OBRA '89), supplemental services are mandated for identified nutrition problems. More recently nutritionists have been listed among those disciplines qualified to provide early intervention services under P.L. 99–457, Part H (1986), and the modifications of the law under the Individuals with Disabilities Education Act of 1991 (IDEA) include a mandate to provide nutrition services. However, despite these facts, not all children at risk have routine access to nutritional care due to barriers which include those enumerated later in the chapter under "unmet needs, service". For this reason, an effort has been under way nationwide since the late 1970s to ensure that nutrition services be available to all children with disabilities or chronic illness. In 1980, according to a baseline survey of 43 of the then-termed state *crippled children's* agencies, only six had state–level nutritionists with full-time responsibilities for these children; 37 did not employ a nutritionist, even part–time or for special programs.[28] As of 1990, a survey of public health nutritionists in 54 official state health agencies reported that 40 (75%) had plans that incorporated nutrition services for individuals served in CSHCN programs.[41] The approaches to service delivery that have been developed vary according to the resources and constraints of the states or localities.[5,13,15,18,24] The purpose of this chapter is (a) to outline the commonalities involved in developing a system for nutrition service delivery, (b) to briefly describe the content of those services, and (c) to identify some currently unmet needs related to research, training, and service provision.

DEVELOPING NUTRITION SERVICES FOR
CHILDREN WITH SPECIAL HEALTH CARE NEEDS

Needs Assessment

Nutrition needs. The first step in developing comprehensive nutrition services is to ascertain what services currently exist and to what degree they are meeting the needs of the targeted children. These needs vary from very complex problems requiring highly specialized interdisciplinary assessment and care* to relatively simple questions of normal nutrition, food purchasing and storage, or information on patient eligibility for government-sponsored food distribution and nutrition education programs.

In conducting a needs assessment, one of the goals is to determine the prevalence of nutrition problems, as well as factors suggesting high nutritional risk within the population. If there has been no coordinated system of service delivery (including data collection) to date, this information may need to be inferred from the types of disorders seen. Fig. 29-1 presents a list of problem areas most often associated with certain diagnostic classes. The problem areas are divided arbitrarily into those related directly to the child and the child's condition and those related to more environmental or caregiver issues.

Several states have begun to collect data describing the prevalence of the most commonly-seen problems. The states in Region IX (AZ, CA, HI, NV), for example, have developed a database to assist in planning for nutrition services. Fig. 29-2 presents some preliminary pooled data which show the prevalence of feeding problems by selected diagnosis.

Once an estimate of patient service need has been established, programmatic considerations must be addressed. These include nutrition program-management needs as well as service-delivery potential within the existing financial constraints of the overall program. Here, information based on the assessment of existing nutrition services and resources can be matched to the estimated needs to identify gaps as well as overlaps in the existing system.

Existing services. A wide spectrum of services is necessary to meet identified nutrition needs. To assess the adequacy of existing services, the following questions are helpful:

1. Do the children served receive nutrition screening as an integral part of the total health screening?
2. Do children identified as being at risk during the screening receive further nutrition assessment?

*References 2, 3, 7, 14, 33, 38, 40, 48, 49.

FIG. 29-1. Percentage of children with feeding problems by selected medical diagnosis.

Disorder	Prevalence Estimates per 1000 (and range)	Child-related — Altered nutrient needs	Altered energy needs/intake	Problem with oral cavity	Nutrient deficiencies	Constipation/diarrhea	Poor appetite	Delayed feeding skills	Malabsorption	Nutrient-drug interactions	Maladaptive behaviors	Caregiver-related — Lack of knowledge	Difficulty understanding diet	Does not limit intake	Inappropriate feeding practices
Asthma	38 (20-35)	•					•			•					
Moderate to severe	10 (8-15)														
Visual impairment	30 (20-35)														
Impairment visual acuity	20														•
Blind	0.6 (0.5-1)														
Mental retardation	25 (20-30)	•		•	•		•			•					
Hearing impairment	16														
Deafness	0.1 (0.6-1.5)														
Congenital heart disease	7 (2-7)		•								•				
Severe congenital disease	0.5		•												
Seizure disorder	3.5 (2.6-4.6)		•					•		•	•		•	•	•
Cerebral palsy	2.5 (1.4-5.1)		•	•	•		•	•		•	•		•		•
Arthritis	2.2 (1-3)	•	•												
Paralysis	2.1 (2-2.3)					•					•		•		
Diabetes mellitus	1.8 (1.2-2.0)		•		•		•					•	•	•	•
Cleft lip/palate	1.5 (1.3-2.0)			•			•				•		•	•	•
Down syndrome	1.1	•	•					•		•	•		•		•
Sickle cell disease	<1.0	•	•		•	•				•			•	•	
Neural tube defect	<1.0	•	•			•	•			•				•	
Autism	<1.0	•	•				•					•			•
Cystic fibrosis	<1.0	•	•	•	•				•						
Hemophilia	<1.0	•	•	•	•										
Acute lymphocytic leukemia	<1.0	•					•		•	•	•	•			
Phenylketonuria	<1.0	•			•						•	•	•		
Chronic renal failure	<1.0	•	•	•	•	•			•	•	•		•	•	•
Bronchopulmonary dysplasia	<1.0	•	•		•	•	•		•	•					
AIDS		•				•	•		•						
Gastrointestinal disorders		•	•		•	•	•	•							

Example of Nutrition Problem and Factors Contributing to High Nutritional Risk

From DHHS Region IX Nutrition Database, 1987-1995, Supported in part by grants MCJ #009079, MCJ #065057 from the Maternal and Child Health Bureau, (Title V, Social Security Act), Health Resources and Services Administration, DHHS.

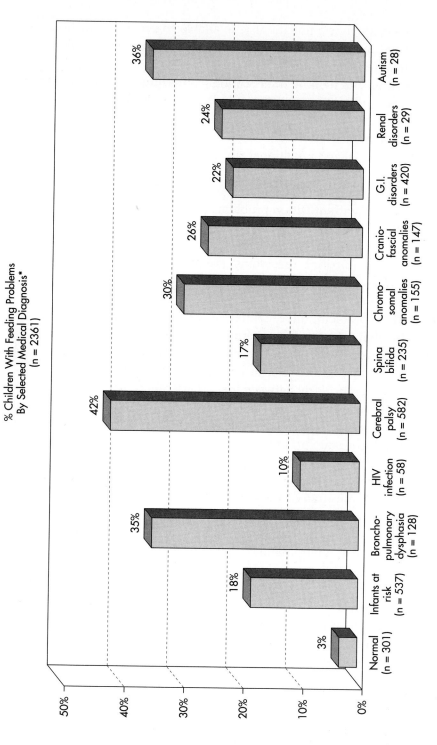

% Children With Feeding Problems By Selected Medical Diagnosis*
(n = 2361)

* Multiple diagnoses possible

FIG. 29-2. Prevalence of certain chronic conditions with associated nutrition-related problems.

From Baer MT, Farnan S, Mauer AM: Children with special health care needs. In Sharbaugh CS, editor: *Call to action: better nutrition for mothers, children and families*, Washington, DC, 1991, Washington DC National Center for Education in Maternal & Child Health.

3. Are there qualified nutritionists available to provide nutrition assessment and intervention? Are there interdisciplinary teams able to assess and treat feeding problems?
4. Is nutrition and feeding intervention (counseling, education, therapeutic diets, feeding therapy, etc.), if indicated, included in the individualized service plan? Is it family centered and culturally appropriate? Is it implemented?
5. Is there specialized nutritional support for children with severe neuromotor dysfunction (e.g., special feeding equipment) or inborn errors of metabolism (e.g., special dietary products)?
6. Do children with nutrition problems receive periodic monitoring of the resolution of those problems? Are children not initially identified to be at nutrition risk regularly rescreened?
7. For which nutrition problems are there established policies and procedures for nutritional care, and to what extent are they being implemented?
8. For which problems have standards for nutritional care been developed and to what extent are they being monitored?
9. Are there community-based nutrition and feeding services available? Is there coordination and referral among individuals and agencies at all care levels, but particularly between the tertiary care centers and the community? Are there gaps in service delivery? Is there duplication of services?

Existing resources. Resources available to support nutrition services may be found within the state program for CSHCN. However, it is also necessary to assess what may be available to children with disabilities or chronic illness through other sources—both public agencies and within the private sector—to avoid costly duplication of service. Relevant questions follow:

1. Are funds available for nutrition services in: (a) the CSHCN Program, (b) early intervention programs under IDEA, Part H; (c) other agency programs (e.g., maternal and child health, developmental disabilities services)?
2. Are nutrition services reimbursable through: (a) Medicaid, EPSDT, (b) private insurance companies? If a child is enrolled in a managed care program, are nutrition services provided (including specialized services)? If not, are they otherwise accessible?
3. Are qualified personnel available for: (a) nutrition screening, (b) nutrition assessment and intervention, (c) feeding assessment and intervention, (d) coordination of nutrition services, monitoring and quality assurance, and data gathering?
4. Are there adequate space, supplies, equipment?
5. Where can personnel obtain specialized training if necessary?

Goals, Objectives, and Activities

Nutritional goals and objectives should be developed from the results of the needs assessment activities and integrated into those of the overall service delivery system. Broad goals may be broken down into specific and measurable objectives, to be achieved within a given time frame, which can then be effectively evaluated.

Setting Priorities

Given the probability that the demands of the total program will exceed its resources, priorities must be set as a matter of policy. Again, these vary from state to state as individual programs determine how best to serve the maximum number of children within their overall service delivery system.

Utilization of Resources

Once the goals and objectives have been decided on and prioritized, steps can be taken toward the utilization of identified community resources to implement the program. This may involve redirecting or augmenting the efforts of service providers within the agency or establishing linkages with, and arranging for financing for, service providers in other agencies.

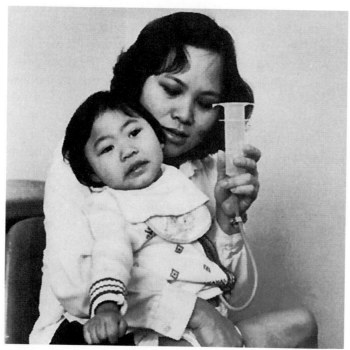

From Pipes PL, Trahms CM: *Nutrition in infancy and childhood,* ed 5, St Louis, 1993, Mosby–Year Book.

Nutrition personnel. In order to provide efficient and effective nutrition services, a public health nutrition director or administrator who functions in a coordinating role at the state level is desirable. Depending on the needs of the state, the director may be full-time with CSHCN or be designated by another agency (e.g., MCH) to assume these responsibilities. This person should be trained and experienced in working with children who have special health care needs, as well as in program development, in order to best assist in program planning, development, implementation, and evaluation.[21]

In addition to the state-level public health nutritionist, others may have a similar function in designated geographic regions, especially in a large state, or in a state with a decentralized health delivery structure. These individuals, in other situations, may serve in a consultant role working with other agency staff; supervise nutritionists, dietitians, or paraprofessionals providing direct service; or even provide some direct service themselves.

Service delivery personnel are, at a minimum, nutritionists with at least a bachelor's degree and who are registered dietitians (RD). They may be assisted by nutrition or dietetic technicians, trained (AA degrees) to work under their supervision.[21] Personnel who will serve children with special health care needs should have further training (master's degree) which includes experience working in an interdisciplinary team.

Other members of the health care team. The discussion of personnel involved in the nutritional care of children with disabilities or chronic illness has so far focused on nutritionists. However, the complex problems presented by these conditions most often require an interdisciplinary approach to their solution. A child may have any combination of medical (physicians), oral structural (dentists, hygienists), neuromuscular (physical therapists, occupational therapists, speech pathologists), or behavioral (psychologists, behavioral specialists) problems that interfere with the intake or utilization of nutrients. Input from these disciplines, as well as from nurses and social workers who can assess the family and community resources, must often form an integral part of the nutrition assessment. Furthermore, it often may be a clinician from another discipline who is the most appropriate person to implement the care plan devised by the team. The nutritionist then becomes a consultant to the primary therapist. By the same token, when nutrition personnel are limited, some other member of the health care team must assume responsibility for assuring the routine use of nutrition screening procedures and, when indicated, referral mechanisms. Furthermore, as parents assume more of a collaborative role with professionals, as well as a greater responsibility for care coordination, they also should become aware of the availability of, and indications for, nutrition services.

Other community nutrition services. Although many states do not yet have a coordinated system for the delivery of nutrition services, with full-time CSHCN nutritionists at both state and local levels, there are many potential resources within the community. If the agency is not yet in a position to employ full-time nutritionists, several types of assistance may be useful in both planning and implementing the delivery of nutrition services. However, it will probably be necessary to assign responsibility for the nutrition component to another member of the agency staff in order to assure effectiveness. Following are suggested resources:

1. To assist with nutrition program planning and development, evaluation, and training, the agency may request consultation in the form of interagency cooperation or contracts from nutritionists in the following positions: public health nutrition directors or consultants in state and local health agencies; nutritionists in programs serving children with, or at risk for, disabling conditions, such as university–affiliated programs, pediatric pulmonary centers, diagnostic and evaluation clinics, high-risk infant follow-up clinics; early intervention programs; regional centers for the developmentally disabled; public health nutrition educators in university settings.

2. To provide direct nutrition services, the agency may establish contracts with the following: nutritionists in programs serving CHSCN (see above); nutritionists in private practice who have received specialized training, such as in university–affiliated programs, nutritionists and dietitians working in local child health programs, such as public health departments, hospitals, Women, Infant and Children Supplemental Nutrition Programs (WIC), Head Start (these professionals may require some in-service training depending on background and experience).

3. To provide specialized therapeutic nutritional management (metabolic disorders, for example) the following professionals would be qualified: nutritionists in programs serving CSHCN; pediatric dietitians in university–affiliated programs or teaching hospitals.

4. To provide food assistance: WIC and Commodity Supplemental Food Program (CSFP); food stamp program; school-feeding and child–nutrition programs; emergency food assistance through various community programs and food banks.

5. To provide assistance with meal planning and food purchasing, storage, and preparation: Cooperative Extension home economists; Expanded Food & Nutrition Education Program (EFNEP) aides for low–income families; nutrition or dietetic technicians and community aides.

In addition, policy decisions must be made regarding specific nutrition services to be reimbursed, under what conditions, and at what level (in-depth assessment, counseling, specialized dietary management); specific formulas, foods, feeding equipment to be reimbursed; qualifications for providers; and standards of care to be implemented.

Implementation Plan

Once resources have been identified, needed inter- and/or intra-agency agreements are in place, and appropriate policies established, a plan for implementation of the delivery of nutrition services can be developed. The plan is sequential with an overall timetable specifying target completion dates for each objective, which may include the following:

1. Staff training
2. Development of a nutrition screening protocol and establishment of clear criteria for referral
3. Development of a nutrition assessment protocol
4. Development of standards of care (which may differ according to the disability)
5. Design of a system for recording and retrieving data on nutrition in order to monitor progress
6. Development of a system of evaluation to measure effectiveness, efficiency, and productivity

DELIVERY OF NUTRITION SERVICES

Although there is no one prescription for the organization or financing of nutrition services, the components of a nutrition service delivery system are more universal. They can be divided into indirect services, or program-management functions, and direct service delivery.

Each state, based on its needs, resources, and the existing CSHCN program structure, must develop its own approach to the delivery of nutrition services.[5,13,15,18]

Program-Management Function

In most settings for purposes of efficiency it is desirable that program management be carried out, or at least coordinated, at the state level. However, the method of translating the following functions into activities may again be variable:

1. Writing the nutrition component of the overall service delivery plan
2. Identifying resources (individuals or agencies) for referrals and serving as a liaison between them in order to avoid duplication of efforts or gaps in services, and providing consultation and technical assistance as needed

3. Developing statewide standards for nutrition screening, criteria for referral for individual assessment, assessment protocol and guidelines for nutrition care
4. Providing workshops or other education programs (in conjunction with university-affiliated programs, whose mandate is training in this area) and printed materials for direct service providers of all disciplines
5. Providing field experience for public health nutrition students
6. Advocating for the nutrition needs of children with disabilities and chronic illness, both within the agency and within the nutrition profession
7. Evaluating program effectiveness
8. Assessing needs for applied research

Direct Service Delivery

The nutritionist, or dietitian, providing direct nutrition services to children with special health care needs is responsible for screening, in–depth assessment, development of a nutrition care plan, provision of care, rescreening or reassessment, and evaluation.[38,16] In some cases, such as screening and provision of nutritional care, particularly if feeding therapy is involved, another professional may actually be carrying out the protocol. However, the nutritionist is trained to design, evaluate, and integrate the various components of an assessment, and should be involved in developing the care plan as well.

Screening and assessment. There are five major approaches to assessment of nutritional status in children; these often require some modification and specialization in the assessment of children with disabilities and chronic illness.[1,6,25] It is beyond the scope of this chapter to present them in the detail found elsewhere[14,33,10,39]; however, they are briefly described below.

Anthropometric. Growth is the best indicator of a child's nutritional status. Therefore careful measurements of height and weight using appropriate and well-calibrated instruments are essential. Measurements over time are especially helpful for children with special needs to determine whether the often substandard height is likely to be due to nutritional as opposed to non-nutritional (normal growth rate) factors.

Estimation of body composition using a combination of skinfold measurements and arm circumference further defines body weight. A child may be underweight for height but still have adequate fat stores, especially if lean body mass is reduced because of an underlying medical problem. The converse also may be true; a child may be overweight if well-muscled but not overfat.

Clinical. Clinical indications of possible nutritional disorders include signs apparent on medical examination of the child, such as abnormal skin or hair conditions. These are rare because they appear only after a prolonged period of nutrient deficiency. They are often quite nonspecific as well and must be substantiated by dietary or biochemical data. The dental examination also may provide information relative to the child's nutritional status. Extensive dental cavities, for example, may result from bedtime bottles or overuse of sweets.

Review of medical records from a nutritionist's point of view would include a search for a history of anemia, recurrent infections, chronic constipation or diarrhea, food intolerances or allergies, pica, and the like. Other relevant historical information includes prenatal maternal weight gain, birth weight, early feeding problems and practices, growth pattern, and laboratory data.

Biochemical. Laboratory assessment of nutritional status, most commonly using fasting serum (or plasma), red or white blood cells, or urine samples, can be used to estimate nutrient stores or preferably the functional capacity of nutrient-dependent enzymes, or to determine the effects of chronic medications such as anticonvulsants or pica. Biochemical methods also are used to diagnose genetic disorders of metabolism that can be treated by diet, such as PKU, or to confirm nutrient deficiencies suspected because of dietary inadequacies.

Dietary. Analysis of a child's dietary pattern can predict and prevent nutrient deficiencies. The method of analysis may range from a simple screening, by food groups, of a 24–hour dietary recall to a computer-facilitated nutrient analysis of a record kept for 3 or more days. Other information pertinent to this analysis includes: child's level of activity; dietary supplements and/or medications; how, where, when, and with whom the child eats; bizarre food habits or inappropriate feeding behaviors; and the cultural/economic constraints on the family's diet as a whole.

Feeding skill development. Children with disabling conditions often exhibit a significant delay in the development of feeding skills. This may be due to neuromuscular dysfunction, resulting in the persistence of primitive reflexes, or to muscle incoordination, which makes positioning, chewing, or hand-to-mouth movement difficult. It also may be due to cognitive delays in a neurologically intact child, leading to infantilization by his caregivers. Assessment of the child's developmental level with respect to these skills, and the child-feeder interaction if there are behavior problems, is essential to developing an intervention strategy and most often requires an interdisciplinary evaluation which includes observation of an actual feeding session.

Developing a nutrition care plan. A nutrition care plan is developed from the integration and interpretation of the results of the five components of the assessment. It is also influenced by input from other members of the health care team, as well as from the parents or caregivers and teacher of the child,

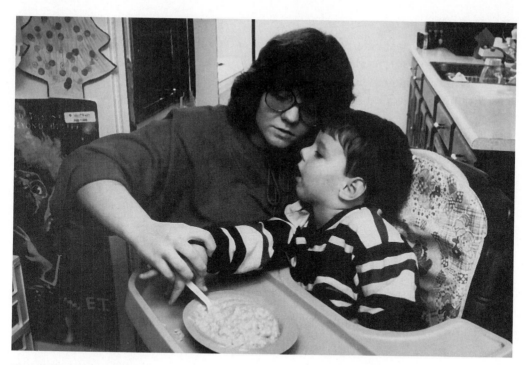

From Pagliarulo M: *Introduction to physical therapy,* St Louis, 1996, Mosby–Year Book.
Photo Credit: Bruce Wang.

as the overall individual service plan is formulated. The nutritionist also builds guidelines into the plan for monitoring progress in achieving the goals, both short and long-term, that the team has prioritized.

Providing nutrition care. The role of the nutritionist/dietitian in providing follow-up may range from direct service delivery, even serving as care coordinator or as a consultant to the care coordinator, to assisting in finding another resource for direct service. In any situation, the monitoring function must be operative.

Rescreening/reassessment. Children in high-risk categories must be rescreened periodically for nutrition problems, even if none is identified at first. Those for whom intervention is indicated must be reassessed at regular intervals to evaluate the success, or lack thereof, of the strategies selected during the development of the individual service plan.

Evaluation. Standards must be set for measuring the efficacy of the intervention strategies so that nutrition care may be made consistent from one clinic to another and so that uniform data may be collected for purposes of quality assurance and determination of cost-effectiveness.[35] Nutrition data should be classified according to diagnosis using standard nutrition problem codes.[11,44]

EVALUATION

Methods for ensuring program quality and evaluating program effectiveness should be developed as an integral part of the implementation plan, both at program management and service delivery levels.[5,31,43] Criteria used have traditionally related to structure, process, and outcome.[45]

Structural criteria relate to the personnel, equipment, and facilities required to carry out the program. Evaluation in this area includes adequacy of staff in terms of both availability and qualifications[42]; appropriateness of equipment, (equipment needed for collecting accurate anthropometric data, effective educational materials); and space, both in offices and in clinics.

Process criteria evolve from the written policies and protocols developed at the program management level during the planning phase. The criteria relate to established activities and procedures used by nutrition care providers at the service delivery level; and as part of the program evaluation, the fact that the criteria are actually being carried out as specified must be documented.

Outcome criteria are the measurable results of the nutrition intervention, based on anthropometric, biochemical, clinical, and dietary data. Ideally, nutrition data collection forms are designed to answer specific questions related to evaluation and based on criteria established as a result of the planning process. For example, if during the needs assessment a large percentage of the children seen in the myelomeningocele clinics is found to be overweight and this is seen as a priority area because of the already limited mobility of such children, an outcome criterion might be a reduction in that percentage as a result of nutrition intervention. Additional and desirable dimensions in evaluating outcome criteria are cost-efficiency and cost-effectiveness studies that provide information leading toward better utilization of resources.

The goal of the evaluation process is to be able, on a regular and ongoing basis, to reassess existing nutrition services. Where goals and objectives are not being met, these criteria should provide clues as to why so that procedures and activities can be altered accordingly. As goals and objectives are achieved new priorities can be set and resources redirected toward meeting those needs.

UNMET NEEDS

Research

Although there has been much progress in the last 25 years in recognizing and responding to the nutrition problems of children with disabling conditions or chronic illness, this is still an underdeveloped area of both basic and applied research. Although quality assurance standards have been developed for some disabling conditions, standards for others are still needed. Most importantly, more data on the benefits of nutrition intervention are needed in order to document its cost–effectiveness. Recently, the Maternal and Child Health Interorganizational Nutrition Group (MCHING) was formed to examine nutrition issues related to maternal and child health, including children with disabling conditions or chronic illness.[37] The background paper on children with disabling conditions or chronic illness, prepared for a national MCHING conference held in 1990, outlines issues and problems related to the nutrition needs of children with chronic illness or developmental disabilities.[8] Examples of specific needs in the area of research include:

1. The role of nutrition in the etiology of growth abnormalities in chronic disorders such as sickle cell anemia, or in babies exposed to drugs, etc.
2. The energy needs of children with decreased lean body mass (such as cerebral palsy, spina bifida, etc.) or who have increased or decreased activity levels.
3. The development of techniques to measure and, where appropriate, disorder-specific reference data to interpret, growth in children whose physical disabilities preclude the use of standardized anthropometry.
4. The development of techniques to accurately predict and measure body composition in children with altered distribution of fat and lean body mass.
5. The differences in energy and nutrient needs of children who are chronically medicated (such as those with a seizure disorder), or those with chromosomal abnormalities (such as Prader-Willi syndrome, Down syndrome, etc.).
6. The effect of nutrition support on treatment outcomes for children with debilitating disorders such as HIV infection and cancer, and the long–term follow-up of the growth and development of high-risk infants.
7. The documentation of the positive effects of early nutrition intervention on the infant's or child's response to other early intervention modalities.

Training

One of the problems resulting from the lack of information about the nutritional needs of this population has been a lack of trained specialists. Many of those at the forefront of the profession pioneered as nutritionists in Title V-funded child development centers and university affiliated programs. The latter are now helping to form a new generation of leaders in the field through long-term preservice training.[4,26] However, although there are now university affiliated programs in nearly every state, the majority do not have the well-developed nutrition component which is mandated only by the Bureau of Maternal and Child Health and not by the Administration on

Developmental Disabilities. Therefore, there is a need to assure that undergraduate and graduate nutrition programs include content and/or field experiences that address the nutrition needs of children with disabilities and chronic illness. Principles of the nutrition care of these children and experiences in the interdisciplinary delivery of that care should be incorporated into dietetic internships and preprofessional practice programs. This is not now the case.[22] Nor are there sufficient inservice and continuing education programs related to the nutrition needs of children with disabilities and chronic illness to compensate for the lack of adequate preservice training. The complex problems of these children and the development of new technology and medications require sophisticated clinical skills and comfort in an interdisciplinary care delivery mode, as well as familiarity with both hospital and community–based resources, in order for the nutritionist to function effectively as a member of the team.

Service

Unmet service needs, however, are of paramount importance at this time. The potential for the delivery of nutrition services, in terms of both the newly–emerging knowledge base and the numbers of well–prepared professionals, far outstrips what exists at present. Some of the barriers which have been identified include[8]:

1. Lack of awareness of the importance of nutrition to the optimal growth and development of children with disabilities and chronic illness.
2. Lack of screening mechanisms to identify nutrition problems while they are still preventable. This is particularly important as the primary care of children with disabilities and chronic illness moves into managed care models where providers may not be aware of the children's special health care needs.
3. Lack of well-established standards of nutrition care upon which to base quality assurance procedures. With the potentially diminishing role of the federal government in the assurance of quality care, it is essential that standards be in place.
4. Failure of discharge planners in tertiary care centers to include a plan for community-based nutrition follow-up.
5. Limited availability of community-based nutrition consultation.
6. Difficulty in identifying funding sources or restricted payment mechanisms, particularly for community-based services where ambulatory care reimbursement for nutrition services is tied to the physician's fee. This appears to be hampering the integration of nutrition services into community-based early intervention programs.

7. Underutilization of existing resources because of unclear eligibility criteria, lack of awareness of existing services or funding possibilities, lack of a referral system to community-based providers.

8. Lack of a state-level nutrition consultant to CSHCN and developmental disabilities programs to serve as coordinator and program planner. This lack has led to fragmentation of, and gaps in, service provision.

Thus much of the unmet service need appears to be due to a combination of financial constraints and a lack of awareness of the part of planners and administrators. It is to be hoped that creative and coordinated planning and programming in the future will help to overcome the present gap between nutrition needs and nutrition services so that all children with disabilities and chronic illness may benefit.

REFERENCES

1. American Dietetic Association: Infant and child nutrition: concerns regarding the developmentally disabled *J Am Diet Assoc 78*:443, 1981.

2. American Dietetic Association: Nutrition services for children with special health care needs. *J Am Diet Assoc 89*:1133-1137, 1989.

3. American Dietetic Association: Nutrition in comprehensive planning for persons with developmental disabilities. *J Am Diet Assoc 92*:613, 1992.

4. Baer MT: University Affiliated Programs: The community role of nutrition components, *Pub Health Curr 28*, 11, 1988.

5. Baer MT editor: Nutrition services for children with handicaps: a manual for state Title V programs, Los Angeles, Calif, 1982, Childrens Hospital Los Angeles, Center for Child Development and Developmental Disorders.

6. Baer, MT: Nutrition assessment of the child with Down syndrome. In DC Van Dyke, DJ Lang, F Heide, S Van Duyne, MJ Soucek editors: *Clinical perspectives in the management of Down syndrome*, New York, 1990, Springer–Verlag.

7. Baer MT, Blyler EM, and Cloud HH et al: Providing early nutrition intervention services: preparation of dietitians, nutritionists, and other team members, *Inf Young Child 3(4)*: 56-66.

8. Baer MT, Farnan S, and Mauer AM: Children with special health care needs. In Sharbaugh, CO editor: Call to action: better nutrition for mothers, children, and families. Washington, DC, 1991, National Center for Education in Maternal and Child Health.

9. Caldwell M: Nutrition services for the handicapped child. *Pub Health Rep 97*:483, 1982.

10. Cloud HH: Nutrition assessment of the individual with developmental disabilities. *Top Clin Nutr 2(4)*:53-62, 1987.

11. Commission on Professional and Hospital Activities: International classifications of diseases 9th rev, *Clin Modif Vol 1*: ICD 9 OM. Ann Arbor, Mich, 1978, Edward Brothers.

12. Dobbing J editor: Early nutrition and later achievement, New York, 1987, Academic Press.

13. Dwyer JT and Freedland J: Nutrition services. In HM Wallace, G Ryan Jr, and A Oglesby editors: *Maternal and child health practices*, ed 3, Oakland, Calif, 1988, Third Party.

14. Ekvall S editor: *Pediatric nutrition in chronic diseases and developmental disorders: prevention, assessment, and treatment*, New York, 1993, Oxford Press.

15. Farnan S: Role of nutrition in crippled children's services agencies. *Top Clin Nutr*, 3, 33, 1988.

16. Fomon, SJ: Nutritional disorders of children: screening, follow-up, prevention. Rockville, Md, 1976, US Department of Health, Education and Welfare.

17. Higgins AC, Moxley JE, and Pencharz PB et al: Impact of the Higgins nutrition intervention program on birth weight: a within–mother analysis, *J Am Diet Assoc 89*:1097, 1989.

18. Hine RJ, Cloud HH, and Carithers T et al: Early nutrition intervention services for children with special health care needs, *J Am Diet Assoc 89*:1636, 1989.

19. Hurley LS: *Developmental nutrition*, Englewood Cliffs, NJ, 1980, Prentice-Hall.

20. Institute of Medicine: Nutrition during pregnancy, Washington DC, 1980, National Academy of Sciences.

21. Kaufman M editor: Personnel in public health nutrition for the 1980's, McLean, Vir, 1982, Association of State and Territorial Health Organizations Foundation.

22. Kaufman M: Are dietitians prepared to work with handicapped infants: PL 99-457 offers new opportunities, *J Am Diet Assoc 89*:1602, 1989.

23. Kennedy ET, Gershoff S, and Reed R et al: Evaluation of the effect of WIC supplemental feeding on birth weight, *J Am Diet Assoc 80*:220, 1982.

24. Kozlowski BW editor: *Meeting nutrition service needs of clients of Crippled Children's Services and supplemental security income disabled children's programs*, Columbus, Ohio, 1980, Ohio State University, Nisonger Center.

25. Kozlowski BW: Cerebral palsy. In Gines, DJ editor, *Nutritional management in rehabilitation*, Rockville, Md, 1990, Aspen.

26. Lucas BL: Interdisciplinary nutrition training: children with special health care needs, *Top in Clin Nutr 5*:24, 1990.

27. Lucas BL: Serving infants and children with special health care needs in the 1990s: are we ready? *J Am Diet Assoc 89*:1599-1601, 1989.

28. MacQueen J: The development of service system models. In Kozlowski BW editor: *Meeting service needs of clients of crippled children's services and supplemental security income disabled children's programs*, Columbus Ohio, 1980, Ohio State University, Nisonger Center.

29. MRC Vitamin Study Research Group: Prevention of neural tube defects: results of the medical research council vitamin study, *Lancet 338*, 131, 1991.

30. National Academy of Science: Healthy people: the Surgeon General's report on health promotion and disease prevention, Washington DC,1979, US Government Printing Office.

31. Peck E: Program planning and evaluating in maternal and child nutrition Final Rep HSMHA-MCH Proj 339, Berkeley, Calif, 1975, University of California, School of Public Health.

32. Pennington BF and von Doorninck WJ: Neuropsychological deficits in early treated phenylketonuric children. *Am J of Ment Defic 89*:467, 1985.

33. Peterson KE, Washington J, and Rathbun JM: Team management of failure to thrive, *J Am Diet Assoc 84*:810, 1984.

34. Pollitt E: Developmental impact of nutrition on pregnancy, infancy and childhood: public health issues in the United States, *Int Rev Res Ment Retard 15*:33-80, 1988.

35. Quality Assurance Committee, Dietitians in Pediatric Practice, American Dietetic Association: Quality assurance criteria for pediatric nutrition conditions: a model, Chicago, IL, 1988, American Dietetic Association.

36. Scott JM, Kirke PN, and Weir DG: The role of nutrition in neural tube defects, *Annu Rev Nutr 10*:277, 1990.

37. Sharbaugh EO editor: Call to action: better nutrition for mothers, children, and families, Washington, DC, 1991, National Center for Education in Maternal and Child Health.

38. Smith MH editor: Guides for nutrition assessment of the mentally retarded and the developmentally disabled, Memphis, TN, 1976, University of Tennessee, Child Development Center.

39. Smith MH, Connolly B, and McFadden S, et al: Feeding management of a child with a handicap: a guide for professionals. Memphis, TN, 1982, University of Tennessee, Child Development Center.

40. Story M: Nutritional needs of adolescents with chronic and handicapping conditions. In RW Blum, editor: *Chronic illness and disabilities in childhood and adolescence*, Orlando, Fla, 1984, Grune & Stratton, Inc.

41. Thompson EB, Bellamy MM, and Kaufman M et al: Capacity of state health agencies to meet nutrition objectives in maternal and child health, *J Am Diet Assoc 90*:1423, 1990.

42. US Department of Health, Education and Welfare: Guide to class specifications for nutritionist positions in state and local public health programs, Rockville, Md, 1971, US Government Printing Office.

43. US Department of Health, Education and Welfare: Guide for developing nutrition services in community health programs, HSA Pub 78-5103, Rockville, Md, 1978, US Government Printing Office.

44. US Department of Health, Education and Welfare: Nutrition problem classification for children and youth, HSA Pub 77-5200, Rockville, MD, 1977, US, Government Printing Office.

45. US Department of Health and Human Services: Preliminary guide to quality assurance in ambulatory nutrition care, HSA Pub 81-51174, Rockville, MD, 1981, US Government Printing Office.

46. Walter T: Infancy: mental and motor development. *Am J Clin Nutr 50*:655, 1989.

47. Walter T, de Andraca I, and Castillo M et al: Cognitive effect at 5 years of age in infants who were anemic at 12 months. *Pediatr Res 28*:295, 1990.

48. Wodarski LA: Nutrition intervention in developmental disabilities: An interdisciplinary approach, *J Am Diet Assoc 85*:218, 1985.

49. Worthington B, Pipes P, and Trahms C: The pediatric nutritionist. In E Allen, V Holm, and RL Schiefelbusch editors: *Early intervention: a team approach*, Baltimore, 1978, University Park Press.

CHAPTER **30**

Genetic Services in the Care of Children with Disabilities

JOHN C. CAREY

The entrance of medical genetic services into the care of children with disabilities and chronic illness is a relatively recent but significant event. The application of human genetics to medicine in general, and to the care of people with disabilities specifically, is crucial because of the important role of genetics in the causation of human developmental disorders. Approximately one third of individuals with developmental disabilities have a genetic disorder or congenital malformation as the primary etiology of the problem.[16] At least 50% of all notable auditory and visual disabilities are caused by a genetic disorder or syndrome.[7,21] Understanding about the causative factors of cerebral palsy has shifted recently from the earlier impression that this symptom complex was primarily due to hypoxic–ischemic encephalopathy to the current understanding that genetic and prenatal causes are paramount.[6] In addition to the importance of these figures, parents of children with disabilities frequently ask questions about the risk of the disorder occurring in future pregnancies. This chapter provides an overview of medical genetics services and their role in the care of people with disabilities.

MEDICAL GENETICS SERVICE

The specialty of medical genetics emerged from the science of human genetics during the past three decades. The clinical discipline of medical genetics developed with improved mortality and morbidity for infectious diseases and with advances in biochemistry and cytogenetics. The field entered mainstream medical practice with the recognition of the American Board of Medical Genetics by the American Board of Medical Specialties in 1992. Genetic services now include clinical programs that involve many facets of the health care delivery system. The box below lists the types and settings of medical genetics services. These services can be broadly divided into the clinical genetics services of diagnosis, management, and genetic counseling services, and genetic screening programs. Although this chapter does not cover the prenatal diagnosis of genetic disorders, references on that topic are provided[10,20].

Types of Clinical Genetic Services and Settings

Center-Based Genetics Clinic

Clinical services
Diagnosis
Counseling
Management

Laboratory Services

Cytogenetics
Clinical biochemistry
Clinical molecular

Specialty Clinics–Multidisciplinary Team Approach

Metabolic clinic
Spina bifida clinic
Hemophilia clinic
Craniofacial clinic
Other single disorder clinics, e.g., neurofibromatosis clinic

Inpatient Consultations

Outreach Clinics

Prenatal Diagnosis Program–Perinatal Genetics

Amniocentesis/CVS clinics
Ultrasound program
Maternal serum AFP/triple screen programs

Teratology Information Services

Genetic Screening

Newborn screening program, follow-up metabolic clinic
Other population screening programs, e.g., Tay-Sachs

Education and Training

Health care professionals
General public

Bernhardt and Pyeritz[5] presented a comprehensive overview of the organization and delivery of clinical genetic services.[5] Most universities in North America include a genetics unit that provides direct care to individuals with genetic disorders and syndromes. In recent years, private genetic services have been established in some areas of the United States; however, these programs usually represent laboratory services rather than direct clinical care. Thus, genetics clinics are still typically based in university or tertiary care settings.

Genetics Clinics

Genetics clinics, whether located in metropolitan areas or in outreach settings, represent the cornerstone of the practice of medical genetics. Families and individuals are referred to these settings for various indications. The box below summarizes the most common indications for referral to a genetics clinic.

The evaluation of a child with developmental delay is one of the most common scenarios in the genetics clinic. The central issue in developmental delay is usually diagnosis. The establishment of a specific and predictive diagnosis of any disability helps in the management of the condition and the counseling

---

Common Indications For Referral To Genetics Clinic

- Evaluation of a person with a developmental or physical disability

- Evaluation of a person with single or multiple malformations; question of a dysmorphic syndrome

- Evaluation of a person with question of an inborn error of metabolism

- Evaluation and counseling for a person with a single gene disorder or consideration thereof

- Evaluation and counseling for a person with a chromosomal disorder including balanced rearrangements

- Counseling for a person at risk for a genetic condition, including questions of presymptomatic diagnosis

- Counseling for a person or family with questions about the genetic aspects of any medical condition

- Counseling for couples with a history of recurrent miscarriages

- Consanguinity in a couple, usually first cousin or closer relationship

- Teratology counseling

- Preconceptional counseling and risk factor counseling, including advanced maternal age and other potential indications for prenatal diagnosis

of the family. The diagnosis of a specific condition provides information regarding cause, natural history, prognosis, and possibly even a specific profile of developmental strengths and weaknesses for the school setting. The box below details the reasons why a specific diagnosis of a genetic condition or syndrome helps the patient, the patient's family, and the practitioner. The diagnosis of Williams syndrome serves as an excellent example of these concepts. This condition is a consistent pattern of malformation involving a specific developmental disability, postnatal growth delays, and a constellation of distinctive dysmorphic features; in addition, just over half of children with Williams syndrome have congenital heart disease, usually supravalvular aortic stenosis.[15] A definite diagnosis of Williams syndrome provides a framework for addressing the care of the child. The medical problems for which children with Williams syndrome are at risk can be looked for in an organized plan of health supervision. Further laboratory tests, such as metabolic studies or an MRI, can be deemed unnecessary since the diagnosis has been established. The specific developmental profile can be shared with teachers and therapists in the classroom and potentially be used for an individual educational plan.[4] Recurrence risk information can be provided to the family in regard to future pregnancies. This need for a diagnosis and the provision of information also applies to other conditions, such as the fragile X syndrome or Prader-Willi syndrome. The importance of making a diagnosis cannot be overemphasized. The establishment of a diagnosis of a common or an uncommon disorder is an important component in the direct care of the child.

Benefits of Diagnosis of a Genetic Condition

1. Recurrence risk in genetic counseling: the recognition of an established disorder of known etiology provides information on cause and heritable aspects of the condition, as well as potential prenatal options for future pregnancies

2. Relative prediction of prognosis: each disorder has its own particular natural history and outcome

3. Appropriate laboratory testing and screening: precise diagnosis eliminates the need for unnecessary tests frequently considered in the evaluation of a child with a potential syndrome; appropriate screening can be planned according to natural history

4. Guidelines for management: knowledge of the natural history of a condition allows for the establishment of guidelines for routine care, including suggestions for educational interventions

5. Family support: in some families the knowledge of a condition helps in dealing with the uncertainty of the situation

---

A new model for the medical care of children with developmental disabilities seems to have emerged from the fields of pediatrics and medical genetics in the last decade.[8,12] The principles of well child care and screening can be applied to the long term management of children with genetic disorders or chronic illness. Knowledge of the natural history of a condition and a critical review of related literature allows the primary care practitioner or specialist to develop a set of routine guidelines for use in the primary care setting, the specialty clinic, or the multidisciplinary team. This approach has been applied to the routine health supervision and anticipatory guidance of children with several syndromes, such as Down syndrome and neurofibromatosis type I.[8] Clinic teams, such as those caring for patients with hemophilia or spina bifida, have been applying these principles for decades. However, the application of these principles to the primary care setting and the emphasis on the role of the primary care practitioner in the orchestration of care is a relatively new concept. Genetics clinics, often in conjunction with multidisciplinary teams, frequently carry out specific care plans. This strategy of team health supervision of people with disabilities represents secondary prevention at its best.

Outreach Clinics

Most medical genetics programs in the United States and Canada have developed a satellite clinic system. In this model, the genetics professionals travel from the centrally-based university center to communities out of the metropolitan area. Epstein et al[11] documented the early history of this model in a Northern California program in 1970. The program for the state of Utah is similar to the one described in California. The Utah Medical Genetics program, as is the case in most states in the U.S., is integrated into maternal child health services and the Children with Special Health Care Needs program in the state Department of Health. The University Genetics Clinic operates as the tertiary level referral center. The outreach clinics in most large communities in Utah function as part of a travelling team of health professionals that visits these communities to provide comprehensive services. The geneticist and/or genetic counselor accompanies the pediatricians, neurologists, nurses, speech and hearing professionals, nutritionists, psychologists, and developmental therapists to the rural communities. In this way, the primary care practitioners in the rural communities operate as a primary level of care while the outreach clinic stands as a secondary level with the university–based genetics clinic representing the tertiary level.

Genetic Counseling

Families who have had a child with a disability of any type often ask questions about the genetic aspects of their child's condition. Genetic counseling is an important component to the care of a family with a child with a disability. The service is usually incorporated into the genetics evaluation and is carried out in the context of the overall diagnosis. In fact, an accurate diagnosis is part of the first task in the genetic counseling model.

An ad hoc committee of the American Society of Human Genetics defined genetic counseling in 1975.[1] This definition is still applicable.

> Genetic counseling is a communication process which deals with the human problems associated with the occurrence or risk of occurrence of a genetic disorder in a family. This process involves an attempt by one or more appropriately trained persons to help the individual or family to: 1) comprehend the medical facts including the diagnosis, probable course of the disorder, and the available management; 2) appreciate the way heredity contributes to the disorder and the risk of recurrence in specified relatives; 3) understand the alternatives for dealing with the risk of recurrence; 4) choose a course of action which seems to them appropriate in their view of their risk, their family goals, and their ethnic and religious standards and act in accordance with that decision; and 5) to make the best possible adjustment to the disorder in an affected family member and/or to the risk of recurrence of that disorder.[8]

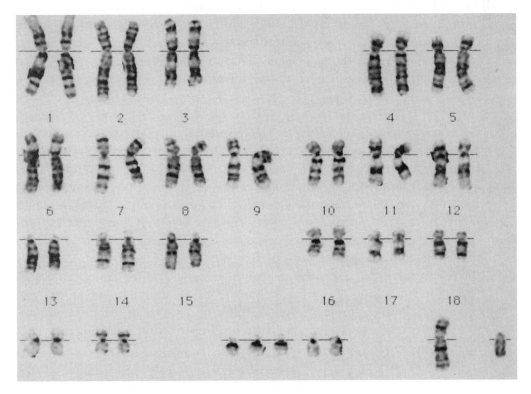

From Jorde, Carey, White: *Medical genetics*, St Louis, 1995, Mosby–Year Book.

A specific diagnosis allows opportunity to acquire information on the etiological and genetic aspects of the condition. Depending on the specific diagnosis and its inheritance pattern, information regarding risks in future pregnancies and options for prenatal diagnosis can be reviewed and summarized. For example, if a child has Down syndrome due to trisomy 21, the recurrence risk for Down syndrome in future pregnancies is discussed; presentation of choices for prenatal diagnosis including chorionic villus sampling or amniocentesis, and their risks, are given. In the case of genetic counseling for a patient who has the fragile X syndrome, the scenario is more complex: X-linked inheritance is explained and screening for family members at risk to carry the gene is offered.

In cases where diagnoses are less clear-cut or a condition is less specific, empiric risk figures are often available. These provide the family a more informed understanding of the possibility of recurrence. The majority of children with developmental disabilities have no obvious etiology or diagnosis even after comprehensive testing. The geneticist can utilize empiric risk figures that have been calculated to predict recurrence risk in a situation of unknown developmental retardation.

Another task of genetic counseling, as outlined in the American Society of Human Genetics definition, is helping families to cope with disorders affecting family members. This is an important role for all professionals who care for people with disabilities. The genetic counseling process is an integral part of the support services needed to provide that care.

Genetic Screening

Genetic screening has been defined as the "search in a population for persons possessing certain genotypes that (1) are already associated with disease or predisposition to disease, or (2) may lead to disease in their descendants."[18]

Newborn screening for phenylketonuria (PKU) is a good example of the first type, while heterozygote screening for autosomal recessive disorders, like Tay-Sachs, or more recently cystic fibrosis, represents an example of the second type. Prenatal diagnosis of genetic disorders and congenital malformations is really a special form of screening. In the case of amniocentesis, the use of maternal age is the screening strategy, and the amniocentesis or chorionic villus sampling is the diagnostic test. Maternal serum alpha–fetoprotein screening in pregnancy for both the occurrence of chromosomal disorders or neural tube defects is another example of the screening approach applied to prenatal care.

Newborn screening. The screening for inborn errors of metabolism in the newborn infant is one of the prototypic examples of secondary prevention in health care. In the United States, newborn screening for various metabolic conditions is a state responsibility. Each state has developed its own program and chosen the disorders for screening. All states in the United States screen for PKU, while most screen for galactosemia and hypothyroidism. The Council for Regional Genetic Services (CORN) has summarized the various state programs in a comprehensive monograph.[14] Some rural states, such as Idaho and Wyoming, have chosen to perform screening by sending samples to a laboratory in an adjoining state that has a larger existing program. Screening for other conditions such as cystic fibrosis or congenital adrenal hyperplasia is done by fewer states either because there is a population with a high risk for a disorder in the region (as in the case of the Yupik Eskimo in Alaska) or because of a particular interest of a medical center in the region.

The Committee on Genetics of the American Academy of Pediatrics has listed the components required to make a decision about newborn metabolic screening.[2] An important ingredient in any screening program is the availability of resources to take care of the disorder once a positive result has been determined. Thus if the necessary specialty clinic is not present in the community, or not accessible and available to carry out the service, the original implementation of such a program in the region should be questioned.

The factors involved in the decision to establish a screening program in any state include the severity of the disorder in question; the sensitivity, specificity, and predictive value of the test; the cost and feasibility of the test; the treatability of the condition; and the availability of follow-up resources.

One class of conditions that has recently been included in many state screening programs in the United States is the hemoglobinopathies, primarily the sickle cell disorders. Though screening of these conditions was at first controversial, the NIH Consensus Development Conference devoted to the discussion of this issue made a firm recommendation of consideration of screening for the hemoglobinopathies.[21]

Carrier detection and heterozygote screening. The development of screening programs for carrier status for Tay-Sachs disease among Ashkenazi Jewish people in North America is the prototype of this strategy. The use of this screening program has led to a decrease in the occurrence of cases of Tay-Sachs disease.

With the development of recombinant DNA techniques and the mapping of many mendelian disorders to their respective chromosomes, heterozygote (carrier) detection and presymptomatic diagnosis using molecular genetics techniques will become available for many more conditions over the next decade. Cystic fibrosis represents the best example of the recent introduction of screening programs. The topic of CF screening is also controversial and has been discussed at length in recent years.[22,23] Given the high frequency of heterozygotes in the Caucasian American population (about 1 in 20) and given the present limitation in the predictive value of the test, most authors on this topic have recommended waiting before institution of such programs. Pilot programs currently exist to delineate the issues surrounding population screening for CF carrier status. Publication of the results of these projects will help in deciding the efficacy of population screening.

The Preventability of Genetic Disorders

The prevention of genetic disease and congenital malformations is a complex and multifaceted topic. Although one of the primary roles of genetic counseling is the prevention of genetic disorders and the lowering of the incidence of such conditions, the principle of nondirective counseling and the ethical tenet of autonomy may cause conflict between individual rights and society's goal of decreasing the occurrence of genetic disorders. If a family has a 50% risk for an autosomal dominant condition of significance (such as Huntington disease or neurofibromatosis type 1), some might state that it is in the best interest of society for this family to limit their offspring. On the other hand, such a statement by a practitioner potentially violates the right of a family to make their own choices regarding reproductive decision making. The traditional primary goal of genetic counseling has been to help the family, and thus the family has made their own decisions about reproduction.

Prevention plays an important role in human genetic services. Prevention strategies have been developed for use at the primary, secondary, and tertiary levels. At the primary level the use of periconceptional folic acid for the primary prevention of neural tube defects has recently been demonstrated.[9,17] This is becoming a routine part of preconceptional and genetic counseling. The administration of the rubella vaccine preconceptionally is another example of primary prevention. Teratogen information services that include discussions of the management of chronic diseases in pregnancy and fetal alcohol prevention projects are other examples of primary prevention. The model of health supervision and anticipatory guidance in children with genetic disorders is to decrease the occurrence of secondary disability, provides a prototypic example of secondary prevention. Newborn screening is also an example of secondary prevention. Tertiary prevention is exemplified by the specialty clinics that care for individuals with chronic conditions and ideally ameliorate ongoing complications; these, of course, are encompassed under the label of rehabilitative services.

CONCLUSION

Genetic services play a significant role in the care of people with disabilities and chronic conditions. Genetics clinics provide consultation on the diagnosis and management of the conditions. Genetic counseling is an important component to the comprehensive care of families in this setting. Genetics professionals are often members of multidisciplinary teams that manage such individuals. Moreover, genetic screening, especially newborn screening for metabolic disorders, provides a prevention strategy for specific conditions.

In this regard, the American Public Health Association presented a position paper with its main objective to "improve the accessibility and availability of quality genetic services."[3] This paper affirmed the important role of genetics services in modern health care delivery.

REFERENCES

1. Ad Hoc Committee on Genetic Counseling: Report to the American Society of Human Genetics, *Am J Hum Genet* 27:240, 1975.
2. American Academy of Pediatrics Committee on Genetics: Newborn screening fact sheets, *Pediatrics 83*:449, 1989.
3. American Public Health Association: Policy statement: genetics and public health. *AJPH 78*:209, 1988.
4. Bennett C, LaVeck B, and Sells CJ: The Williams elfin facies syndrome: the psychological profile as an aid in syndrome identification, *Pediatrics 61*:303, 1978.
5. Bernhardt BA and Pyeritz RE: The organization and delivery of clinical genetics services. In Hall JG, editor, *The Pediatric Clinics of North America*, Philadelphia, 1992, W.B. Saunders Co.
6. Blair E and Stanley FJ: Intrapartum asphyxia: a rare cause of cerebral palsy, *J Pediatr 112*:515, 1988.
7. Carey JC: Genetic aspects of sensory disabilities. In Heller BW, Flohr LM, and Zegans LS, editors, *Psychosocial interventions with sensorially disabled persons*, Orlando, Fla, 1987, Grune & Stratton, Inc.
8. Carey JC: Health supervision and anticipatory guidance for children with genetic disorders (including specific recommendations for trisomy 21, trisomy 18, and neurofibromatosis 1). In Hall JG, editor, *The Pediatric Clinics of North America*, Philadelphia, PA, 1992, W.B. Saunders Co.
9. Cunningham GC: California's public health policy on preventing neural tube defects by folate supplementation, *West J Med 162*:265-267, 1995.
10. DeCherney AH and D'Alton ME: Prenatal diagnosis. *NEJM 328*:114, 1993.
11. Epstein CJ, Erickson RP, and Hall BD, et al.: The center-satellite system for the wide-scale distribution of genetic counseling services, *Am J Hum Genet 27*:322, 1975.
12. Hall JG: The value of the study of natural history in genetic disorders and congenital anomaly syndromes, *J Med Genet 25*:434, 1988.
13. McKusick VA: *Mendelian inheritance in man*, ed 11, Baltimore, Md, 1994, The Johns Hopkins University Press.

14. Meaney FJ and Riggle, SM: The Council of Regional Networks for Genetic Services (CORN): Newborn screening report: 1990, Project #MCJ-361011 from the Maternal and Child Health Program, Maternal and Child Health Bureau, Health Resources and Services Administration, United States Department of Health and Human Services. Available through Susan M. Riggle, CORN Data Coordinator, Genetic Disease Branch, 2151 Berkeley Way, Annex 4, Berkeley, CA 94704.

15. Morris CA, Demsby SA, and Leonard CO, et al: Natural history of Williams syndrome: physical characteristics, *J Pediatr* 113:318, 1988.

16. Moser HW, Ramer CT, and Leonard CO: Mental retardation. In Emery AEH, Rimoin DL, editors: *Principles and practice of medical genetics*, Vol 1, New York, 1990, Churchill Livingstone.

17. MRC Vitamin Study Research Group: Prevention of neural tube defects: results of the Medical Research Council vitamin study, *Lancet* 338:131, 1991.

18. National Academy of Sciences: Genetic screening: programs, principles and research, National Academy of Sciences, Washington, DC, 1975.

19. Newborn screening for sickle cell disease and other hemoglobinopathies, *JAMA* 258:1205, 1987.

20. Simpson JL and Golbus MS: Genetics in obstetrics & gynecology, Philadelphia, PA, 1992, W.B. Saunders Co.

21. Warburg M: Congenital blindness. In Emery AEH, Rimoin DL, editors, *Principles and practice of medical genetics*, Vol 1, New York, 1990, Churchill Livingstone.

22. Wilfond BS and Fost N: The cystic fibrosis gene: medical and social implications for heterozygote detection, *JAMA* 263:2777, 1990.

23. Wilfond BS and Nolan K: National policy development for the clinical application of genetic diagnostic technologies: lessons from cystic fibrosis, *JAMA* 270:2948, 1993.

CHAPTER **31**

Mental Health Services

SUZANNE M. BRONHEIM

There is almost universal recognition that mental health services are an important component of a comprehensive system of care for children with special health care needs (CSHCN) and their families. There is also almost universal frustration with the lack of success many families, medical care givers, and mental health professionals have experienced in trying to make this component work effectively. Families are often insulted that mental health services are even offered to them or, when they have requested them, they have not found professionals who truly understand their particular life circumstances. Medical caregivers often feel frustrated, because the mental health professionals have not been able to "fix" the problems that their patients exhibit or because services are scarce in the community. Finally, mental health professionals often experience difficulty dealing with these families because the families have not willingly sought their services and are resentful that they must see a "shrink."

Many of the problems in making mental health services work stem from current limitations and misconceptions about the role of mental health services for CSHCN and their families. One problematic view is that mental health services are only used to treat those who are mentally ill or who have significant coping problems. Another unfortunate assumption is that mental health services always mean traditional psychotherapy, in which the professional and patient meet for treatment in the professional's office, and that this treatment is only necessary when a patient's problems become overwhelming. These misconceptions tend to have an adverse effect on families' willingness to accept mental health services, on the appropriateness and effectiveness of the mental health services offered to this population, and on the availability and funding of such services. To develop effective mental health services for CSHCN and their families, the role of mental health services for this population must be expanded. A comprehensive, community-based approach to providing mental health services to chronically ill and disabled children must include a far broader view than currently exists of what mental health professionals can offer to children, families, and other professionals on the team.

THE ROLE OF MENTAL HEALTH SERVICES ON THE CARE TEAM

The first purpose of mental health services for this population should be increasing the coping capacity of children and families and decreasing the traumatic effect of illness and medical treatments for them. Many children and families face their medical problems with coping skills that have served them well in other situations. However, the specific stresses that can accompany medical care are new to these families; these stresses may include dealing with frightening information about a child's health, dealing with painful and at times potentially dangerous treatments, finding time to attend numerous appointments or provide special care for a sick child, and overcoming financial burdens. Families need to know how to negotiate the medical care system, how to help their children cope with pain and fear, how to handle people in the community who are not accepting of a child with differences, how to keep informed about medical treatments, how to parent a child whose development may not be typical, and how to seek resources that reduce stress on the child and family.

Mental health professionals can step in at the beginning to offer support services to help families learn to apply their own coping strategies to this new set of demands on the family. This supportive help is not therapy designed to help people with psychopathology, but rather services to expand families' natural support systems and help them gain the knowledge needed to cope effectively with a child's illness or disability. Mental health professionals can deliver such services directly or can ensure their existence and quality by offering training and consulting to parents who organize and run such services themselves. By enhancing families' coping abilities and helping them expand their skills and knowledge, many problems can be prevented.

In addition to increasing the child's and family's ability to cope with the stresses of medical programs, mental health professionals should play a role in decreasing the psychologic trauma of medical procedures, hospitalization, and hearing "bad news." Mental health professionals can work directly with children to decrease anxiety about procedures and help with pain control,

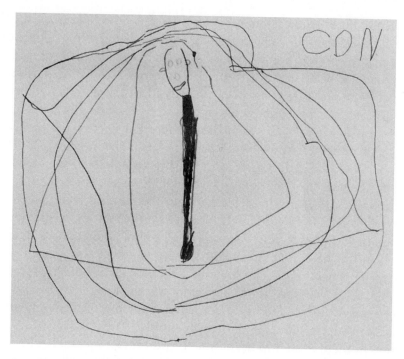

From Clunn: *Child psychiatric nursing,* St Louis, 1991, Mosby–Year Book.

thereby reducing the emotional trauma they experience. Mental health professionals can also educate their colleagues about how best to approach the process of caregiving in a manner that decreases the emotional effect on a family, consulting with both the family and colleagues to accomplish this goal. For example, if a mental health professional learns that a family copes most effectively by always seeing the bright side of things (while at the same time completing all recommended treatments), the mental health professional can help the caregiving team adapt to this style; efforts to make the family more realistic will only serve to alienate them, increase their distress, and may lead to problems in compliance later. Such consultation can also lead to changes in procedures and schedules to reduce trauma for children and families. For example, children who are ill often feel that their lives are controlled by others. Giving these children as many choices as possible about their lifestyle and medical care (within appropriate limits) may reduce their resistance to situations where they cannot have any say. Again, none of these services are traditional therapy, yet they are all legitimate—in fact, primary—ways in which mental health professionals should serve as part of the care team for CSHCN.

Mental health professionals also have a pivotal role to play in enhancing the effectiveness of medical treatments. Again, the types of services offered in this vein are not traditional therapy services but are instead an application of the principles of mental health practice and research to the particular problems faced in providing care to chronically ill and disabled children. Compliance is often a problem when medical treatments may be unpleasant, interfere with life activities, and continue for long periods of time. The mental health professional can work with families and medical staff to design behavior therapy approaches to increasing compliance, thereby enhancing the effectiveness of treatment. A psychologic assessment of a child's intellectual abilities and learning styles can help the medical team design teaching approaches to self care and self monitoring that are more likely to be successful. In addition, techniques such as relaxation, biofeedback, imagery, and hypnosis can help regulate blood pressure,[2] affect the amount of insulin needed by diabetics,[1] lessen the need for powerful pain medication,[5] and even improve tolerance for treatment of burns or other wounds.[3] Although never a substitute for medical treatments, the input of mental health professionals can support and enhance such efforts.

Finally, there is an important role for traditional mental health services in treating CSHCN who are having emotional difficulties. This treatment, however, must be framed within the context of the effect of the illness or disability on the child or family. This is discussed further in the section on training later in this chapter.

CONSIDERATIONS AND OBSTACLES TO PROVIDING MENTAL HEALTH SERVICES

Developing a comprehensive model of mental health services for CSHCN and their families has been an often frustrating challenge, particularly at the community level. While specialty teams and clinics in teaching hospitals may have instituted such a model, it is rare that such an approach is implemented effectively in the community. Considerations and obstacles to developing the role of mental health services within a community-based service system are described below.

Structure

To develop a comprehensive approach to mental health services for CSHCN, there should be a rethinking of the structure of delivery of such services. Mental health professionals must not be tied to one office with patients coming to them at appointed times. These caregivers must be free to be in the hospital or in the physician's office to consult and provide onsite supports to families and children. They should be involved from the beginning—introduced as an integral part of the care team from the diagnostic process on, rather than being some distant resource that families are sent to when they have problems. Changing the structure of the delivery model is essential.

Training

There are a number of training issues related to setting up within a community mental health services to serve chronically ill and disabled children. Some of these relate to mental health professionals themselves. Frequently, mental health professionals have not had the training needed to add to their expertise that extra layer of knowledge about CSHCN and their families. They may not realize the immense demands on a family's time and resources; they may have no idea about the course of the child's disease or its prognosis. As a result they may not be able to appropriately treat the needs of these children and their families. In addition, many illnesses and their treatments have considerable effect on behavior and emotions. Medications used for treating psychiatric disorders may be contraindicated because of medical conditions or other treatments. Appropriate mental health services must consider these factors, yet most training programs for mental health professionals do not emphasize these skills. Without some training relating to this subject, however, there is often a problem with the appropriateness of services.

Supporting continuing education programs for mental health professionals on topics in this area could be one solution to this problem. For example, a local mental health agency or professional organization could sponsor speakers and workshops taught by professionals familiar with pain control or other aspects of providing mental health services for CSHCN. Because many professionals need to earn continuing education credits for licensure, this type of event could be attractive. A less formal approach could be "brown bag" lunch discussions in which mental health professionals could discuss readings pertaining to specific CSHCN issues. Guest consultants could be invited to teaching staffings, meetings to discuss the diagnosis and treatment plans for specific children who have a chronic illness and need the input of mental health professionals.

Medical caregivers must also be trained to understand the expanded role for mental health professionals and to make referrals for mental health services in a way that will enhance families' acceptance of such recommendations. Holding teaching staffings of specific children in the community served by mental health professionals can help train medical personnel about mental health issues and at the same time alert mental health professionals about issues related to the child's health problems.

Finally, families need to be educated about the many roles mental health professionals can play as part of the treatment team so they will not view the appearance of these caregivers as a sign that the team thinks they are "crazy." Without such training it will be almost impossible to overcome the problems that have stymied the system in the past.

Funding

There need to be changes in the approach to funding mental health services that support a more comprehensive system. The funding of mental health services is generally linked to the traditional models of outpatient psychotherapy or inpatient treatment. Private and public third-party payers rarely reimburse for support or preventive services, often do not pay for assessment, and may not even consider a mental health service as a medical treatment. At times only certain types of mental health providers are reimbursed. Funding for clinics is also often tied to the number of clients seen in therapy and does not account for time used in prevention or in the consultation/training of medical caregivers needed for a complete approach. As a result, these nontraditional types of services are often inaccessible because there is no way to pay for them. Payment for mental health services also should not be contingent on the child or family having a psychiatric diagnosis, as is now frequently the case. Lastly, there must be some funding resources that can pay for services to the system such as consultation and training to improve the delivery models. Without these types of changes in funding strategies, comprehensive services cannot be put into place.

Availability

Availability of mental health services for CSHCN and their families is a critical issue in many communities. This is not a surprise because there is a shortage in this country of mental health professionals who are specially trained to deal with children. Even generally trained professionals are often clustered in high–population-density areas and thus are not available in many communities. It is estimated that there are not enough trained mental health professionals to deal with children who have significant emotional problems; therefore it is understandable that resources to provide a comprehensive set of services to a population not classified as emotionally disturbed are scarce.[4]

Even where there are mental health services available in a community, access to those services to provide a comprehensive approach to CSHCN and their families may not exist. In response to the paucity of mental health services many communities have had to prioritize who has first call on those services. Typically, those who are chronically mentally ill, suicidal, or in severe crisis take precedence; the needs of children with chronic illness and disability come very low on the priority lists. Thus families may find themselves on long waiting lists for services. Working with institutions that train mental health professionals and providing practicum placements working with CSHCN and their families can help make services available and accessible in the community for little cost. Collaboration with other efforts to help children and families, such as early intervention programs, substance abuse programs, juvenile justice services, and family support and protective services may be useful. These groups may have mental health services available to their constituencies, and these mental health services, may be able to serve CSHCN and their families as they come through these services and systems. Finally, working with local employers who provide health care benefits to many community members can be fruitful. If benefit packages include reimbursement for mental health services at a level that can give families access to care, then the community will have a better chance of attracting mental health professionals to practice in the area. Additionally, some large employers now have programs that provide counseling services and advice about getting family support services in the community. Training those service providers about the needs of CSHCN and their families may develop another set of resources, particularly for delivering some of the more preventive types of mental health services described in this chapter.

Acceptability

Acceptability of mental health services is often a sticking point in making a system work. Many families still attach a stigma to seeing a "shrink" and may not want to be seen going to the mental health clinic or the therapist's office. In addition, families often view this type of referral as a rejection by the medical professionals. They feel they are being told, "You are too much trouble so we're sending you away to these other people." Unfortunately, many medical professionals share the view that mental health services are for "crazy" people and reflect this sense to patients referred. When mental health professionals are not involved from the beginning, and when families are only referred to them when problems become overwhelming, acceptability of mental health services will be low. Changing the structure of the system as described above—so that services are offered from the start as an integral part of the care program—and helping families, health care workers, and mental health professionals adopt new attitudes should help to mitigate this problem considerably. Co-location of mental and medical health services and collaborative funding of programs that bring these services together can also increase the acceptability of psychologic care.

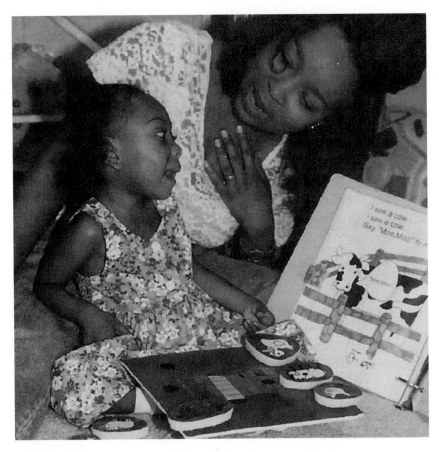

From Case-Smith J, Allen AS, Pratt PN: *Occupational therapy for children*, ed 3, St Louis, 1996, Mosby–Year Book.

CONCLUSION

While mental health services are a key component of serving CSHCN and their families in the community, these services have historically been poorly integrated into the care team. Misunderstandings about what mental health services are and what they can offer these children and their families are at the root of the difficulty. The current structure of mental health services, the need for appropriate training, the lack of availability of services, and the funding issues have all played a role in the failure to successfully integrate mental health services into the community system of care. Successful strategies for developing mental health services for CSHCN and their families will require interagency planning, programming, and funding of this type of care as part of a coordinated systems-development effort.

REFERENCES

1. Agras WS: The behavioral treatment of somatic disorders. In Gentry W, editor: *Handbook of behavioral medicine,* New York, 1984, Guilford Press.
2. Herd JA: Cardiovascular disease and hypertension. In Gentry W, editor: *Handbook of behavioral medicine,* New York, 1984, Guilford Press.
3. Tarnowski K et al: Pediatric burn injury: self versus therapist medical debridement, *J Pediatr Psychol* 12:567, 1987.
4. U.S. Congress, Office of Technical Assistance: *Children's mental health: problems and services, a background paper,* OTA-BP-H-33, Washington, DC, 1986, U.S. Government Printing Office.
5. Varni J, Katz E, and Dash J: Behavioral and neurochemical aspects of pediatric pain. In Varni J and Russo D, editors: *Behavioral pediatrics,* New York, 1982, Plenum Press.

CHAPTER **32**

Early Intervention

ELIZABETH S. RUPPERT

THE HISTORY OF EARLY INTERVENTION

Early intervention has become a synonym for the law enacted by the United States Congress entitled "Education of the Handicapped Act Amendments of 1986."* Today virtually every community in the U.S. has been affected by this concerted national and local effort designed to promote a system for the benefit of children with disabilities, birth to age 3, and their families. The system's foundation rests upon the policy that the United States Government will provide financial assistance to states to meet the following objectives:

    1) to develop a statewide, comprehensive, coordinated, multidisciplinary, interagency program of early intervention services for infants and toddlers with disabilities and their families

    2) to facilitate the coordination of payment for early intervention services from federal, state, local, and private sources

    3) to enhance a state's capacity to provide quality early intervention services and expand and improve existing early intervention services being provided to infants and toddlers with disabilities and their families.*

However, early intervention is much more than a federally funded program; early intervention is a body of knowledge initially based on experiential reports that revealed that some children with delays and disabilities could function better because of education in infancy and early childhood. For example, in 1910 Maria Montessori, an Italian physician, developed an inter-

*PL 99-457. 100 Stat 1149-1159

ventional education program for the poor children in the slums of Rome. The result was that some of the children who were considered to be at risk for retardation became capable, curious, and self sufficient.[5] In the 1940s and 1950s intervention reports written by the John Tracy Clinic in California and the Lexington School for the Deaf in New York City reported successes with the early introduction of amplification and parent education. Deaf children diagnosed before age 2½ scored significantly higher on intelligence exams than did their deaf peers who began treatment after 30 months of age.[4] Thus some of the effects of sensory deprivation could be ameliorated by amplification and parent-child education.

However, it was Head Start that made early intervention a political and social force. In the fall of 1964 during the Lyndon Johnson administration the concept of Head Start evolved as a prekindergarten educational experience designed to permit poor children to be as prepared for entry into school as were their middle-class peers. Head Start became a comprehensive child development program with child health and nutrition, child motivation, parent participation, and preparation for school as the major program goals. Although some studies of Head Start revealed long-term benefits in school performance, the Westinghouse study[10a] showed no sustained rise in IQ. Fortunately, the metaanalysis study completed in the late 1970s revealed positive outcomes that included significant improvement in progression through school, social adjustment, and family functioning.[11]

The political success of Head Start was not the direct result of well-planned scientific studies but rather the result of the compelling elements of this nurturing, nonthreatening community-action program for the benefit of children and their families. In 1987 Shonkoff and Hauser-Cram[9] published the results of 31 selected studies that used early intervention for children younger than age 3. Results indicated that these infants and toddlers with biologically-based disabilities did demonstrate enhanced developmental progress because of early intervention. Intervention programs that used structured curriculum and planned parent involvement resulted in better child outcomes. When programs linked the parent's role to the services given the child, developmental progression was better than if the intervention was solely child-focused or the parent program was isolated from the child's.[9]

An understanding of protective and risk factors in a child's environment was reported by Sameroff et al[7] from a longitudinal study of 215 families. The study examined 10 variables including maternal mental health, anxiety, education and occupation, family social support, and stressful life events. They found that the higher the number of risk factors, the lower the competence of the child. Although no single risk factor was either always present or always absent among children with cognitive difficulties, children with four or more risk factors were 20 times more likely to have marginal cognitive functioning than children with less than four risk factors.[7] Thus it is clear that a child's early development is complex and is enhanced or impeded by both biological and environmental influences. For this reason early interventionists must assess both the infant and his or her family before implementing a planned, structured curriculum that promotes positive, ongoing parent-child interaction.

Mandated Services for Children with Disabilities

Federal policy has been a strong tool to help meet the needs of young Americans. The Education for All Handicapped Children Act of 1975 established a "right to education" for children with disabilities between ages 6 and 18. A few years later The Preschool Incentive Grant Programs lowered the ages of eligible children to include 3, 4, and 5 year olds. PL 99-457 mandated that states serve handicapped 3, 4 and 5-year old children with disabilities and it established an early intervention system for infants and toddlers—Part H of the legislation. The findings that influenced its policy formulation were the following: (1) a child's development will not be as delayed as it would be if left unattended until age 6 or older, (2) the capacity of a family to meet the needs of infants and toddlers with disabilities will be enhanced, (3) over time children and their families will use less costly specialized educational services, the likelihood of institutionalization will be minimized, and these children will have enhanced opportunities to live socially integrated within their community.

The Individuals with Disabilities Act (IDEA)* provides grants to states to support the planning of service systems and the delivery of services, including evaluation and assessment. Funds are provided through the Infants and Toddlers Program (Part H of IDEA) and through the Preschool Program (known as Section 619 of Part B of IDEA) for services to children age 3 to 5.

IDEA stipulates that early intervention be provided to infants and toddlers with disabilities who have developmental delays (as measured by appropriate diagnostic instruments) in one or more of the following areas: cognitive development, physical development, speech and language development, psychosocial development, or self-help skills, or who have a diagnosed physical or mental condition with a high probability of resulting in developmental delay. The law also allows states at their discretion, to serve children who are at risk of having substantial developmental delays if early intervention

*Individuals with Disabilities Act, Public Law 102-119, 1991.

services are not provided. This system of early intervention services is provided under public supervision by a lead agency appointed by the state's governor, and advised by a state interagency coordinating council.

The specific early intervention services must meet the standards of the state and must include: (1) early identification, screening, and assessment services, (2) medical services only for diagnostic or evaluation purposes, (3) health services necessary to enable the infant or toddler to benefit from the other early intervention services, (4) family training, counseling, and home visits, (5) special instruction, (6) speech pathology and audiology, (7) occupational and physical therapy, (8) psychological services, and (9) case management services. It is worth emphasizing that the early intervention services are family centered (home visits, family training and counseling) and that the pivotal role of the family is respected and supported.

Finally, the law requires that each infant and toddler with disabilities and their families receive an individualized family service plan (IFSP). The IFSP is a written document developed by a multidisciplinary team that includes parents or guardians and that promotes comprehensive and coordinated service delivery to the child and his or her family in a timely fashion with specified services delivered by specified providers with projected outcomes to be measured at specified intervals. A case manager is named and assists the team in accurately stating the family's strengths and needs and is responsible for implementing the IFSP and coordinating with other agencies and persons. Finally, the IFSP must include the steps supporting the transition of the child to the services of the mandated Preschool Program to the degree that such services are appropriate (needed by the child and desired by the family).

The IFSP is a well-designed roadmap to promote service coordination. It is essential that the infant's medical diagnosis be included in the IFSP because medications, surgery, and prognosis can all significantly affect a toddler and his or her family. A word of caution—if an infant or toddler qualifies for early intervention services but has never had a comprehensive medical assessment, it should be done immediately. Accurate medical diagnosis is a fundamental factor in promoting the development of infants and toddlers and their families. The IFSP fosters cross-disciplinary communication and should prevent duplication and omissions while promoting the family as the center of all services.

THE ROLE OF PROFESSIONALS

Each discipline has a specific knowledge base and a certain group of practice skills and attitudes. This unique set of skills and knowledge specific to a discipline should continue unchanged. However, today with the challenges of early intervention each professional must realize that a single professional cannot and should not function alone as the omniscient and omnipotent professional for a child and family. A toddler with cerebral palsy, for example, needs skilled orthopedics, physical therapy, and occupational therapy. In addition, however, this child's hearing, vision, nutrition, and cognitive development need evaluation, and the family needs help understanding and accepting the child's disability and how it affects his or her development. Equally important is understanding how this family functioned prior to the child's diagnosis, supporting their adaptations, and allowing the family to build its own individualized and personalized plan. Thus the number one role of everyone involved in the care of the child is to "commit to the system including, at least the parents, public health sector, private health sector, mental health providers, and the education system."[1] Each has something significant to offer but must do so in context and in concert with others. Each stakeholder must be willing to participate with the family's case manager in the development and implementation of the IFSP. For example, attendance of all service providers at significant IFSP meetings is ideal; however if it is not possible for a professional to attend a certain meeting, then that person should communicate with the case manager before the IFSP meeting to

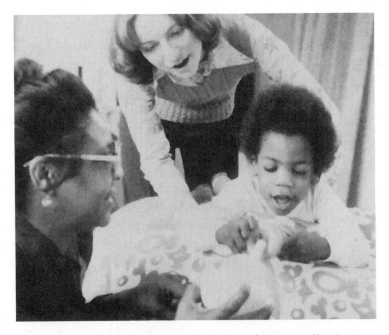

A visiting occupational therapist works with local staff to bring specialized skills to a small community hospital.

From Worley JS: Occupational therapy. In *Introduction to health professions*, ed 3, St Louis, Mosby–Year Book.

ensure inclusion of each discipline's plan for treatment, observations, and concerns. Thereby, good communication is timely and open among parents, providers, and the case manager. Although certain agencies have traditionally provided case management services, it is essential that the person identified in the IFSP as the central case manager be used as the lead service coordinator and advocate for family and child. To have multiple case managers who bypass the identified IFSP case manager is destructive to coordination and wastes precious professional time. Parents can be overwhelmed by having too many case managers. Parents soon see that collaboration among professionals requires commitment, practice, and mutual respect.

Professionals must also play an advocacy role that encourages the development of comprehensive, community-based service systems that are staffed by adequately prepared care providers. Look at your professional interests and skills and decide if you are suited to the challenges of early intervention. Are there professional skills that need strengthening? Does your community, professional organization, or agency provide updated training about early intervention and your state's system? Encourage your peers and your local university to include more training for early childhood educators, doctors, psychologists, business people, and legislators about family-centered, community-based, coordinated care.[2,6]

THE IDEAL E I SYSTEM

Ideally, the first phase of the early intervention system should begin with prevention. Prevention via education might include the implementation of a family-life education curriculum in schools that promotes an understanding of the developmental stages of life and promotes the acquisition of knowledge and skills about parenting, the value of accessing prenatal care and family planning, and the risks associated with the use of drugs, alcohol, and unprotected sex. A coalition of community leaders with EI professionals and parents as key players in this ongoing education program could better prepare these parents of tomorrow.

Identifying all infants and toddlers with developmental delay and those at risk for developmental delay is fundamental to the EI system. Known risk factors and conditions must be used to identify children in the newborn nursery, hospital pediatric units, and ambulatory visits in public and private settings. Some elements of tracking should be a part of the system to ensure ongoing care and monitoring. No child should be lost to follow-up care who has a disability or is at risk of developing one.

Parental concern about a child's development is a green light for action. If a mother is concerned about her baby's delayed speech, her concern should be acknowledged and an appropriate comprehensive assessment should follow.

For example, a toddler with delayed speech may be mentally retarded, hearing impaired, or may have a mother with depression. A comprehensive evaluation is essential because diagnosis will directly affect educational programming. Parental concern about delayed development triggers more evaluations than any other single activity, planned or unplanned, again demonstrating how important it is to bring parents in as partners in the EI system.

Another key element in the system is the development of a community team or teams.[10] From this team can come (1) quality in evaluation, (2) complete knowledge of local resources, (3) openness in communication with a central intake and referral system in place, (4) trust and respect of the role of parents and of a single case manager, (5) benefits of shared care, (6) identification of weaknesses or deficiencies in the community, and (7) advocacy and conflict resolution.

Teams of people who work together to support families in their natural care-giving and decision-making roles for their special-needs child will be very effective. Turfisim and professional isolation will progressively lessen as community-based teams work collaboratively to implement the mission of EI.

BEST PRACTICE MODELS

Finally, what specific interventions are most effective? If an infant is sensory deprived (visually and/or auditorially), diagnosis during the first 6 months of life followed by surgery, spectacles, hearing aids, and intensive communication training will result in better function than if diagnosis and intervention are deferred until age 2 or later. Programs that foster a high degree of family participation in intervention enhance child development. Center-based intervention programs are feasible for infants and toddlers and are beneficial for development of low birthweight, premature infants and for infants and toddlers from lower socioeconomic status.[6] All children could benefit from having a medical home but it is especially beneficial for the 6% of the birth to age 3 population who are delayed or disabled. The ideal medical home includes:

- preventive care including but not restricted to immunizations, health care supervision, and patient and parental counseling about health and psychosocial issues
- access to care 24 hours a day, 7 days a week, 52 weeks of the year
- continuity of care
- identification of the need for subspecialty consultations and referrals and knowing where these can be obtained
- interaction with school and community agencies to be sure health needs are met
- maintenance of a central record and database containing all pertinent information about the child, including hospitalization

This medical home concept can work synergistically with the IFSP process and community teams. Quality child protective services, family preservation services, and quality child/day care are also essential elements to a community-based comprehensive system.[2,8,10]

The challenge now is to continue the momentum of the EI system as we know it today and to have the intellectual integrity to conduct carefully constructed outcome-oriented research that will further define what program elements are most effective for which families. All Americans must take responsibility for supporting young children and their families. The Carnegie report of 1994[2] challenges all community leaders to develop a local plan for young children and to implement the plan based on local strengths. The Head Start approach and neighborhood family child center are models that show promise. Whatever the model, our future depends on how well young children are nurtured and their families are supported.

REFERENCES

1. Bureau of Maternal and Child Health and Resources Development, American Academy of Pediatrics: *Establishing a medical home for children served by Part H of Public Law 99-457*, Washington, DC, 1989, The National Center for Networking Community Based Services.
2. Carnegie Corporation of New York: *Starting points*, New York, 1994.
3. Cicirelli VG: The impact of Head Start: an evaluation of the effects of Head Start on children's cognitive and affective development, Report presented to the Office of Economic Opportunity, Rep No PB 184 328, Washington, DC, 1969, Westinghouse Learning Corporation.
4. Meadow-Orlans KP: An analysis of the effectiveness of early intervention programs for hearing-impaired children. In Guralnick MJ and Bennett FC, editors: *The effectiveness of early intervention for at-risk and handicapped children*, Orlando, Fla, 1987, Academic Press Inc.
5. Orem RC: *Montessori today*, New York, 1971, GP Putman's Sons.
6. Ramey CT et al: Infant health and development program for low birth weight, premature infants: program elements, family participation, and child intelligence, *Pediatr* 89:454-465, 1993.
7. Sameroff AJ et al: IQ scores of 4-year-old children: social-environmental risk factors, *Pediatr* 79:343-350, 1987.
8. Schorr LB: *Within our reach: breaking the cycle of disadvantage*, New York, 1988, Doubleday/Anchor Books.
9. Shonkoff JP and Hauser-Cram P: Early Intervention for disabled infants and their families: a quantitative analysis, *Pediatr* 80:650-658, 1987.
10. Sia CCJ: The medical home: pediatric practice and child advocacy in the 1990s, *Pediatr* 90:419-423, 1992.
10a. Westinghouse Learning Corporation and Ohio University: The impact of Head Start: an evaluation of the effects of Head Start on children's cognitive and affective development, vols 1 & 2, Report to the Office of Economic Opportunity, Athens, Ohio, 1969, Westinghouse Learning Corporation and Ohio University.
11. Zigler E and Muenchow S: *Head Start*, New York, 1992, Harper Collins Publishers, Inc.

CHAPTER **33**

Preschool Programs:
The Search for Quality Services

JOHN T. NEISWORTH
LISA A. SCHNEIDER

Never before have America's preschool children with special needs had greater developmental services and opportunities. Not long ago parents of infants and preschoolers with disabilities experienced confusion and exclusion. The extra and early needs of their children were not addressed in systematic or thorough ways, and early help was typically at family expense. However, the times are rapidly changing and now parents and children are entitled by public law to quality, professional services.

Recently early intervention became a federal entitlement. The entitlement program first appeared in 1987 through passage of PL 99-457. Subsequently the legislation was reauthorized and combined with other special education legislation thereby creating the Individuals with Disabilities Education Act (IDEA). Part B of this legislation was written for preschoolers (children ages 3 to 5). For eligible children IDEA guarantees much of the same rights that school-age children enrolled in special education receive. That is, every eligible child is entitled to a free and appropriate education. (It should be noted that the term *early intervention* originally referred to birth to age 2 or 3 but is currently used to describe infant, toddler, and preschool services, i.e., birth to age 5.) Some of the services now available at public expense are screening, eligibility assessment, parent education, home visits by early childhood specialists, enrollment in preschool programs, and the services of various specialists—depending on documented needs.

For a preschool-age child a team of family members, professionals, and paraprofessionals plan and work together so that the child can benefit from a specially designed program. Services may include specialized instruction, speech pathology, physical and occupational therapy, counseling, medical diagnostic services, parent counseling and training, psychologic services, transportation, and school health services. Although nursing services are not central to actual delivery of services, the role of the nurse as a team member is critical for some children and families in each of the following steps of the early intervention process:
- referral for screening/assessment
- preschool placement and program planning
- delivery of services

REFERRAL

The identification of children eligible for early intervention often begins when children receive health services or screenings at hospitals, in pediatrician's offices, at clinics, or through home health care programs. Considering the critical role of health services in the referral process,[9] nurses often are in an excellent position to identify children who may need early intervention. A nurse's involvement in referral is probably the most common and often the first contact made in the early intervention process. The referral process involves identifying a child who needs help, sharing this information with the child's family, and finding an early intervention provider.

Identifying Children for Referral

Children are eligible for preschool-age early intervention when they show evidence of developmental delay or disability. If a disability is used for eligibility it must adversely affect educational performance and fall within one of 15 categories subsumed within the following five groups:
- Sensory impairments such as vision and hearing impairments, including deafness and blindness and dual sensory impairments (deaf-blindness)
- Physical impairments such as orthopedic and other health impairments and traumatic brain injury
- Language and/or social difficulties including autism, specific learning disabilities, speech and language impairments, and serious emotional disturbances
- Mixed types of disabilities such as traumatic brain injury and multiple disabilities
- Cognitive challenges, including mental retardation

Parents and professionals frequently agree to use the developmental delay category rather than the disability categories. *Delay* has less severe connotations than *disability* and is often the actual case; that is, a child's attainment of developmental milestones may just be on a slower schedule. A delay can be caused by environmental, medical, or social factors. The delay category also is often chosen because a disability diagnosis (e.g., mental retardation) is not definitive at an early age and certain disability diagnoses can only be established after serial assessment and intervention efforts.[2] When a disability is evidenced through assessment and clinical judgment, then a disability label may be warranted, especially when such a label is required for insurance/medical reasons. The stigmatizing and often inaccurate labeling of children must be weighted against whatever benefits accrue from a disability designation. Finally, the term *developmental delay* offsets the educational performance requirement of legislation for children who have had no educational history.[4]

Children can be identified for referral through interviews with families, record reviews, and developmental screenings. Much information about a child's development can be gleaned simply by asking families if they have any concerns about their child's development. Families are typically in the best position to comment and can be accurate reporters of development.[5] So if a parent believes that his or her child shows delay, most likely the child needs attention and a referral should be made.

Although interviews can be sufficient, sometimes parents are unsure whether or not their children have a developmental disability. Thus a formalized system of documenting a diagnosis is available. If no diagnosis can be estimated a developmental screening is warranted. Developmental screenings generally involve checklists that, once completed, reveal a child's developmental level. A 20% to 25% degree of delay usually qualifies a child for services. Parents and professionals can perform the screening by observing the child and recording the child's present level of skills. The medical profession often relies on the Denver Developmental Screening Instrument.[7] Other screening devices (and there are numerous ones available) that are considered more thorough and accurate although more time consuming include the Early Screening Inventory,[11] the Early Screening Profiles,[10] numerous parent questionnaires, and composite screening instruments developed by various organizations to meet certain requirements (e.g., Head Start community screening efforts).

During the screening process remember again that parents probably are in the best position to present and/or comment on screening items. Parents have good rapport with their child to perform items on the screenings. When a child does not perform an item for the professional screener it is appropriate to check with the parent and to believe the parent's answer.

Documentation about the child's diagnosis or scores on screening instruments helps the family to work with a service provider. The documentation provides concrete information about the child's developmental status and what services are needed. With this information families can become the first specialist helping with their child's development.

Sharing Information with Families

After discovering that a child may need to be referred for more detailed assessment or specialized services, it is important to share the information with the family. Most parents are already aware of their child's developmental status. Parents involved in developmental screenings also can have a keen understanding of their child's developmental level.

Even though parents may be familiar with their child's development, the information sharing process is a sensitive time for families. Parents need to know accurate information in a way that is understandable. They also need to know positive features of their child's development. Parents often equate hearing bad news about their child's developmental status or disability with the death of a loved one. Too often well-intentioned professionals focus on the diagnosis and attempt to ensure that the parent understands the problem. The trauma of hearing about a developmental disability can be lessened if positive statements about the child are made and parents know where to find help.

Finding a Service Provider

Before providing parents with information, professionals should know about their regional early intervention system. Inquiries can be made about early intervention programs at state and local levels. To identify how the system operates in the local area, contacts can be made to state departments of health, human services, and education. One of these departments is responsible for early intervention programs in your state and can provide information about local providers through a directory of early intervention services; each state is required to have such a directory. Preschool providers may be private agencies, public school districts, or special education units.

Local contacts also can be made by telephoning school districts and agencies such as ARC, Easter Seals, and United Cerebral Palsy. Inquires can be made about the early intervention system and also about the Local Interagency Coordinating Council (LICC). LICCs are mandated so that families, providers, and decision makers can work together to make recommendations for early intervention policy. The membership for the LICC comprises families, service providers, and representatives from state departments. With some work on the telephone and through LICC meetings parents can attain an indepth understanding of the system.

To find an appropriate provider it is important to determine what services are offered, how parents access services, and the reputation of the program. Public programs are free to families but private programs often require a fee for services and often the family's medical insurance is billed for therapies. If a referral to a private provider must be made, the family must be advised concerning costs and the ramifications of using insurance money (a family can lose insurance benefits by using too much therapy time for early intervention).

ENTERING THE EARLY INTERVENTION SYSTEM

After a referral is made there is a formal process for obtaining services. The responsible agency arranges for a multidisciplinary team evaluation (MDE) and an Individualized Education Plan (IEP) meeting. The process proceeds in the context of assuring that due process rights are applied.

Multidisciplinary Team Evaluation (MDE)

Eligibility for educational/developmental services should be accomplished through nondiscriminatory assessment by a multidisciplinary team evaluation (MDE). The MDE is conducted to determine whether a child is eligible, what services are deemed necessary, and where services will be offered (the child's placement).

To conduct the evaluation the team comprises at least two qualified professionals who use at least two assessments. The term *qualified* implies that the professional is certified, licensed, or meets other professional standards. The professionals are selected to address the child's main area(s) of need. For children who are medically involved a nurse can be a member of the team. Once an evaluation is conducted the team writes and then reviews the report with the family. The report can contain recommendations for educational, psychologic, medical and nursing services, and routines that the child needs during early intervention.

Also discussed at the MDE meeting is the issue of placement. Placement involves *where* the child is to receive services and is often the issue of most concern to families. As much as possible the placement must occur in the least restrictive environment (LRE). That is, children should receive services in the same settings as peers who have typical development. LRE is based on the notion that children can remain in typical settings while receiving intervention. Removing a child from a typical setting can be an infringement of his or her civil rights.

Individualized Education Plan (IEP)

Appropriateness of programming is specified by the IEP. The IEP contains the prescription for specially designed intervention for the child, including the type and intensity of services as well as yearly goals and objectives.

Today many early intervention providers write an Individualized Family Service Plan (IFSP) instead of an IEP. The IFSP includes the IEP as well as a designation of support that the family needs so the child can benefit from early intervention. (An IFSP is required for infant programs, but is not mandatory for preschoolers.)

Nursing services may be included in the plan if the child needs nursing to derive benefits from early intervention. However, this issue is controversial and has received much attention through litigation. If the child does not require nursing services an alternative role for a nurse is to help the family prepare for the IEP meeting. This can be accomplished by asking the parents what they want the child to achieve and what help can be provided so the child can succeed in the setting selected—optimally a typical setting.

Due Process

Parents who are having problems with a service system may contact the original referral source. It is important to know that the IDEA highlights the value of families and their due process rights. Before any decision about a child and early intervention services, parents must receive notification and give informed consent. That means that parents must consent before professionals identify their child as eligible for services, write an IEP, place their child in a program, provide services, or initiate a change in service. When there is an unresolvable disagreement parents can request an independent evaluation and/or a due process hearing. Increasingly, parents are demanding more appropriate and effective services. As a general rule, professionals should attempt to work through issues and accommodate parents. However, if a workable solution cannot be obtained within a reasonable period of time, the family should be referred to an advocacy agency so they have help in getting an impartial hearing and procuring their rights.

PROVIDING SERVICES

Preschoolers can be enrolled in several kinds of programs, depending on developmental needs, family and professional needs, family and professional judgments, and program availability. Not all states or localities offer the same range of options, and sometimes parents who relocate can be disappointed at what is or is not available in their new hometown.

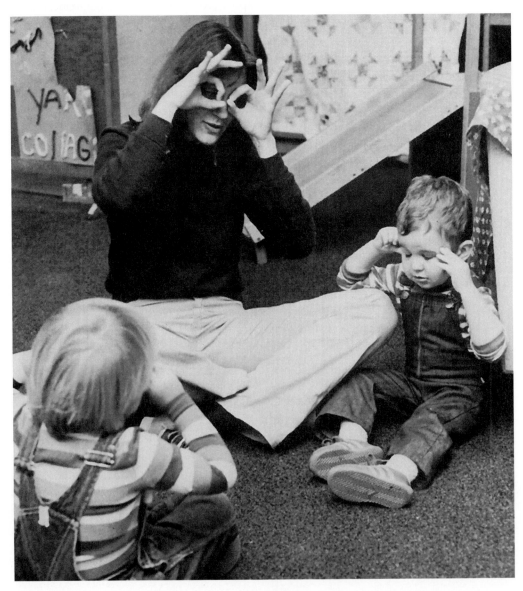

From Weizer MG: *Group care and education of infants and toddlers*, St Louis, 1982, Mosby–Year Book.

Service Models

Services can be provided in the child's home, a preschool center, in both the home and center, or in a clinic or hospital. Using the concept of least restrictive environment, children should be enrolled in the same settings as their typical peers. Exclusive home-based models are usually not appropriate unless the preschooler would be in jeopardy if enrolled in a center. Usually preschoolers with special needs should be enrolled in inclusive preschool centers where children with a range of developmental levels are enrolled.[10] Such inclusive preschools are considered optimal placements because they foster social integration and normalization. The principle of normalization[13] refers to the use of progressively more normal methods and materials to achieve progressively more developmentally normal (typical) goals. Currently it is often difficult to locate an inclusive preschool within reasonable proximity of the family. In the past most preschool programs have been provided by private agencies and comprised only children with special needs (e.g., United Cerebral Palsy, Easter Seals Society, Association for Retarded Citizens). Fortunately, however, many private agencies and school districts are rapidly moving toward inclusive enrollments. Staffing for such inclusive preschools may include an itinerant (consulting) special educator, the regular early childhood educator, and several allied professionals. Specialists may also visit the center to work with selected children and plan therapy activities that can be carried out by the teachers. Speech/language specialists, physical and occupational therapists, school psychologists, nurses, and social workers may all be involved on a regular or temporary basis. These onsite therapies woven into the child's day are usually preferred over "pull out" services.

Quality Service Indicators

Several professional organizations have formulated recommended or "best" practice guidelines for delivering services to preschoolers and their families. The Council for Exceptional Children, Division for Early Childhood (CEC/DEC),[6] the National Association for the Education of Young Children (NAEYC),[3] the National Association of School Psychologists (NASP),[12] the American Speech and Hearing Association (ASHA),[1] and other organizations are prominent in advocating for excellence and ethics in early intervention practices. In particular, DEC has published recommended practices for 14 areas related to early childhood services, including almost 40 recommendations pertinent to home, center, clinic, and hospital-based programs. Although the several organizations provide varying recommendations, at least four major practice dimensions are common to all; preschool services should be (1) family centered, (2) cross disciplinary, (3) normalizing, and (4) developmentally appropriate.

Family-centered refers to both the focus and decision making for services. The family is seen as the unit of concern because the child must be treated in the family context. Further, parents (or surrogates) are empowered to be primary decision makers. When family-centered practices are taken seriously services become family-directed, demanding high levels of understanding and collaboration between parents and professionals. Obviously, cultural sensitivity and related concerns are also embodied in a family-centered approach.

Cross-disciplinary practices are those that call for collaboration among professionals. Early childhood services require the coordination of multiple disciplines. Much has been written about multi, inter, and transdisciplinary teams. Whatever approach or model is used it is clear that quality service delivery demands the orchestrated services of collaborative professionals who work together in the interest of the family. It is important to look for assessment and service teams that are cross disciplinary.

Normalization is a recurrent standard emphasized by prominent professional organizations. What this means for preschool programming must be understood and carried out as intended by the normalization principle. Children should be provided with materials, instructional strategies, and social/physical circumstances that are as close to normal (i.e., typical) as possible and that at the same time foster progress. Sometimes procedures and materials must be atypical, contrived, or prosthetic to help a child learn and thrive. For example, explicit, contrived prompts and highly structured lessons may sometimes be needed to incite motivation and promote progress. The principle of normalization (like least restrictive environment) does not prohibit the use of atypical arrangements, but such circumstances should be accompanied by a plan to move gradually toward more normal arrangements.

Serious adherence to normalization includes concern for following Developmentally Appropriate Practice (DAP) guidelines.[3] Essentially, DAP encompasses the same features as normalization and promotes a child-as-initiator, active learner view. Early special education experts have examined the issues associated with DAP versus some of the highly structured, teacher-directed instruction common in special education.[15] Essentially, the professional advice is that preschool programs should follow developmentally appropriate practices except when these procedures are insufficient to guarantee child progress. Again, it seems that normalization guidelines subsume the issues under discussion.

The appendix on pp. 355 to 358 displays specific recommendations (quality indicators) for preschool programs. The indicators are applications of the major principles in the preceding discussion and offer a way to appraise placement options for children ready to go to preschool. Use of the indicators can help professionals and parents find a quality preschool program for children who need, deserve, and have the right to developmental help.

APPENDIX

Preschool Quality Indicators[8]

Although not a complete list, the following items provide a systemmatic way to appraise the features of a preschool program that includes features related to children with special needs. For each item give the program a score of 3, 2, or 1, using the following guidelines: 3 = yes, standard is clearly fulfilled; 2 = partly fulfilled; and 1 = not satisfactory on this standard.

Some quality indicators may be more important than others for a given child or family, so absolute is not as important as a consideration of program strengths and weaknesses. (The highest total score is 111, the lowest program score is 37.)

CONCERN	QUALITY INDICATOR	SCORE (1, 2, or 3)
Physical Arrangements Safety	Excellent use of safety features in the design of room and equipment; safety is stressed in the curriculum; children are well supervised during play time.	
Furnishings	Furnishings are appealing and comfortable; appropriate for all ages attending; excellent adaptations to accommodate persons with disabilities. Furnishings lend themselves well to overall educational program.	
Personal space	Personal space is available and is used to potential in classroom activities.	
Attractiveness	Very attractive environment; attractiveness is manipulated to direct attention to program-relevant features. Room invites exploration but is not cluttered.	
Accessibility	Classroom is barrier free.	
Cleanliness	Environment is very clean and uncluttered.	

continued

Basic Care Needs	
Toileting	Separate diapering area; tables and adequate supplies of diapers (cloth and disposable); child-sized bathrooms close by; training potties; well-adapted facilities for children with disabilities.
Nutrition	Nutritious snacks; adequate portions; regular schedule; exceptional dietary need taken into consideration; meals used as teaching time (life skills).
Clothing	Extra clothing/underwear; changes used as teachable moments; dress is proper for outside play.
First aid	Well-supplied medical kit; staff well trained in first aid procedures; exceptional children's needs taken into consideration.
Access to medical needs	Safe supplies with much variety; materials neatly displayed and stored; accessible to children.
Materials	
Art equipment	Safe supplies with much variety; materials neatly displayed and stored; accessible to children.
Play equipment	Many toys; variety across age ranges; displayed to encourage play and ease in clean-up.
Books and tapes	Many books with a variety of age appropriateness and subjects; very accessible and displayed in eye-catching manner.
Nap provisions	Cots or other comfortable provisions made; each child has own blanket; privacy is maximized.
Gross motor equipment	Equipment is safe; wide variety is available.
Adaptability	Material accessible to all children; good opportunities for sensory stimuli across modalities.

continued

Age appropriate	Equipment at appropriate levels that allows for safe and enjoyable play while giving the opportunity to develop.	
Curriculum (Fine motor, gross motor, language, self-care, social skills, cognitive)	Curriculum area has well-defined individual goals; materials are completely adequate to support goal attainment; planning is excellent among staff and objectives are reinforced across curriculum; planning takes into account the maintenance, fluency, and generalization of skills; proper reinforcement schedules are used; all gains are systematically documented; curriculum is comprehensive in scope.	
Activities		
Variety	Good balance of active and passive activities; frequent changes of types of activities available but with disability needs taken into consideration; activities very child centered; allows for exploration and experimentation.	
Structured play	Structured play built into curriculum; areas set up for play but with clearly stated developmental goals; structured play planned daily; reinforces other curricular goals.	
Transition time	Transitions well planned and orderly; children know expectations; extra activities planned for those who finish early.	
Free play	Fair variety of toys; set time for free play; children allowed to choose but with staff joining in when invited; more than one of most popular toys available to prevent disputes; staff alert to possible problems.	

continued

Scheduling	Staff aware of time-order activities; activities planned well ahead of time but children are also aware of schedule of activities; parents informed of special events.	
Dramatic	Dramatic play built into curriculum; planned to occur several times per week; great deal of variety of dramatic activities; integrated play with other areas of curriculum.	
Adult/Interpersonal		
Parent relations	Good communications with parents/caregivers; frequent conferences encouraged (place and procedure readily available); parents are welcome to observe.	
Child interactions	Staff anticipates children's needs and effectively interact with children at all times.	
Staff coordination	Staff communication is organized and effectively transferred to instructional activities; staff works as a coordinated team at maximum efficiency.	
Adult areas	Adult space available and comfortable; time for staff breaks built into schedule to maximize morale and staff efficiency.	
Supervision	Good supervision at all times; staff members aware of child's location and needs.	
Preparation	Lessons are very well organized. Excellent preparation and follow-through are obvious.	
Professional development	Opportunities such as reading materials, professional consultants, and inservice training available on site; time allocated for attending seminars.	

REFERENCES

1. American Speech and Hearing Association: The roles of speech-language pathologists in service delivery to infants, toddlers, and their families, *ASHA 32*, 1990.

2. Bagnato SJ and Neisworth JT: *What is convergent assessment? Assessment for early intervention: best practices for professionals*, New York, 1991, The Guilford Press.

3. Bredekamp S, editor: *Early childhood teacher education guidelines*, Washington, DC, 1987, National Association for the Education of Young Children.

4. Developmental delay: questions and answers: *Communicator 17*(4):1-2, 1991.

5. Diamond KE: The role of parents' observations and concerns in screening for developmental delays in young children, *Topics in Early Childhood Special Education 13*(1):pp 68-81, 1993.

6. Reference deleted in pages.

7. Fratenburg Wand Dodds J: *Denver-II Developmental Screening Test*, Denver, 1990, Denver Developmental Metrics.

8. Froman B, Rourke M, and Buggey T: Preschool Rating Scale, Unpublished manuscript, 1992, Pennsylvania State University.

9. Handen BL, Mandell F, and Russo D: Feeding induction in children who refuse to eat, *Am J Dis Child 140*:52-54, 1991.

10. Harrison P et al: *Early screening profiles (ESP)*, Circle Pines, Minn, 1990, American Guidance Service.

10a. McLean M and Odom S: *Early intervention–early childhood special education recommended practices*, Austin, Tex, 1996, Pro.Ed.

11. Meisels SJ and Wiske MS: *Early screening inventory (ESI)*, New York, 1988, Teachers College Press.

12. NASP/APA: Preschool practices, problems and issues, *Preschool Interests 2*(3):1-11, 1987.

13. Nirje B: The normalization principle. In Kugel RB and Shearer A, editors: *Changing patterns in residential services for the mentally retarded*, Washington, DC, 1976, President's Committee on Mental Retardation.

14. Vincent L et al: A behavioral-ecological approach to early intervention: focus on cultural diversity. In Meisels S and Shonkoff J, editors: *Handbook of early intervention*, New York, 1990, Cambridge University Press.

15. Wolery M, Strain P, and Bailey D: Reading potentials for children with special needs. In Bredecamp S and Rosegrant T, editors: Reading potentials: appropriate curriculum are assessment for young children, vol 1, Washington, DC, 1992, NAEYC.

CHAPTER 34

Special Education

ELEANOR W. LYNCH
DOUGLAS B. FISHER

All educators share a similar goal—to help students acquire the skills and knowledge to become informed, productive citizens. Although special educators work with students who may be gifted or disabled from infancy through young adulthood, this chapter focuses particularly on the role of special education for students with disabilities from age 3 to 21.

PL 94-142 and its current amendment, PL 101-476, define special education as "specially designed instruction, at no extra cost to the parent, to meet the unique needs of a handicapped child."[20] From this and other legislation (e.g., PL 98-199, PL 99-457, PL 102-119, and Section 504 of the Rehabilitation Act of 1973) five primary differences separate special education from regular education: (1) curriculum, (2) focus on the individual learner, (3) instructional processes and procedures, (4) emphasis on evaluation of student progress, and (5) the extent of parental involvement.

CHARACTERISTICS OF SPECIAL EDUCATION

Curriculum refers to content or what is taught. Although curricula vary from district to district and state to state, there is a generally agreed upon set of skills that are taught at each grade level. The curriculum in special education programs usually deviates in breadth, depth, and/or content from the regular academic curriculum. For example, a student with mild mental retardation may be taught basic arithmetic skills such as adding, subtracting, multiplying, and dividing but may not be introduced to higher level mathematics such as algebra or geometry. The curriculum for students with more severe disabilities often differs in content. Students may be taught the math needed to use coins in vending machines or to make purchases from a local store but they may not be taught formal arithmetic. This type of curriculum, which focuses on teaching life skills that the person can use now and in the future, is referred to as a functional curriculum[8] and is frequently used in programs for students with more severe disabilities.

A second difference between general and special education is the focus on the individual student. PL 101-476, Individuals with Disabilities Education Act (IDEA), mandates that each student receiving special education services have an Individualized Educational Plan (IEP). Following assessment of the student's current level of performance, the interdisciplinary IEP team, which includes the student and his or her appropriate family members, develops goals and objectives that are the focus during the next year of instruction. Unique IEPs are developed for each student receiving services or support through special education to ensure that instruction is tailored to the individual's needs.

For many students in special education to achieve the goals and objectives that were developed by the IEP team the instructional process must be modified. Some students need only to be taught at a slower pace with more opportunities to practice, others may need material sequenced into smaller steps, and still others may require very systematic teaching that includes direct instruction and immediate reinforcement of correct responses.[13]

Although all teachers measure student progress, special educators are especially concerned with the student's rate of learning and skill acquisition. When a student has learning difficulties there is not time to waste on methods that do not work. Daily or weekly measurement of the student's progress can alert the teacher to needed changes in the program methodology or provide documentation that the skills have been mastered and the student can begin work on a new objective.[15]

Finally, there is a considerable degree of parent involvement with students in special education. IDEA requires that parents be included in the decision-making process and on the IEP team. Consequently parents are seen as partners in education and their priorities for their child's education are included in the instructional program.[19] As a result of this partnership, special educators must be particularly sensitive to the changing definition of families and family diversity.[9]

THE PURPOSE OF SPECIAL EDUCATION

Improving students' performance has always been a goal of the field of special education, but it is only recently that successful performance in the mainstream of home, school, and community has been emphasized for all students with disabilities, regardless of their level of cognitive ability. The Regular Education Initiative (REI)[21,23] and the full inclusion model of service delivery[6,18] both emphasize the importance of teaching students with disabilities in the same schools and classrooms as their peers of the same chronologic age. This shift in thinking represents a significant change in the way that services are conceptualized and delivered for those students with the most severe disabilities or those with the most intensive support needs. Students who used to be in special centers or schools are now being included in their neighborhood schools. This change has brought general and special educators together to examine ways to teach all children more effectively.

THE SPECIAL EDUCATION PROCESS

Special education programs are quite variable in the curriculum that is taught and the instructional procedures that are used. This variability is essential because of the range of student needs that must be met. For example, a college-bound 17 year old with a specific learning disability needs different supports than a 17 year old who has limited cognitive skills and limited mobility. Regardless of the type of program, all students will have an IEP developed by an interdisciplinary team. IEP development is a process that includes assessment of the student, program planning, placement, program implementation, and program monitoring. Parents frequently become partners in their child's education, providing opportunities at home and in the community for the practice of skills taught at school.

Throughout the IEP process parents' and students' rights are protected. Parents have access to all school records about their child, and records must be maintained and stored according to strict rules of confidentiality. If at any point in the process parents and school personnel cannot agree on the program or placement, the parents have the right to challenge the school through a due process hearing.

The first step in the process of IEP development is assessment of the student. By law the parents must give permission for the assessment, the student must be assessed by a multidisciplinary team, the assessment instruments must be unbiased, reliable, and valid for the purpose for which they are being used, and the tests must be administered in the language normally used by the student. No single test can be used as the basis for decision making, and the assessment must be comprehensive, examining all aspects of a student's disability.[15]

After the assessment the IEP meeting is convened. The meeting must include a school system representative who is charged with supervising the

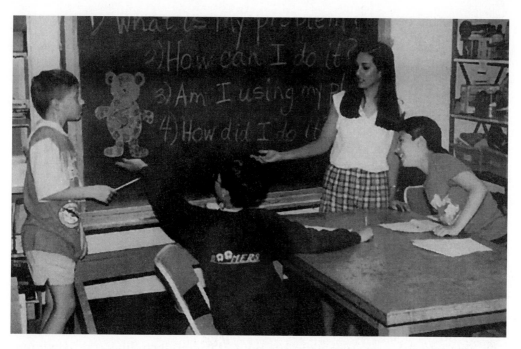

From Paul R: Language disorders from birth through adolescence: assessment and intervention, St Louis, 1995, Mosby–Year Book.

proceedings, the student's teacher or teachers, one or both parents, the student when appropriate, and a member of the assessment team or someone familiar with the assessment procedure and findings. It is the team's responsibility to develop the written IEP document that will serve as the plan of instruction. An IEP must contain the following: (a) the student's present levels of educational performance, (b) a statement of annual goals and short-term objectives, (c) specification of the special education and related services (e.g., transportation, physical therapy, counseling, assistive technology, etc.) that are to be provided, along with a statement about the student's extent of participation in regular education programs, (d) the date that the services are expected to begin and the probable duration of the services, and (e) objective criteria for determining on an annual basis whether or not the short-term objectives have been met.[20] Each student's IEP is reviewed at least yearly to evaluate progress, determine whether services should be continued, and determine what (if any) modifications are needed. Although the IEP is not a formal contract between the school and the family, it serves as an agreement about what is to be taught, the setting in which it is to be taught, the additional services that will be provided, and how progress will be evaluated.

APPROACHES TO SPECIAL EDUCATION: THEORY AND PHILOSOPHY

The field of special education draws on numerous theories to determine its approach to teaching and learning, and as with any professional discipline the influence of various theories has changed as each has been empirically tested. The theories that have withstood empiric scrutiny continue to be applied in developing and implementing special education programs and services. Behavioral learning theory, first in the form of applied behavior analysis and more recently in the form of systematic instruction, has had a profound effect on the field of special education.[3] Through the application of this theory in the home, in classrooms, and on the job, researchers have clearly demonstrated that all students, regardless of their apparent limitations, can and do learn. Systematic instruction, as defined by Snell and Brown,[17] refers to a process that uses frequent and systematic measurement of student progress to develop and modify instruction. This data-based approach to helping students learn, master, remember, and appropriately transfer their learning to new situations is a hallmark of high-quality special education.

A second approach that is currently being used is based on literature related to teaching effectiveness.[3,16] The research on effective teaching has identified several principles that promote learning including: (a) maximum emphasis on academic work or the skills to be learned, (b) direct control of the teaching and learning process and environment, (c) high expectations for student learning and behavior, (d) student accountability and responsibility for learning and behavior, and (e) a learning environment that is not negative in action or effect.[13,22] Teachers who create classrooms that reflect these principles are far more likely to have positive outcomes with all students.

A third approach that has been determined to be effective in improving learning among students with mild learning disabilities is strategy training.[2] Work by Alley and Deshler[1] using the Strategies Intervention Model includes three components: (1) curriculum, (2) instruction, and (3) organization. The curriculum component comprises the various strategies that are taught to students, such as strategies related to specific tasks, social skills, or motivation. The instructional component includes procedures that are used to teach those strategies to students, and the organizational component addresses the ways in which the school setting can be adjusted to accommodate these procedures. Although this system is complex, it has been demonstrated to be effective in increasing students' performance.

In addition to the theories that have shaped special education programs and services, philosophic perspectives have also been critical in formulating best practices. Those perspectives have included the belief that all individuals, regardless of their abilities, share civil and human rights. This belief is the cornerstone on which PL 94-142 was built and it continues through amendments to that law that guarantee free and appropriate public education services to students with disabilities. The normalization movement[24] also continues to influence practice. Educating all students in their neighborhood schools alongside their nondisabled peers and preparing students for competitive employment opportunities are both outgrowths of a philosophy of normalization. Most recently in special education programs and services for infants, toddlers, preschoolers, the belief in the importance of family-professional partnerships has been reaffirmed.[9,14,23]

Theory, research, and philosophic perspectives are all important in designing and implementing high-quality special education programs and services. As research informs theory and as beliefs and values about people with disabilities evolve, so too will special education.

TRENDS IN SPECIAL EDUCATION

Several trends have influenced special education in the past decade, and those trends will continue to shape the field into the 21st century. Four of those trends—early intervention, increased emphasis on curriculum and instructional methodologies, transition planning, and schooling that includes all students in meaningful ways—should be highlighted for their effect on the field of special education programs and services and on the lives of students who receive those services.

With the passage of PL 99-457 in 1986 the mandate for a free and appropriate public education for children with disabilities was extended downward to include children age 3. This legislation required that public schools take responsibility for providing special education programs, services , and supports to children with disabilities beginning at age 3. By the 1992 school year those services were to be in place in all states. In addition, this legislation encouraged states to initiate planning for a comprehensive, coordinated, multi-agency service system responsive to the needs of children with disabilities from birth through age 2 and their families. This portion of the law (PL 99-457, Title I, Part H) allowed states to determine which agency would take the lead in planning for a comprehensive early intervention system. This legislation underscored the importance of early intervention for children with disabilities and their families and represented an important trend that is supported by education law. As of 1995 all of the states and territories had developed and begun to implement early intervention programs for infants and toddlers.

A second trend relates to the increased emphasis on curriculum and instruction in all areas of special education. For students with mild disabilities the emphasis has been on instruction. As described in an earlier section of this chapter, systematic instruction and strategy training have been used very successfully with students with mild learning disabilities. For students with more severe disabilities both curriculum and instruction have been emphasized. The curriculum has moved from one based on normal development to one based on functional skills—those skills and behaviors that are important in the current environment and those that are predicted to be important in future years.[4] For example, using instructional time to teach 15-year-old students with disabilities to stack blocks in a special class does not reflect a functionally appropriate curricular objective; however, teaching those same students to put away dishes during a nutrition class or to wash dishes for a school job in the cafeteria would be functionally appropriate if those skills are required in their current home environment or are predicted to be needed in the near future.

The emphasis on functional curricular objectives has also led to changes in instructional settings and methods. Although systematic instruction that relies on data-based decision making is still used, it is done in more complex situations. For example, systematic instruction used to be applied to teach specific skills on a one-to-one basis in the classroom; now those procedures are applied in small group settings in the home, community, general education class, or on the job. Teaching a student cause and effect can be done in a cooperative group in which the student with disabilities operates a switch to turn on a tape recorder or water sprayer for a ceramics table.

Transition planning has assumed major importance in all areas of special education. Although transition planning is often thought of in terms of students' transition from school to higher education or the world of work, there are many transitions that precede transition into young adulthood. For some children in special education the first transition occurred several months after birth when they were sent home after a long stay in the neonatal intensive care unit. For others the first transition occurred when they entered a school- or center-based early intervention program at 12 or 18 months of age. The transition from preschool to kindergarten or from grade school to middle school, junior high, or high school also presents challenges for children with disabilities. To help students succeed as they encounter the increased demands of a new environment, teachers, family members, and other professionals work with the student to plan for and make the transition.

The current emphasis on inclusive schooling has had a major effect on students in special education programs, particularly those with more severe disabilities. As previously noted, general and special education have begun to work more closely to fully integrate students with disabilities into the mainstream of home, school, and community life. Adapting the general education curriculum, training students in social skills, and maximizing opportunities to be with chronological age peers while still addressing the student's own needs represents a new approach to special education service delivery.

These trends have already made considerable differences in the way that students with disabilities are viewed, the way that teachers (both general and special educators are trained), and the way that special education services are designed and delivered.

UNMET NEEDS

During the late 1980s and early 1990s considerable gains were made in the design and delivery of special education programs and services. However, despite such gains a number of needs are still unmet. Services for children from birth to age 3 is an area in which services are still developing. Although the mandate that services be provided for 3- to 5-year-old children is now in place, services for infants, toddlers, and their families are in their own infancy in many areas of the country and many of the provisions of the law are far from being fully and comprehensively implemented.[10] Until programs and services for all young children are available, needs will not be met.

Providing appropriate special education services to students from diverse cultural and linguistic backgrounds also continues to be a need. As the demographics of the United States change and the number of students from nonwhite and Hispanic families increases, there is an increasing mismatch between special educators and the students that they teach.[11] By the year 2000 nearly one third of the children under age 18 are projected to be from nonmajority families.[7] One of the major challenges of the next century will be to find appropriate ways to assess and provide services for students with disabilities who are nonEnglish speaking or who have limited English proficiency.

A final unmet need is integrally related to those previously discussed. Throughout the United States there is a shortage of teachers including a serious shortage of trained special education teachers. Nationally, it is estimated that as many as 30% of special education teachers do not meet the certification criteria in their states, and these shortages are predicted to continue.[12] Until adequate numbers of trained personnel enter the field, few of the other unmet needs can be addressed.

SUMMARY

Special education is a broad field that includes a wide range of programs and services. Although this chapter focuses on students with disabilities, special education incorporates the full range of exceptionality, from individuals who are gifted and talented to those with intensive support needs. Just as the students vary, so to do the programs and services that are offered. Minor adaptations in the curriculum or method of instruction are suitable for some students, while other students require considerably greater adaptations. Like all professional disciplines, special education is developed through philosophy, research, and practice. These combine to make special education a field that responds to today while improving practice for the future.

REFERENCES

1. Alley GR and Deshler DD: *Teaching the learning disabled adolescent: strategies and methods*, Denver, 1979, Love Publishing.
2. Ariel A: *Education of children and adolescents with learning disabilities*, New York, 1992, Merrill.
3. Brophy JE and Good TL: Teacher behavior and student achievement. In Wittrock, editor: *Handbook of research on teaching*, ed 3, New York, 1986, Macmillan.
4. Brown L et al: A strategy for developing chronological age appropriate and functional curricular content for severely handicapped adolescents and young adults, *Journal of Special Education* 13:81-90, 1979.
5. Bruder MB and Nikitas T: Changing the professional practice of early interventionists: an inservice model to meet the service needs of Public Law 99-457, *Journal of Early Intervention* 16:173-180, 1992.
6. Calculator SN and Jorgensen CM: *Including students with severe disabilities in schools*, San Diego, 1994, Singular.
7. Children's Defense Fund: *The state of America's children, 1991*, Washington, DC, 1991, Children's Defense Fund.
8. Falvey MA: *Community-based curriculum*, Baltimore, 1989, Paul H. Brookes.
9. Hanson MJ and Lynch EW: Family diversity: implications for policy and practice, *Topics in early childhood special education* 12:283-306, 1992.
10. Hanson MJ and Lynch EW: *Early intervention: implementing child and family services for infants and toddlers who are at risk or disabled*, ed 2, Austin, Tex, 1995, PRO-ED.
11. Hanson MJ, Lynch EW, and Wayman KI: Honoring the cultural diversity of families when gathering data, *Topics in early childhood special education* 10:112-131, 1990.
12. Hume M: Shortage of special educators, *Education Daily*, pp 1-2, April 3, 1989.
13. Lewis RB and Doorlag DH: *Teaching special students in the mainstream*, ed 4, New York, 1994, Macmillan.
14. McGonigel M, Kaufmann R, and Johnson B, editors: *Guidelines and recommended practices for the individualized family service plan*, ed 2, Bethesda, Md, 1991, Association for the Care of Children's Health.
15. McLoughlin JA and Lewis RB: *Assessing special students*, ed 4, Columbus, Ohio, 1994, Merrill.

16. Rosenshine B and Stevens R: Teaching functions. In Wittrock MC, editor: *Handbook of research on teaching*, ed 3, New York, 1986, Macmillan.

17. Snell ME and Brown F: Instructional planning and implementation. In Snell ME, editor: *Instruction of students with severe disabilities*, New York, 1987, Macmillan.

18. Stainback S and Stainback W: *Curriculum considerations in inclusive classrooms*, Baltimore, 1992, Paul H. Brookes.

19. Turnbull AP and Turnbull HR: *Families, professionals, and exceptionality: a special partnership*, ed 2, Columbus, Ohio, 1990, Merrill.

20. U.S. Office of Education: Implementation of Part B of the Education for the Handicapped Act, *Federal Register* 42:42474-42518, 1977.

21. Wang MC, Reynolds MC, and Walberg HJ: Integrating children of the second system, *Phi Delta Kappan* 70:248-251, 1988.

22. Weil ML and Murphy J: Instruction processes. In Mitzel HE, editor: *Encyclopedia of educational research*, ed 5, New York, 1982, Free Press.

23. Will M: *Educating students with learning problems, a shared responsibility: a report to the Secretary*, Washington, DC, 1986, U.S. Department of Education, Office of Special Education and Rehabilitative Services.

24. Wolfensberger W: *The principle of normalization in human services*, Toronto, 1972, National Institute on Mental Retardation.

CHAPTER **35**

Transitions from
Adolescence to Adulthood

PAMELA LUFT
FRANK R. RUSCH

The year Mary was in my class was the first time she had been able to
attend school for more than 2 days a week. She was 14. At least twice a year
she would miss a month or more but never long enough to engage home-
bound instruction. Academic programming for her had been almost impossible. Her skill attainment was extremely scattered and there were huge
developmental gaps. Her language patterns were immature and she could
not always make her needs and wants known. Mary's social interaction
with peers consisted of insults designed to get their attention, followed by
bewildered tears when they eventually sought revenge. She consistently
tested in the high normal intelligence range but was performing at primary
grade levels. It was all very discouraging.

American youth with special needs have the same aspirations as all other
youth. They wish to live, work, and recreate in the community with their
friends and family. They want to be part of the American dream. Unfortunately, history suggests that many of them do not find jobs, live independently, or find desired opportunities for recreation.

Over the past 2 decades major changes have taken place in the delivery of
educational and social services to persons with special needs.[9] Specifically,
the era of specialized and isolated service delivery is over. Further, the passage of transition legislation signals a recognition of the lifelong needs of individuals with disabilities and the beginning of an integrated programs model.

As a result many young adults with disabilities are now able to live, work, and play in our towns and cities, just as many of us expected to do when growing up. This legislation defines transition from school as:

> a coordinated set of activities for a student, designed within an outcome-oriented process, that promotes movement from school to post-school activities, including postsecondary education, vocational training, integrated employment, continuing and adult education, adult services, independent living, or community participation.[6]

In this chapter we examine transition with reference to (1) four legislative acts that affect transition services, (2) seven legislated implementation mechanisms, (3) seven outcome areas, and (4) a social system for evaluating services to transitioning youth.

TRANSITION LEGISLATION
PL 94-142

Universal provision of services to students with special needs began in 1975 with PL 94-142, the Education of All Handicapped Children Act. Every special education child is guaranteed educational services in the least restrictive environment generally determined as the local school district. Additionally, all special services are documented on an Individualized Education Program (IEP), an annual plan that is designed by parents, school personnel and, when appropriate, the student. Services are guaranteed through rights of due process and parents have the authority to challenge school decisions and placements.

This act marked a trend toward increased decision-making power for parents and consumers with disabilities. At the same time the IEP meetings initiated many of the collaborative planning practices that now characterize service provision to individuals with disabilities, including mandated transition services.

IDEA

Taking PL 94-142 a step further, the Individuals with Disabilities Education Act (IDEA) of 1990, addresses problematic discontinuity of services and preparation for adult services. IDEA mandates that transition planning for special education students begin no later than age 16 and be documented on students' IEPs. This planning must list interagency links and responsibilities for each team member, the student and parents, the school, and other service agencies involved in achieving the transition outcomes.

This legislation addresses specific categories of special education students. For example, both the orthopedically impaired category and the other-health impaired category include students with chronic medical conditions[4]; however, the health problems associated with these chronic impairments are not the characteristics that make a child eligible for services.[2] In general, unless a child has a condition that adversely affects educational progress, he or she is not included.

Section 504

Many children ineligible for IDEA may receive services under Section 504 of the Rehabilitation Act of 1973. In accordance with this piece of legislation these students receive personal and assistive technology interventions if they have a physical or mental impairment that limits one or more major life activities.[1] Amendments passed in 1986 and 1992 have increased opportunities for supported employment (community employment with monitoring and support), expanded independent living programs, and streamlined the transition from high school into rehabilitation programs.

ADA

The Americans with Disabilities Act (ADA) of 1990 is the most recent major legislation to expand transition opportunities for individuals with disabilities by addressing their rights. This bill guarantees access to employment and community facilities and mandates reasonable accommodations to achieve this. As a result, regardless of private or public status, all community postsecondary training, employment, and recreation facilities now must be available for transition services and activities.

Through guaranteed access and accommodation, these four pieces of legislation have secured educational, personal, and transition services for special education students with special needs and have expanded transition opportunities. A student like Mary, from the beginning of the chapter, qualifies for special education services because of her significant academic delays. Because she is 14 a transition plan is not required; however, because of her health and attendance problems her IEP should begin addressing independent living and future career choices and remediating her academic and social skill deficits.

In the following section we examine the mechanisms that are incorporated into IDEA to ensure that the following critical outcomes stipulated in the transition definition are addressed: provision of educational activities, integrated employment, independent living, and community participation.

TRANSITION MECHANISMS

Based on current educational best practices, IDEA includes seven provisions designed to promote the identification and achievement of appropriate transition outcomes:

1. Transition services must be based on the needs, preferences, and interests of individual students.
2. IEPs will include statements of needed transition services beginning no later than age 16.
3. School and adult services will coordinate efforts to promote movement into post-school activities.
4. Coordinated, community-based experiences and instruction will be used to develop employment and adult living skills.

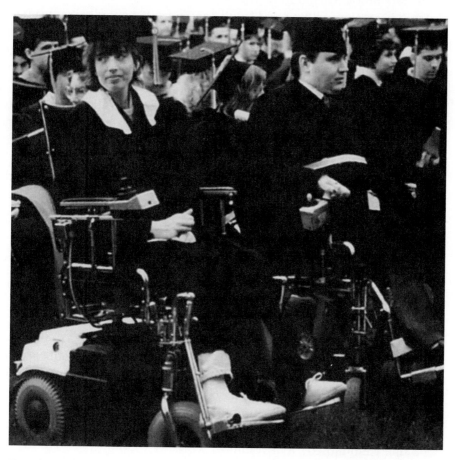

From Payne and Hahn: *Understanding your health,* ed 4, 1995, St Louis, Mosby–Year Book.

5. Transition needs will be individually determined and include postsecondary education, vocational education, vocational training, integrated employment, continuing and adult education, adult services, independent living, and community participation as needed.

6. Evaluation of transition services will be based on student outcomes in the postschool and community environments.

7. The educational agency will be responsible for monitoring and assuring delivery of appropriate transition services.

Such coordinated and collaborative planning is particularly valuable for students with complex needs requiring multiple service specialists. The interactive team process assists these specialists in managing the various systems and disciplines involved[7] and prepares all team members for periodic acute health care problems and more chronic needs.[12]

Mary has severe asthma and could benefit from a coordinated team effort to reduce the effect of this condition on her academic achievement and to prepare her for future transitions. Team members would include Mary (at age 16 if not before), her parents, her teacher, the school nurse, adult service agency representatives (such as the Department of Vocational Rehabilitation), her medical specialist or family doctor, and an adult-education or community college representative, as appropriate. An important transition activity would be to introduce her to the personnel and agencies she will come in contact with when moving from student or pediatric services to adult services. The IEP team should form the basis for a long-term personal support network as Mary becomes increasingly independent. Mary's school would monitor the transition responsibilities until she graduates and would reconvene the IEP meeting if goals are not met.

While legislation mandates these seven practices to ensure interagency cooperation and collaboration, the specific nature of transition outcomes are less well defined. In the next section we look at a series of desired outcomes that need to be addressed in transition planning.

TRANSITION OUTCOMES

A number of options have been suggested for addressing the outcomes contained in the transition definition.[6,12] For example, the California State Department has divided transition outcomes into the following seven categories[3]:

1. Employment—ranging from competitive employment (work in the community), to supported employment (community work that is routinely monitored), and volunteer work

2. Training and education—vocational services and agencies, school work experiences, and postsecondary education or training programs

3. Financial/economic—wages and benefits, income taxes, social services, insurance, and money management
4. Recreational—use of leisure time, sports and fitness, and stress management activities
5. Social relationships—socialization and friendships encompassing work acquaintances and close friends, personal relationship skills and support systems, and requisite communication skills
6. Independent living—home management and maintenance, consumer services, community awareness, survival and safety skills, personal management, health services (medical, dental, mental), sexuality and family life, adult rights and responsibilities, and advocacy and legal services
7. Residential—remaining in the family residence, shared living, independent living, supervised group living (dormitories), and residential care facilities

Choices within each of these categories are based on individual student needs and preferences. For example, Mary's training and education category would address developmental gaps, and specific social interaction interventions would be listed under social relationships. The independent living category would include steps toward increasing her responsibility for health and other decisions, and employment would identify potential careers and preparatory work experiences that Mary will need.

An annual meeting cannot address all of the ongoing information, support, and service needs of both students and their families, however. In the following section we examine some of these needs and the solutions generated by using a social systems perspective. A multiple systems approach defines problems broadly and produces more expansive solutions and potentially an entire environment that is more responsive and supportive of an individual and family with unique needs.

ISSUES AND SOLUTIONS

Rappaport[8] introduced a systems-level approach to examine and resolve social problems. This same approach was used to address the needs of students and workers with disabilities in 1985.[10,11] This social systems framework consists of the following four reciprocal and interactive levels:

1. Student and family—the target or focus of interventions and programming
2. Program—the group or agency responsible for implementing the interventions
3. Interagency—the network of agencies collaborating with the primary program in delivering services

4. Community—the services and opportunities available such as employment, recreation, and transportation

We will use this system to identify issues at every level for Mary and her family and for an additional student, Alan. Only by addressing all four levels and the unique interactions and contributions of each, can we adequately understand the needs presented by these students and their families.

> Alan had recurrent headaches, a periodic complaint thought to be associated with his scoliosis. Just 21 years old, he had started a training program as a new client of the Department of Vocational Rehabilitation. However, he was neglecting to call in to report that he was ill and he missed an important meeting with his rehabilitation counselor. This behavior was a surprise because only 2 months earlier he had successfully completed a 1-year career and training program in a supervised apartment setting and had been quite responsible. If it had not been for his mother dragging him to the next meeting with his counselor he would have been dropped as a rehabilitation client and left without further training or support services.

Student and Family Level

Mary's family is very supportive of her health care needs. Because an aunt also has severe asthma the family is acquainted with both her routine and acute needs. In addition, the aunt is a source of emotional support and encouragement for both Mary and her family.

The family has expressed concern about the costs of Mary's health care, however. Their income level exempts them from a number of public programs yet is insufficient to cover all costs. Consequently they are reluctant to seek medical services as often as needed. They hope that someone at the school can help them.

Alan's family is also supportive but is frustrated that he no longer listens to their advice. Consequently they have asked for assistance in enabling Alan to make responsible decisions, especially with respect to realistic timelines, employment, and financial support. They are willing to support him until he leaves home if he is willing to contribute toward this move.

Alan and his girlfriend wish to get married soon and both families support their decision. However, Alan is having difficulty fitting his dreams with reality. For example, he is unconcerned about being unemployed and believes that his brother will give him his former house when his brother moves. Further, when making career choices Alan tends to overestimate his physical endurance, which is limited because of his scoliosis. Alan needs help in a way that will further his growing independence and self-determination.

Program Level

Mary's IEP team will develop educational goals to address developmental gaps, social skills training, and increased opportunities for interacting with peers. Although only 14, Mary needs to take increasing responsibility for monitoring her own health, using her medications appropriately, and seeking information from her doctor.

Mary's school program includes introductory work-exploration activities, giving her opportunities to interact with co-workers and supervisors. Specific career training and residential options will be addressed as she gets older. The school is not able to provide Mary's family with information or resources concerning financial assistance. Instead they plan to contact other agencies that may be of more help.

Alan was a special education student because of severe learning disabilities. He is now receiving training through the Department of Vocational Rehabilitation and can continue to do so provided that he fulfills his obligations with them. If not he will be left to his own and his family's resources. Although possibly an effective lesson in real-life consequences, it is not cost effective if Alan remains unemployed, supported by either welfare or Supplemental Security Income. Once individuals with disabilities are without work, unemployment rates increase over time.[5] As a result Alan's compliance with his rehabilitation program is becoming a critical life decision and one that must be addressed at other levels.

Interagency Level

Mary's IEP team members are pursuing information about financial support available through other agencies. Also her medical specialist may know of a parents' group that could assist Mary's family in identifying financial resources in the community and in addressing other issues as Mary moves into adulthood. Further, a patient support group puts Mary in touch with other peers, thereby improving her social skills and offering opportunities to share some of her own frustrations.

Mary's team wants to know specifics about Mary's prognosis, symptoms they should be aware of, and possible interventions to reduce Mary's absenteeism. This information will influence career decisions, especially regarding the "health" of potential work environments and the physical demands of the job. Mary's parents have agreed to ask the aunt to meet with the team because she is a potentially useful resource in guiding future decisions.

Alan's rehabilitation counselor has invited members from his former IEP team to assist Alan and his family with timelines and decision-making strategies. At some point the team may wish to do joint planning with Alan's girlfriend, also a rehabilitation client, to help the couple develop realistic goals and plans.

The team has some concern about Alan's headaches. If they are indicative of a deterioration in his overall health they may affect future career and support services needed. On the other hand, the headaches may be symptomatic of Alan's anxiety over his new adult status and independence. In this case he needs constructive reassurance; a mutually developed sequential plan that is reviewed periodically may provide him with a sense of structure without compromising his sense of self-direction. Additionally, Alan's medical specialist may know of a support group that could help Alan learn about and cope with his physical limitations and make realistic yet optimistic life choices.

Community Level

The financial dilemmas facing Mary's family are not unique; health care for families in this country generally depends on the parents' employment. Assistance programs frequently set low-income–level criteria. Mary's health care costs are higher than average. Along with her current school absenteeism they could present significant barriers to employment. Thus without changes in current policy Mary may not be able to get the insurance or the job she needs to be able to pay for her health care. Financing health care for individuals with disabilities is an issue that must be resolved at the policy and legislative level. It will require information and action by consumers, their families, and their advocates.

Although Alan was fortunate to have been in a supervised apartment-living and career program, he would still benefit from additional training and opportunities in a program with gradually decreasing supervision and support. His former school has considered opening such a program for graduates but needs interagency and state-level help to secure the facility, train and certify the staff, and write the grant. The school has made initial state-level contacts but is currently involved in a district-wide program review and therefore has not had time to pursue this issue.

Unlike many individuals with disabilities, Alan is fortunate to be eligible for vocational rehabilitation services. Funding is allocated locally and resulting services vary with each locale. Further, counselors are evaluated based on numbers of clients placed in employment, an ineffective way to deal with the diverse needs of individuals with disabilities now guaranteed access to employment and community participation and who currently represent the majority of individuals receiving rehabilitation services. Individuals determined to be ineligible or who lose their eligibility for services have no other rehabilitation agency to turn to. Without training options and assistance in finding employment, their only option is to seek public assistance—a burden for tax payers that only worsens over time.

Individuals at all levels of the social system need to provide local-, regional-, and federal-level decision makers with specific information about problems and suggestions for change. The legislation guaranteeing access has ever-broadening effects. At the same time, however, it is making more apparent the tremendous gaps in services that currently exist and the need for a unified and consistent service delivery system, particularly after an individual reaches adulthood.

CONCLUSION

This chapter examines various issues related to transition, all of them pointing to the need for service professionals and the entire community to work together to ensure full participation and independent living for young adults with disabilities. In many instances we need to identify solutions that extend beyond our own professional or programmatic resources and involve all four levels of the social system. As a result of growing collaboration we, as team members, will increasingly be asked to function as facilitators or knowledgeable advocates rather than as experts. In addition, our roles will change toward assisting individuals with disabilities in making their own decisions and in supporting them in these decisions. Only by working together will the time come when individuals with disabilities are truly empowered to lead their own lives in a community that is increasingly accepting and supportive.

REFERENCES

1. Arizona Department of Education: Section 504: a challenge for regular education. In *AZ-TAS themes and issues: a series of topical papers on special education*, Phoenix, 1991, The Department.
2. Biehl RF: *Handicapped children and youth: a comprehensive community and clinical approach*, New York, 1987, Human Sciences Press, Inc.
3. California School for the Deaf-Riverside: *Individual transition plan*, Riverside, Cal, 1992, Author.
4. Kendall RM: *Unique educational needs of learners with physical and other health impairments*, East Lansing, Mich, 1991, Center for Quality Special Education Disability Research Systems, Inc. (ERIC Document Reproduction Service No. ED 342 186).
5. Mithaug DE et al: *Why special education graduates fail: how to teach them to succeed*, Colorado Springs, 1988, Ascent Publications.
6. NICHCY (National Information Center for Children and Youth with Disabilities): *Transition summary*, New York, 1993, The Center.
7. Pacer Center: *Speak up for health: young people with chronic illness and disabilities speak about independence in health care* [videotape], St. Paul, Minn, 1992, Armour Productions.
8. Rappaport J: *Community psychology: values, research, and action*, New York, 1977, Holt, Rinehart, and Winston.
9. Rusch FR et al: *Transition from school to adult life: models, linkages, and policy*, Sycamore, Ill, 1992, Sycamore Publishing.
10. Rusch FR, Enchelmaier JF, and Kohler PD: *Employment outcomes and activities for youths in transition, career development for exceptional individuals* 17:1-16, 1994.
11. Rusch FR and Mithaug DE: Competitive employment education: a systems-analytic approach to transitional programming for the student with severe handicaps. In Lakin CK and Bruininks RH, editors: *Strategies for achieving community integration of developmentally disabled citizens*, Baltimore, 1985, Paul H. Brooks Publishing Co.
12. Wehman P: *Life beyond the classroom: transition strategies for young people with disabilities*, Baltimore, 1992, Paul H. Brookes Publishing Co.

CHAPTER **36**

Vocational Preparation for Students with Disabilities

CAROLYN MADDY-BERNSTEIN

Vocational-technical education is in a unique position to assist students with disabilities to become productive citizens. According to findings of the National Longitudinal Transition Study of Special Education Students,[10] students with disabilities who are enrolled in vocational-technical education:

- stay in school longer
- have better attendance
- are more likely to attend postsecondary vocational education
- have a job after 2 years

DEFINITION OF VOCATIONAL EDUCATION

In the Carl D. Perkins Vocational and Applied Technology Education Act of 1990,* Congress defined vocational education as:

> organized educational programs offering a sequence of courses which are directly related to the preparation of individuals in paid or unpaid employment in current or emerging occupations requiring other than a baccalaureate or advanced degree. Such programs shall include competency-based applied learning which contributes to an individual's academic knowledge, higher-order reasoning, and problem-solving skills, work attitudes, general employability skills, and the occupational-specific skills necessary for economic independence as a productive and contributing member of society.

*Carl D. Perkins Vocational and Applied Technology Act, 1990, Public Law 101-392.

While earlier definitions of vocational education concentrated on preparing conventional students for work, the Perkins legislation requires that vocational education programs are of the size, scope, and quality to be effective; integrate academic and vocational education programs through a coherent sequences of courses; and provide equitable participation for special populations.

This broader definition of vocational education is in part a response to the national school reform effort and also an attempt to restructure vocational education to be more responsive to the needs of business and industry. Reformers note that all students—especially students who are members of special populations—learn more by participating actively in the learning process. Cooperative learning, a reality in vocational education programs since its conception in the nineteenth century, is also reaffirmed in reform efforts. Vocational educators are quick to point out that new educational strategies such as cooperative learning and applied learning have long been the backbone of good vocational programs. Indeed, vocational education laboratories are ideal environments for such learning.

The broadened definition provided in the Perkins Act also emphasizes the need to educate all segments of the population. The greatest portion of labor force entrants over the next decade will consist primarily of those who have been underserved by our education systems in the past: women, minorities—many of whom will have limited English proficiency—and other at-risk groups, including those with disabilities.[5] We must ensure that these new members of the work force are well prepared if we are to continue to be a world economic power.

STAGES AND AGES

For students with disabilities to gain the most from vocational programs, educators, parents, businesses, and the community must work together with them to plan educational programs that lead to a productive life. There should be an emphasis on strengths and abilities, not disabilities. Students must understand and appreciate their abilities, interests, and values. Furthermore, they need to have high self-esteem, know their career options, and be able to make good decisions. A one-time, 1-year or even 2- or 3-year process is insufficient to make this happen. Rather, the process must be ongoing and infused throughout the curriculum beginning in the student's early years with career exploration and progressing through vocational assessment to job preparation and placement.

Career Exploration

Career exploration and self-assessment should begin in preschool and kindergarten (earlier if possible) and last through adult education. The need for continuous assistance in career development is well documented.[1,7,12] Opinions about ourselves and how we relate to various occupations are formed at a very young age, beginning in infancy. It is critical for students with disabilities to understand the world of work, to have realistic expectations of job demands, and to be exposed to positive nonstereotyped role models. Indeed, role stereotyping is so pervasive that the school must work collaboratively with business, the home, and the community to assure all students equitable choices.

In 1989 the National Assessment of Vocational Education (NAVE) found that females with disabilities were much more likely to be enrolled in low-paying, service-occupational education programs than their male counterparts. Similar findings were noted for youth who are disadvantaged. It is imperative that the school, home, business, and community actively intercede using proven career intervention methods to assist students to reach their full potential. The interventions must take place throughout their school years and beyond. Some techniques include the following:

- identifying successful role models
- conducting student tours of industry and business, especially where there are role models at work
- requiring all teachers to continually relate their subject matter to a variety of careers
- encouraging students to volunteer
- arranging for internships/shadowing experiences
- encouraging students to work after school and in summer
- arranging cooperative work experiences during the final years of school

To assure students of equal opportunity careers it is imperative that relevant career materials and activities be formally infused into all facets of the curriculum. At the same time educators must overcome personal biases that have too frequently barred students from the education they might have chosen if given the opportunity.

Vocational Assessment

Although vocational assessment is required by federal mandate for students who are members of special populations, the scope and depth of the assessment is not defined. Practitioners must determine the process and the content of the assessment. The trilevel Texas model[8] is accepted nationally as a viable format.

Level I vocational assessment. This first level of the model is designed to gather preexisting student information. Information on attendance, grades, previous testing scores, previous work experience, prevocational classes, and special considerations for placement in educational programs should be available. As a rule students with disabilities have extensive test data that is often sufficient without further testing. Student, parent, and/or teacher interviews may also be used to obtain information during Level I.

Level II vocational assessment. During the second level additional information is gleaned from further assessment through paper-and-pencil–type assessment instruments, performance tests, and measures of dexterity, spatial ability, eye-hand coordination, strength, and/or perceptual abilities. Level II assessments are usually administered by teachers and/or counselors in the school.

Level III vocational assessment. This final level is a comprehensive process used only when the school needs more placement information than can be obtained from Levels I or II. The Level III assessment may last from a few hours to several weeks and involves abilities assessment through structured exploratory exercises or simulated occupational tasks/work samples. A trained vocational evaluator should administer the Level III assessment.

The vocational assessment process will vary according to individual needs. Although there can be benefits from group assessment (e.g., achievement tests, interest surveys), vocational assessment techniques are usually highly individual and do not lend themselves to mass testing. The expense for Level III assessment may be significant, but is well worth the effort when correctly done.

Program Placement

Program placements should be based on the expressed goals of students. In turn, the students' goals should be based on their knowledge of self and the world of work. A placement committee (maybe the Individualized Education Plan committee) comprising the student, parent, vocational teacher, counselor, resource teacher, and other pertinent professionals should be formed. The involvement of the vocational teacher is central to the student's success.

The placement committee should have access to the vocational assessment report identifying specific abilities, vocational aptitudes, and interests. The assessment report should include suggested support services that the student will need to succeed in a given vocational program. It is very important that the evaluator, counselor, psychologist, or teacher responsible for compiling the assessment report and recommendations understand vocational education. He or she should be very familiar with the competencies required for completing vocational programs and should make recommendations based on that knowledge. Students who enter vocational programs based on the recommendation of professionals who have little understanding of the complexities of the program are at high risk for failure.

Job Preparation

Vocational education has a variety of delivery systems. Some of these systems include programs in public high schools, area vocational technical schools, private vocational schools, state and private schools for students with specific disabilities, and postsecondary institutions such as community colleges. In the future the trend for full inclusion of all students may alter some of these systems, such as the alternative school. In addition to inschool programs there are cooperative work programs for secondary students and on-the-job training programs offered by industry.

Ideally the curriculum for most vocational programs is based on competencies business and industry have agreed are necessary for workers to have. An auto mechanics curriculum would undoubtedly include a competency area of brake repair, cosmetologists would learn competencies for cutting hair, and computer programmers would learn computer languages. Competency-based vocational curriculum provides an excellent opportunity for secondary and postsecondary students with disabilities to plan customized training programs. For example, students who are interested in auto mechanics may not realistically expect to complete all the competencies included in that program area but could learn those related to a specific, specialized area (e.g., a quick lubrication technician or a tire technician). A customized vocational program placement must:

- be arranged in cooperation with the program area instructor
- be detailed in the Individualized Education Plan (IEP)
- have carefully identified the competencies needed for a specific entry-level job

Because many competency-based vocational education programs work on the "open entry/open exit" principle, it is feasible to extend the program completion time to whatever is needed for the student to master the required competencies. Some school personnel are resistant to customizing programs for students with special needs, but more and more vocational programs are becoming accessible.

Creating a seamless progression from secondary to postsecondary vocational education has also been accomplished through articulating programs between secondary education and community colleges with competency-based curriculum serving as the bridge. Students are then able to transition easily into a thirteenth or fourteenth year of school without duplicating learning. The articulation agreements also serve as a catalyst for pursuing postsecondary education.

VOCATIONAL PROGRAMS THAT WORK

In 1989 20 components of good vocational programs serving students with special needs were identified in a survey conducted by the National Center for Research in Vocational Education (NCRVE)[9] (see the box below).

Annually the National Center's Office of Special Populations (OSP) conducts a national search for exemplary vocational programs serving students with special needs. The following describes three of the programs identified.[2]

Vocational Tracker Program (Utah)

Salt Lake City's Granite School District supports the transition of individuals with disabilities into work and future life through a unique program called

---

Components Of Exemplary Programs

Program Administration

Strong administrative leadership and support
Sufficient financial support
Staff development
Formative program evaluation
Summative program evaluation

Curriculum and Instruction

Individualized curriculum modifications
Integration of academic and vocational curricula
Appropriate instructional settings
Cooperative learning experiences

Comprehensive Support Services

Assessment of individual's vocational interests and abilities
Instructional support services
Ongoing career guidance and counseling

Formalized Articulation and Communication

Family/parent involvement and support
Notification of both students and parents regarding vocational opportunities
Vocational educator's involvement in individualized planning
Formalized transition planning
Intra- and interagency collaboration

Occupational Experience

Work experience opportunities
Job placement service
Follow-up of graduates and nongraduates

the Vocational Tracker Program. Paraprofessionals known as vocational trackers individualize placement needs of students and business, monitor student progress, and help them to build independence on the job. Trackers accomplish these objectives through (a) assisting students to develop appropriate job and social skills, (b) gaining access to community-based work sites for their students, and (c) providing job coaching to help ensure success. Parents play an integral part in every phase of the program.

Currently 16 trackers housed in the Granite School District's 10 high schools provide a wide array of services to more than 1200 students with disabilities. Business and agency partnerships have been developed over the 6 years of the program's existence with more than 350 businesses and a large number of agencies now participating. Initially funded through special education funds, the program is now supported through Job Training Partnership Act (JTPA), Carl D. Perkins Vocational and Applied Technology Education, and local funds.

New River Valley Community College (Virginia)
Learning Achievement Program for the Learning Disabled (LEAP)

Initiated in 1984, the Learning Achievement Program for the Learning Disabled (LEAP) annually serves more than 125 students with learning disabilities through the New River Community College. The unique program attracts students from around the state who enroll and/or attend a summer preparatory program designed to help them succeed at New River Community College or other colleges of their choice. During this phase students learn how to tape lectures, obtain taped textbooks, or arrange for special testing accommodations. They are also helped to understand their problem in relation to the college community, their rights, and how to interact with teachers and others who may not understand their problem.

During the school year students receive varying degrees of assistance depending on expressed need. Services include counseling, tutoring, mentoring, job placement, and other needs as they arise. All staff, including vocational instructors, are extremely responsive to student needs and difficulties.

Because the LEAP staff has provided inservice activities to help the faculty and staff understand and teach students with learning difficulties, the entire campus is sensitized to the special needs of students with learning disabilities. All staff—faculty, learning lab staff, counseling staff, job placement coordinators, and even the president of the college—take great pride in the accomplishment of students with learning disabilities who have been in the program. LEAP staff also provide inservice activities to personnel at other Virginia community colleges and high schools.

Lake Washington Technical College
Electronic Manufacturing Support Services Program (Washington)

While the Electronic Manufacturing Support Specialist Program is open to all students who attend Lake Washington Technical College, many students who are members of special populations have been extremely well served in the program. At any one time class members may include nontraditional students, students with limited English proficiency, those who are academically and/or economically disadvantaged, students with disabilities, and those who have no special needs. Because the program uses an entirely individualized, competency-based, open-entry, open-exit format, students work at their own pace. Upon entry each student works with the instructor to design a customized training plan. Instruction includes life skills (e.g., responsibility, commitment) and employability skills (e.g., interviewing, resumé writing, job search process).

The program is run like an industry shop with students serving in various roles, including supervisor. Projects are organized around the cooperative learning concept. Once students grasp basic competencies they may opt for internships or cooperative work experience programs to gain on-the-job experience. There is a strong network of area employers who serve as models for students, donate funds and equipment to keep the shop up to date, and most importantly, hire program completors. The 1991 to 1992 placement rate was 88%.

IMPORTANT RELATED LEGISLATION

The amount of federal legislation affecting the vocational education of students with special needs is indicative of the national interest and the critical need to assist people with disabilities. The following is a review of the Carl D. Perkins Vocational and Applied Technology Education Act of 1990, the major legislation on the topic.

Background

Although the Vocational Education Act of 1963 did not provide funds for students with special needs, the law required that those students should have access to vocational training programs. The Vocational Amendments of 1968 separated special-needs learners into two categories of *handicapped* and *disadvantaged* and required 10% of the basic state grant funds to provide services for students with disabilities and an additional 15% of the state grant for those who are disadvantaged.

In 1976 Congress mandated 10% of the funds authorized under the Vocational Education Act of 1976 be set aside to support additional costs required for supporting students with disabilities in vocational education programs; 22% was mandated to be set aside for students who are disadvantaged. The law, which often referenced the Rehabilitation Act of 1973 and the Education for All Handicapped Children's Act, attempted to mainstream vocational education programs (e.g., students were to be placed in the least restrictive vocational education environment).

The Carl D. Perkins Vocational Education Act of 1984 required that persons with disabilities and those who are disadvantaged must have equal access to quality vocational programs. The act also required that students with special needs receive vocational assessment, equal access to recruitment, enrollment, placement, guidance and counseling, and be informed of the school's vocational offerings before the ninth grade. The act set aside 10% of the basic state grant for students with disabilities and 22% of the state grant for students who are disadvantaged. In all, 57% of each state grant allotment was earmarked for special-needs populations.

Findings from the National Assessment of Vocational Education (NAVE), a study mandated by the Carl D. Perkins Vocational Education Act of 1984, found that despite previous federal mandates, serious inequities still existed for special groups participating in vocational programs.[4] This finding, coupled with the fact that less populated geographic areas received only trivial funds under the 1984 vocational education legislation, led Congress to draft a reauthorization bill that reshaped vocational education legislation. Thus the Carl D. Perkins Vocational and Applied Technology Education Act of 1990 targeted money to areas with the largest concentration of special populations and required that programs be of the size, scope, and quality to be effective.

Special Populations Defined

Even among public school teachers, misconceptions about who make up special populations are more the rule than the exception. Many perceive "special populations" as students with disabilities who qualify under the IDEA. The Perkins Act expands the definition to include:

> individuals with handicaps, educationally and economically disadvantaged individuals (including foster children), individuals of limited English proficiency, individuals who participate in programs designed to eliminate sex bias, and individuals in correctional institutions.*

Provisions

The Perkins Act of 1990 is in part the congressional response to findings from research reports that have triggered an alarm among the business community and educational leaders across the nation. *Workforce 2000,*[5] *The Forgotten*

---

*Carl D. Perkins Vocational and Applied Technology Act, 1990, Public Law 101-392.

Half: Pathways to Success for America's Youth and Young Families, Final Report,[11] and *America's Choice: High Skills or Low Wages!*[3] have documented the dreadful consequences of continued neglect of the educational, social, and economic needs of the nation's poor students, especially minorities, with limited English proficiency, and those with disabilities.

To ensure the prudent implementation of the law by states and local education agencies receiving funds, Section 118 of the Perkins legislation requires each state to ensure that students who are members of special populations will:

- have equal access to vocational recruitment, enrollment, and job placement activities
- be provided with equal access to the full range of vocational programs including cooperative education and apprenticeship programs and guidance and counseling
- be provided vocational education in the least restrictive environment
- afford all the rights and protections guaranteed under section 504 of the Rehabilitation Act of 1973 to students with disabilities who do not have an IEP
- have programs coordinated by vocational education and vocational rehabilitation representatives
- have information on vocational programs, eligibility requirements, specific courses, special services available, employment opportunities, and placement information. This information will be provided before the time they are eligible for vocational education (and no later than the beginning of the ninth grade)

The Perkins Act requires all recipients of the funds (local educational agencies, area technical schools, consortia, and postsecondary institutions) to:

- assist students who are members of special populations to enter vocational education programs and to assist in fulfilling the transitional services required under the Individuals with Disabilities Education Act (IDEA)
- assess special-needs students with respect to their successful completion of vocational education programs in the most integrated setting possible
- provide supplemental services to students who are members of special populations including:
  - curriculum modification
  - equipment modification
  - classroom modification
  - supportive personnel
  - instructional aids and devices

- provide guidance, counseling, and career development activities conducted by professionally trained counselors and teachers
- provide counseling and instructional services designed to facilitate the transition from school to postschool employment and career opportunities

Participatory Planning

The Perkins Act requires recipients of funds to establish procedures so that parents, students, teachers, and area residents concerned will be able to directly participate in local decisions that affect the program. Furthermore, the act requires recipients to give technical assistance to ensure that such individuals are given access to information about the procedures.

Other Related Legislation

Kochhar and Deschamps[6] illustrate the relationships between three pieces of national legislation created to enhance the lives of special populations. While the Individuals with Disabilities Act reaffirms the national effort to provide an equitable general education for students with disabilities, the Perkins Act mandates equal vocational education for special populations, and the Americans with Disabilities Act grants equal employment opportunities to persons with disabilities. ADA also ensures that public accommodations will be accessible, including public transportation, and requires employers to make reasonable accommodations for employees with disabilities to allow them the same benefits and privileges enjoyed by other employees.

Kochhar and Deschamps[6] point out that just as the IDEA and Perkins Act compliment and support each other, the ADA legislation supports the Perkins Act of 1990. The four areas of mutual support include assurances of equal access, transition, supplementary services, and guidance and counseling.

CONCLUSION

All advocates for students with disabilities should be aware of pertinent legislation, workforce preparation needs, and current educational practices that enhance the education and lives of students with special needs. Our vigilance will assist us in knowing when education systems are practicing good pedagogy and implementing federal and state mandates.

REFERENCES

1. Brown D and Brooks L: *Career counseling techniques*, Needham Heights, Mass, 1991, Allyn and Bacon.

2. Burac Z and Maddy-Bernstein C: TASPP names 1992 exemplary vocational special needs programs, *TASPP Bulletin*, Champaign, Ill, University of Illinois at Urbana-Champaign, 4:1, 1992, pp 1-3.

3. Commission on the Skills of the American Workforce: *America's choice: high skills or low wages!* Rochester, NY, 1990, National Center on Education and the Economy.

4. Hayward BJ and Wirt JG: *Final report: handicapped and disadvantaged students: access to quality vocational education*, vol 5, Washington, DC, U.S. Department of Education, National Assessment of Vocational Education, 1989.

5. Johnston WB and Packer A: *Workforce 2000: work and workers for the twenty-first century*, Indianapolis, 1987, Hudson Institute.

6. Kochhar CA and Deschamps AB: Policy crossroads in preserving the right of passage to independence for learners with special needs: implications of recent changes in national vocational and special education policies, *Journal for Vocational Special Needs Education* 14:9-19, 1991.

7. Kokaska CJ and Brolin DE: *Career education for handicapped individuals*, Columbus, Ohio, 1985, Charles E. Merrill Publishing Company.

8. Patterson RE and Mikulin EK: *Guidelines for serving members of special populations in vocational and applied technology education*, Austin, 1992, Texas Education Agency.

9. Phelps LA and Wermuth TR: Effective vocational education for students with special needs: a framework, Berkeley, Calif, 1992, National Center for Research in Vocational Education, University of California at Berkeley.

10. Wagner M: *The benefits of secondary vocational education for young people with disabilities: findings from the national longitudinal transition study of special education students*, Menlo Park, Calif, 1991, SRI International.

11. Wermuth TR and Coyle-Williams M: National recognition program for exemplary vocational education programs serving special needs populations, *TASPP BRIEF*, Champaign, Ill, University of Illinois at Urbana-Champaign, 1:3, 1989.

12. William T. Grant Foundation Commission on Work, Family, and Citizenship: *The forgotten half: pathways to success for America's youth and young families*, Washington, DC, William T. Grant Foundation Commission on Work, Family, and Citizenship, 1988.

13. Zunker VG: *Career counseling: applied concepts of life planning*, ed 3, Pacific Grove, Calif, 1990, Brooks/Cole Publishing Company.

CHAPTER **37**

Assistive Technology

GLENN E. HEDMAN

Assistive technology involves the application of technology and engineering principles to increase the independence of individuals with disabilities. This can be achieved through the use of devices made for the entire population, devices made for a specific group of individuals having similar abilities, or devices that are designed and fabricated specifically for use by one individual.

The modern field of assistive technology is the result of a 20-year evolution. During the early 1970s the United States federal government began the funding of rehabilitation engineering centers (RECs). Usually located at major universities, the RECs each focused on specific areas of assistive technology (e.g., seating, wheelchair design, augmentative communication, etc.). RECs were able to devote their resources to the design and fabrication of new devices and evaluate prototype effectiveness with clients in their own laboratories. Work at the RECs resulted in the transfer of successful technology to the private sector for mass production and the stimulation of other work by professionals at other locations.

As more products made their way to the private sector and became commercially available, client evaluations for appropriate technology began to be performed by professionals from disciplines other than engineering, including occupational therapists, physical therapists, and speech/language pathologists. This initiated a change in the term *rehabilitation engineering* to *rehabilitation technology*. Then as the application of technology grew in educational and vocational settings, the term *assistive technology* became preferred to *rehabilitation technology*, which was felt to imply a medical model or the application of technology to address only medical issues.

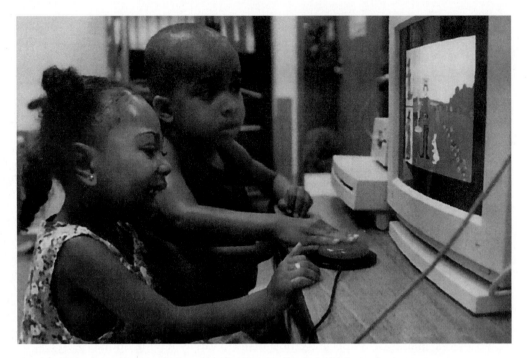

From Case-Smith J, Allen AS, and Pratt PN: *Occupational therapy for children*, ed 3, St Louis, 1996, Mosby–Year Book.

Today the term *assistive technology* covers many areas of work, including accessibility, augmentative communication, computer access, environmental control, mobility, orthotics, prosthetics, and seating. Although many of these have been introduced during the past 20 years, orthotics and prosthetics have existed for a much longer period of time and have well established identities within the medical and rehabilitation communities. For a discussion of orthotic and prosthetic devices and applications the reader is referred to the article by Michael[3] noted at the end of this chapter.

DESIGN FACTORS

Assistive technology devices should meet the same criteria for good design as devices in other areas, including:

- effectiveness
- appropriate size and weight
- durability
- serviceability
- aesthetics
- economics

Many individuals initially think of sophisticated devices such as voice-input computers or voice-output communication aids when the word *technology* is used. However, low-tech devices and adaptations such as reachers and adapted eating utensils are just as much a part of the field as is high-tech equipment. Finding the simplest level of technology to match an individual's abilities with the task needing to be performed is essential to the successful application of assistive technology and is the value that a qualified professional brings to the process. The problem-solving process of an assistive technology evaluation first considers the use of commercially-available equipment, then modification of commercially-available equipment, and only lastly the custom design and custom fabrication of a device.

Seating

To be able to be seated without pain or the development of pressure sores is a basic need. The field of assistive technology has produced several methods of addressing seating needs but all can be considered within three basic categories: (1) linear/planar, (2) modular-contoured, and (3) custom-contoured.

Linear/planar. These seating systems employ flat seat and back cushions that are sized and positioned according to a client's measurements. They consist of a firm support foundation such as plywood or plastic covered by a foam layer. The foam layer material and thickness varies depending on the use of the cushion (as a seat or back) and the need for pressure distribution. Linear/planar seating systems may also include lateral hip blocks, lateral trunk supports, and equipment to position the individual's lower extremities, upper extremities, or head.

Modular-contoured. This second category of seating system is used when there is the need for some contour to the profile of the seat or back cushion. These systems use cushions that have a generic curve and do a better job of distributing sitting pressure than do flat cushions so that adequate blood flow to the skin can be maintained and pressure sores avoided.

Custom-contoured. Custom-contoured seating systems are used when the cushions need to be made to the exact contours of the individual. These may be needed to address pressure sore problems or the existence of fixed scoliosis.

A basic engineering principle is the inverse relationship that exists between pressure and area; increasing the area of support reduces the pressure at a client's skin. Linear/planar seating systems have foam that takes on the shape of the user. Although effective for many individuals, linear/planar seating systems may still result in localized areas of relatively high pressure and shear forces that can restrict skin blood flow and produce pressure sores.

Modular-contoured seating systems provide a greater area of support and result in lower pressures. However, because they have a generic curve the distribution of pressure is still somewhat uneven. Custom-contoured seating system cushions, made to the exact contours of the user, distribute support to a wider area, thus minimizing the pressure.

Custom-contoured cushions can be produced through the use of chemical kits, enabling the cushion to be made in the clinical setting, or through the use of seating simulators where a mold is produced and sent to a manufacturer for fabrication. Once the customized cushions are received from the manufacturer, they can be attached at the appropriate angles on the individual's mobility base. Seating simulators can also be used to evaluate the effectiveness of linear/planar and modular-contoured seating systems.

An appropriate, properly positioned pelvic stabilizer is also essential to the proper function of any seating system. This is usually a nylon seatbelt-type strap positioned at a 45-degree angle with respect to the seat tubes of the mobility base. Other types of pelvic stabilizers, such as contoured padded bars anchored to the sides of the seating system or mobility base, may be used when more support is needed.

Hybrid systems often offer the most cost-effective combination of seating system components. An example of a hybrid system would be a custom-contoured seat, modular-contoured back, and linear/planar lateral trunk supports and headrest.

Proper seating systems can give an individual with a disability the opportunity to be upright for long periods of time and perform upper-extremity activities with much greater efficiency because of the support provided by the components. Children with disabilities usually have definite opinions on the relative comfort and the aesthetics of a given seating system.[5]

Mobility

The ability of an individual to move from place to place independently is important for functional and play activities. After an appropriate seating system has been produced it is commonly positioned on a mobility base. Evaluation for the most appropriate mobility base requires both the consideration of the child's abilities and the environment in which the mobility base will be used.[1]

Design work done at the University of Virginia REC and by various wheelchair manufacturers has resulted in a wide array of manual mobility bases from which to choose. Materials used in the construction of these commercially available wheelchairs include aircraft-quality steel tubing, aluminum, titanium, and plastic composites, and many are available in a variety of colors. This has enabled the overall weight of wheelchairs to be reduced while their aesthetics have improved.

The use of a powered mobility base should also be considered. It is now generally agreed that powered mobility can be appropriate for children as young as 24 months. The concern that the use of powered mobility might inhibit a young child's progress toward other mobility goals appears unfounded. The general feeling is that a child's desire to be mobile will not be stifled and that use of a powered mobility base will only help children become more excited and interested in mobility in other forms.

Powered mobility bases offer a variety of control options, including a standard joystick, lap tray switches, head switches, foot switches, puff-and-sip control, and ultrasonic systems. The most appropriate type should be determined only after an opportunity to try the controller in a powered base that has a seating system providing adequate support for the evaluation.

Augmentative Communication

The ability to communicate with others is another important function of life. Devices that may be recommended in this area range from low-tech communication booklets and binders to high-tech battery-powered, voice-output communication aids. The more sophisticated the device, the greater the number of communication messages that are available, the greater variety of input methods that may be used to operate the device, and the more options there are for the type of output (e.g., voice-output, print, LCD).

Environmental Control

Environmental control technology includes the adaptation of devices already in an individual's environment, the introduction of new devices to manipulate or control those existing devices, and the use of new devices to perform a given task.

The installation of a lever attachment to the control button of a fan or toy represents one type of adaptation of an existing device. If adaptation of existing devices is not appropriate, the use of an environmental control unit may enable the individual to operate lights, fans, radios, or other appliances using a central transmitter. This transmitter can communicate with receiver modules via the existing house wiring or through ultrasonic signals. In other situations the introduction of a new piece of equipment to perform the same function as an existing device is most appropriate. For example, the replacement of a standard touch-tone telephone with a big-button telephone and a handset supported on a gooseneck may enable an individual with poor fine motor skills to independently make and receive telephone calls.

The use of adapted toys can not only enable a child with a disability to control a toy for play, but can also demonstrate a cause-effect relationship that may be exercised in the use of an environmental control unit. In addition, the switches and switch locations found to be appropriate for use of the adapted toy may also be used to operate the environmental control unit, as noted by Langley.[2]

Computer access. Computer access is an area sometimes considered within the spectrum of environmental control. A wide range of commercially available computer access equipment exists, from low-tech keyguards that increase accuracy in typing, to alternate keyboards that match with a child's motor skills, to high-tech alternate input methods such as head control or voice input.

Accessibility

Architectural changes to the home or school environment to improve access are usually simple in nature and benefit other individuals using the same space. Examples of useful accessibility components include ramps or vertical platform lifts to provide a path of travel between grade and a first-floor level, lever profiles or attachments to doorknobs, and grab bars, cantilevered sinks, and roll-in showers in bathrooms. Consideration of the difference in abilities of children with disabilities and adults with disabilities is important when recommending environmental changes.[6]

DELIVERY OF ASSISTIVE TECHNOLOGY

Although the amount of assistive technology that is commercially available is impressive, a user cannot benefit from the technology until it is acquired. It is the process of assistive technology service delivery that helps ensure that individuals receive the most appropriate equipment, that it is set up properly, and that it serves individuals over the length of time anticipated. Assistive technology service delivery consists of three phases: (1) evaluation, (2) implementation, and (3) follow-up.

Assistive technology service providers have a wide variety of backgrounds, including engineering, occupational therapy, physical therapy, speech/language pathology, and more recently, rehabilitation technology. The setting in which evaluative services are provided are as varied as the backgrounds of the providers. The Rehabilitation and Assistive Technology Society of North America, an association for the advancement of rehabilitation and assistive technologies, classifies the different types of assistive technology service providers as:

- durable medical equipment (DME) suppliers
- departments within a comprehensive rehabilitation program
- technology service delivery centers in a university
- state-agency–based programs
- private rehabilitation engineering/technology firms
- local affiliates of a national nonprofit disability organization
- miscellaneous types of programs, such as volunteer groups and information resource centers

Some of these providers have the capacity to deliver services in the community through the use of mobile units. This is not only more convenient for the consumer but also permits evaluation in the environment where the equipment will be used.

A key feature of successful Assistive Technology delivery programs is comprehensive evaluation. Most of the models listed in the previous pages use a multidisciplinary approach to do this. The specific disciplines required to perform a comprehensive evaluation vary depending on the type of technology being evaluated and prescribed. The way in which each model achieves multidisciplinary evaluation also varies. For example, a DME supplier may use only an engineer and/or fabrication technician and may need to supplement their services through collaboration with therapists from local schools or rehabilitation facilities. However, all needed disciplines may be present on the team of a technology service delivery center at a university.

After delivery of an assistive device it is important that the consumer, parents, siblings, teachers, and other appropriate individuals receive training in its use. The cost involved in providing this training is not always reimbursed by third-party payers, however. If training is not funded and as a result not provided, there is significant risk that the device will be misused or unused and the cost of the device wasted.

Assistive technology devices also commonly need some measure of adjustment or modification after issuance. This is to be expected because the exact matching of a device to a given individual's abilities and needs may be difficult during a relatively brief implementation visit. Quality assistive technology service delivery programs characteristically provide follow-up to make needed adjustments a few weeks after the issuance of each device.

Another factor that needs to be considered by the consumer, service provider, and third-party payer is the expected duration of use of the device. Few devices can be expected to last or be appropriate forever. An assistive technology device will remain appropriate only as long as it matches the abilities of the consumer with the task needing to be achieved. Thus when the

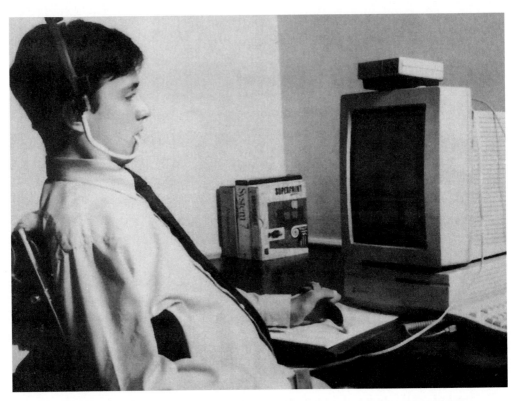

From Cook AM and Hussey SM: *Assistive technologies: principles and practice*, St Louis, 1995, Mosby–Year Book.

abilities of the consumer change or the tasks needing to be performed change, new technology must be considered. Discontinuing use of the original device should not be thought to mean an unsuccessful implementation of that piece of technology. Rather it should be seen as evidence of growth and the development of the consumer's further independence.[4]

CONCLUSION

The field of assistive technology is evolving and expanding in the number and type of service providers involved, the ways in which services are being provided, and the spectrum of devices available to consumers. Assistive technology includes both sophisticated and low-tech devices and it is in finding the simplest, most appropriate solution to meet an individual's need that characterizes a quality service. It must be remembered that assistive technology is only a tool designed to enable individuals with disabilities to achieve their goals. It is the spirit of the consumer that is ultimately responsible for the successful accomplishment of those goals.

REFERENCES

1. Deitz J et al: Pediatric power wheelchairs: evaluation of function in the home and school environments, *Assistive Technology 3* (1): 24-31, 1991.
2. Langley MB: A developmental approach to the use of toys for facilitation of environmental control. In Hedman G, editor: *Rehabilitation Technology*, 1990, Binghamton, NY, Haworth Press.
3. Michael J: Pediatric prosthetics and orthotics. In Hedman G, editor: *Rehabilitation technology*, Binghamton, NY, 1990, Haworth Press.
4. Phillips B and Zhao H: Predictors of assistive technology abandonment, *Assistive Technology 5* (1): 36-45, 1993.
5. Ryan S et al: *Toward obtaining useful consumer feedback from young children with physical disabilities*, Proceedings of the 16th Annual Conference on Rehabilitation Technology, Las Vegas, 1993.
6. Seeger BR and Bails JH: Ergonomic building design for physically disabled young people, *Assistive Technology 2* (3): 79-92, 1990.

CHAPTER 38

Respite Care: Support for Families in the Community

JENNIFER M. CERNOCH
ELIZABETH E. NEWHOUSE

Becoming a parent is usually a joyous occasion; however, it also can be very stressful. Changes within the family unit through the birth or presence of a new child many times alter the dynamics of family functioning, causing stress to be present.[2] Parents may feel the need to create new schedules, to increase household duties, to increase financial resources, and to decrease leisure time. Because of these and other family pressures, all parents need an occasional break from the responsibilities of caring for their children. All parents need time to relax with one another, to run errands, to work, to keep appointments, to respond to emergencies, and to take much needed vacations.

For many families everyday activities can become even more stressful when accessible and affordable child care options are not available. Typical support systems such as extended family members, neighbors, babysitters, or other persons within their social support network may not be available to accomplish these daily activities.

Families of children with disabilities or chronic illness are faced everyday with the reality that their social support networks may not be available to them. These families must meet the usual demands placed on all families but are additionally challenged with the unique stresses associated with parenting a child with disabilities or chronic illness. The increased time needed for caregiving activities, the burdensome financial costs, ongoing concerns about health needs, and the prolonged dependency of a child with disabilities on a family are all indicators of increased stress levels in families of children with disabilities and chronic illness.[18] Thus the need for social and family support services to relieve some of these stresses and to help families adapt and cope with everyday activities is especially critical for families of children with disabilities and chronic illness.

DEFINITION AND NEED FOR RESPITE SERVICES

Families of children with disabilities and chronic illness most often identify respite care as a priority service to maintain family stability and unity. In a review of the literature from the 1970s and early 1980s, Cohen and Warren[4] cite numerous studies and statewide needs assessments that indicated that respite was a vital and necessary service for families to maintain long-term survival. In the 1990s the need for respite services has not diminished, as shown by two statewide surveys in Maryland and Texas.[8,14] In Maryland more than 600 families within a 2-year period were denied respite services because of the overall statewide demand for services. In Texas a survey completed by 223 families of children who are medically fragile indicated that the most frequently and ardently voiced need among these families was more respite services; the need for respite services was mentioned by families more than twice as often as the need for any other single support service.

Respite has been traditionally defined as, "a system of temporary supports for families of individuals with disabilities which provides the family with relief. 'Temporary' may mean anything from an hour to three months. It may mean, 'periodically or on a regular basis'. Respite can be provided in the client's home or in a variety of out-of-home settings."[22] Programs and service options that have developed from this definition have focused on the family or caregiver as the primary beneficiary of services. This has resulted in a philosophic shift from the traditional disability services in which the client has predominantly been the individual with disability. There continue to be service options specifically designed to meet the needs of individuals with disabilities, such as schools, recreation programs, therapy, and intervention programs that provide relief to the family as a secondary benefit.

For the past 10 to 15 years respite has become a predominant service within family support systems across the country. By 1989 41 states had developed programs designed to give families support. Family support programs are designed to provide whatever services are necessary to maintain and enhance a family's capability of providing care at home to an individual with disabilities.[12] These family support programs traditionally have been developed to serve families and individuals with disabilities. It has only been recently that family support and respite services have expanded to include families of children with chronic illnesses and complex medical conditions, families of children at risk of abuse and neglect, families of young adults with disabilities, and families of elderly individuals in need of support services. In 1994 the 103rd Congress adopted the following expanded definition for respite services as part of PL 103-252: "Respite services means short-term care services provided in the temporary absence of the regular caregiver (parent, other relative, foster parent, adoptive parent, guardian) to children who meet one or more of the following categories: (A) the children are in danger of abuse or neglect; (B) the children have experienced abuse or neglect; and (C) the children have disabilities, or chronic or terminal illnesses. Services provided within or outside the child's home shall be short-term care, ranging from a few hours to a few weeks of time, per year, and be intended to enable the family to stay together and to keep the child living in the child's home and community."* This expanded definition has set policy implications to support families and children in the home rather than institutional care as in the past.

BENEFITS OF RESPITE SERVICES

Numerous research studies have been published regarding the benefits or outcomes of respite services to families. Summaries of these research studies have indicated that, overall, respite reduces stress in families, improves family functioning, decreases social isolation within the family unit, enhances positive attitudes about children with disabilities, and decreases the likelihood of out-of-home placements of children.[4,10] More recent studies have supported these general outcomes and have also found that the provision of respite services has somewhat of a lasting effect (from 3 days to a few months) on reducing maternal stress levels and increasing coping mechanisms.[3,16] In addition, Sherman's[19] recent study indicates a trend toward a decrease in the number of hospitalizations of children with chronic illness after the provision of in-home respite services for families. All of these empiric studies have shown positive outcomes for the provision and utilization of respite services. However, the most important aspect regarding outcomes of respite services is what families perceive as the benefits of respite services.

In a national survey conducted among subscribers of *Exceptional Parent Magazine*, families reported that they were essentially pleased with the respite services they were receiving. In particular, families were pleased with the individuals who were providing respite services. However, families did report substantial problems with coordinating respite services. These prob-

---

*Public Law 103-252, Title II: community-based family resource programs, 42 USC 5116, 1994.

lems were primarily in areas where families were not active partners in the planning and implementation of services. One final result of this national survey was that families wanted to be able to exercise control over the services that affect their home life and they wanted to play a substantive role in forming or reforming the system of services in a way that was responsive to their needs.[11] Additional data obtained through national site visits and family interviews also found positive reactions to the benefits of respite services, particularly the relief that it provides families from caregiving responsibilities.[9] The benefits of respite services to families are extremely positive, but more importantly they provide the needed relief for families to continue to keep their child at home in a loving and nurturing environment.

A second area of benefit of respite services has been documented through research with siblings of children with disabilities. Just as parents are many times stressed with the caregiving responsibilities of a child with disabilities, siblings also share many of these stresses. Parents of children with special needs often do not have time to spend with their other children and many of these children may be denied access to extracurricular activities because of the time demands of the child with disabilities. In addition, siblings often face behavioral and emotional adjustments to the child with disabilities. All of these factors are important to consider when providing respite services. Siblings can benefit from respite services by being an active participant in the planning of the service and an excellent source of information regarding care needs.[15] Siblings also can be respite providers to other families of children with disabilities through specialized training courses adopted for adolescents.[5]

A third area of benefit of respite services has been documented through parental report regarding positive outcomes for children with disabilities and chronic illness. Through anecdotal information parents have reported that respite services have allowed their child with disabilities an opportunity to meet new individuals, to learn socialization skills through out-of-home respite services, and to develop trust in others as caregivers.[19] This benefit is of primary importance to families because their primary concern is the overall welfare of their child; families will not use respite services if the welfare of their child or the quality of services is not top priority.

A final benefit of respite services has been documented from a state policy perspective. In a recent study conducted by the Virginia Department of Social Services,[21] the number of disrupted foster family placements was reduced because of the provision of respite services. Foster families caring for children with disabilities were more likely to continue caregiving responsibilities when respite services were available to them. This resulted in the children spending longer durations of time in the same foster family. In addition, the provision of respite services enhanced the recruitment of new foster families within the system. The benefit of receiving respite services was viewed as a positive factor in expanding the foster family base.

All of these studies and reports have shown the positive benefits of respite services from different perspectives. However, two underlying premises still need to be addressed in the development of respite services. First, the need for respite services must be addressed to fully understand the benefits to families. In all of the above cited reports and studies, families continued to request additional respite services to meet their needs. Because of inadequate financial resources, a lack of providers, or other variables, many programs have not been able to meet the true respite needs of families. Given the positive benefits and outcomes with the limited amount of respite services that currently exist, what would truly be the effect on family stability and unity if abundant services were available to meet the needs of families? Second, the respite service delivery system must be designed with active participation and planning from families. Respite services must be accessible and affordable to families, and families must have control over the delivery of services. These variables are paramount to the successful delivery of respite services and overall family satisfaction and positive outcomes with respite services.

GUIDELINES AND MODELS OF RESPITE SERVICES

The design and delivery of respite services have changed dramatically over the past 25 years. Respite programs developed in the 1970s were predominantly designed for families of children with mental retardation as part of the deinstitutionalization movement. These programs were developed primarily in urban areas where resources were more available and the services were based on the needs of the system rather than on the families' needs. Services were provided either in the family's home by trained providers or in out-of-home settings such as large institutions. With changes in federal laws, advances in medical technology, and family advocacy efforts, the respite service delivery system began to change. Currently, respite services are more varied, more geographically dispersed, more user friendly for families, more accessible to families of children with disabilities other than mental retardation, and more prevalent within social policy reform and state systems. Even with these differences and advances, however, the need for expansion of respite services is still great.

The Access to Respite Care and Help (ARCH) National Resource Center for Respite and Crisis Care Services[6] has developed a set of *National Respite Guidelines* to assist service providers in expanding and developing quality services and to help families have some means of discerning the quality of their respite options. The guidelines provide general information in seven major areas including family involvement, care needs of the child, care providers, community involvement, service delivery, administration, and evaluation. These guidelines have been widely distributed and have proven beneficial to local communities, states, and families in the design and delivery of respite options and consequently in the expansion of respite models. In addition, these guidelines incorporate the latest trends and changes that are important for the expansion and utilization of respite services.

The respite models of the 1990s are similar in design to models developed in the past; however, changes have occurred in the planning and delivery of respite services. Traditional respite models currently in use include:

- In-home models—home-based services; sitter companion services; parent-trainer services.
- Out-of-home models—family care homes or host family services; day care or center-based services; foster home settings; residential facilities; parent cooperative services; respitality services; hospitals.[1]

In any of these models, friends and relatives, volunteers, and/or paid trained providers (ranging from unlicensed trained providers to registered nurses) can provide respite services to families. The type of provider used in various models is dependent on many factors such as family comfort level with the provider, availability of providers, level of need and/or disability of the child, and liability issues of the agency or program. Respite models that have incorporated all of these factors are highly successful in meeting the needs of families.

Within the last few years local communities and states have changed the focus of respite model development in three primary areas. First, initiatives have been taken by programs to include parental input in the design and delivery of services. Using parents as trainers, building trust within families, asking families their needs, and providing flexible and affordable services have all been critical variables for the development of successful respite services. Families will not use respite services if they do not feel comfortable with the service and if the service does not meet their needs. Building trust with the family is probably the key ingredient in a successful respite program.[13]

Second, respite programs that allow families flexibility and choice and control over their provider have higher use rates than programs who do not allow these factors. Families prefer to make the same respite or sitter arrangements for their child with disabilities as they do for their other children. In addition, they prefer someone that they know to provide the service, if not, someone who is clearly seen as being their employee.[11] Being family centered, family focused, and family controlled is one of the positive changes within respite model development that has gained national attention. Many respite programs and family support state systems offer families vouchers or cash subsidies to purchase their own respite services through family members, friends, volunteers, or paid providers. This allows families to determine the level of care needs of their child and to maintain the flexibility within their own home situation.

The final major change that has occurred in respite program development is the focus on generic supports for families. Respite programs of the past were designed as specialized services for children without much integration within the community. Current respite programs are focusing on providing services to families within the broader aspect of communities such as general day care centers, churches, and recreation programs. As an example, some religious communities have extended their ministries to include respite services as part of the daily activities of the congregation. In Georgia one religious community offers a one-on-one weekend recreation program for children with and without disabilities. The integration and inclusion of children with disabilities within this program have been highly successful.[7] Other community services also can play a major role in providing family respite services in the areas of training providers, adapting facilities, increasing resources, collaborating between agencies, and changing attitudes. The use of generic community resources not only provides respite to the family but also allows the child with disabilities the opportunity for recreational, vocational, and social pursuits.[17]

The changing evolution of respite services to meet the individual needs of families and to provide quality services within diminishing resources is a challenge to local communities, states, and the federal government. This challenge will continue as the need for respite services increases.

CONCLUSION

This chapter focuses on the needs, benefits, and service design systems of respite options for families of children with disabilities and chronic illness. It has been estimated that children with chronic health problems comprise about 10% to 15% of the population of children from birth to age 18 in the United States and that about 10% of these children have a severe chronic illness that impairs their ability to perform a major activity of daily living.[20] As the population increases, as medical technology advances to save the lives of more children, as violence in our society increases, and as families choose to keep their children at home in a loving and supportive environment, the need for respite services will only continue to increase. Our society must focus on this need to support families and to provide all children with a safe and nurturing environment.

From a social policy perspective, the support of all families must be paramount and private and public resources must be redirected to allow families the choice and control over their own lives. Families who care for a child with disabilities or chronic illness are ordinary people who accomplish extraordinary things—they think of possibilities rather than certainties, they look beyond the constraints of program policies and procedures, they imaginatively ferret out services in the community, and they advocate for the development of needed services that do not exist. Respite must be an integral part of this system to give families strength to continue to survive. As one family member expressed:

> I still cry, grieve, deny and feel anger over my child's condition. And over the loss of my marriage. And over the pain and loss my other children endured. I carry all of those feelings forward with me. However, gloom and doom are not my style. I'm not sure when it happened, when I decided to steer myself, my child and my family in the direction of life and living, not illness, disability and dying. But, I replaced fear with knowledge, dependency with experience, and intimidation with confidence. Instead of viewing medical caregivers as 'gods and saviors,' I allowed them to return to the human race. I also worked on making things right at home. We became a family with a special need, not a special need with a family.[8]

REFERENCES

1. ARCH National Resource Center for Respite and Crisis Care Services: *Starting a Respite Care Program*, Chapel Hill, NC, 1993, ARCH National Resource Center for Respite and Crisis Care Services.
2. Boss PG: Normative family stress: Family boundary changes across the life span, *Family Relations* 29(4): 17-22, 1980.
3. Botuch S and Winsberg BG: Effects of respite on mothers of school-age and adult children with severe disabilities, *Mental Retardation* 29(1), 43-47, 1991.
4. Cohen S and Warren RD: *Respite care: principles, programs and policies*, Austin, Tex, 1985, Pro-Ed.
5. Edgar EB, Reid PC, Pious CC: Special sitters: youth as respite care providers, *Mental Retardation* 26(1), 33-37, 1988.
6. Edgar M and Uhl M: *National respite guidelines*, Chapel Hill, NC, 1994, ARCH National Resource Center for Respite and Crisis Care Services.
7. Gaventa B: Respite care: an opportunity for the religious community, *Exceptional Parent* 20(4): 22-26, 1990.
8. Gray I: *Children in Texas who are medically fragile: their families' voices*, Austin, Tex, 1993, Texas Respite Resource Network, Texas Planning Council for Developmental Disabilities.

9. Huntington K and Langmeyer D: Summary of 1992 site visits to crisis nurseries and respite care programs, *ARCH National Resource Center Factsheet 30*:1-6 1993.

10. Intagliata J: Assessing the impact of respite care services: a review of outcome evaluation studies. In Salisbury CL and Intagliata J, editors: *Respite care: support for persons with developmental disabilities and their families*, Baltimore, 1986, Paul H. Brooks Publishing Co.

11. Knoll J and Bedford S: Respite services: a national survey of parents' experience, *Exceptional Parent 19*(4):34-36, 1989.

12. Knoll J et al: *Family support services in the United States: an end of the decade status report*, Cambridge, Mass, 1990, Human Services Research Institute.

13. Miller S: Respite care for children with developmental and/or physical disabilities: a parent's perspective, *ARCH National Resource Center Factsheet 4*:1-2, 1992.

14. Montgomery County Government, Department of Family Resources Division on Children and Youth: *Respite care: a supportive and preventative service for families—a statewide survey of provider organizations and parent experiences*, Rockville, Md, 1990, The Department.

15. Powell T and Ogle PA: Brothers and sisters: addressing unique needs through respite care services. In Salisbury CL and Intagliata J, editors: *Respite care: support for persons with developmental disabilities and their families*, Baltimore, 1986, Paul H. Brooks Publishing Co.

16. Rimmerman A: Provision of respite care for children with developmental disabilities: changes in maternal coping and stress over time, *Mental Retardation 27*(2): 99-103, 1989.

17. Salisbury CL: Generic community services as sources of respite. In Salisbury CL and Intagliata J, editors: *Respite care: support for persons with developmental disabilities and their families*, Baltimore, 1986, Paul H Brooks Publishing Co.

18. Salisbury CL: Parenthood and the need for respite. In Salisbury CL and Intagliata J, editors: *Respite care: support for persons with developmental disabilities and their families*, Baltimore, 1986, Paul H. Brooks Publishing Co.

19. Sherman BR: *Impact of home-based respite care on families of children with chronic illnesses*, Children's Health Care 24(1):33-45, 1995.

20. United States Department of Health, Education, and Welfare: *Health: United States 1990*, DHHS Pub No PHS 88-1232, 1990.

21. Virginia Department of Social Services, Commonwealth Institute for Child and Family Studies/Virginia Treatment Center for Children: *Respite care for foster families*, Richmond, Vir, 1991, The Department.

22. Warren RD and Dickman IR: *For this respite, much thanks: concepts, guidelines and issues in the development of community respite care services*, New York, 1981, United Cerebral Palsy Associations Inc.

CHAPTER 39

Home Care for Children with Technologic Needs

ARTHUR F. KOHRMAN

JOANNA KAUFMAN

Most care of children, whether well or sick, occurs in the home or in a non-medical setting. Parents have always provided care for routine childhood illnesses and injuries; hospitalization is a relatively rare event for children. Increasingly, the population of children who are hospitalized fall into two categories: (1) those who require a relatively brief medical or surgical intervention, and (2) those with chronic disease or disability. Of the latter group there is a small but growing number of children who are dependent on or assisted by technology for survival and for whom that dependence may continue for months, years, or for the child's lifetime. For some of these children the length of their lives will be determined by the success of the technologic intervention and devices on which they depend.

In recent years many such children have been moved from the hospital to the home or other community setting as it has become apparent that permanent or extended hospital care is not in the best interest of the child, the family, the institution or society. There is a tendency to label this effort as a "new" home care movement, but in fact the only new attribute is the intensity of the experience. The severity of the medical problems with which children are now being sent home has increased as the resultant responsibilities for the caretakers and families have intensified. The advancements of modern medicine have allowed complex medical care to reach into the home; increasingly, living rooms and bedrooms have become places where children receive care previously restricted to hospitals. Intravenous antibiotics, oxygen tanks, and ventilators now accompany children as they leave the hospital.[11] As parents build simulations of intensive care units within their homes, they take on new and challenging roles as administrators and monitors of advanced technologic equipment. The severity of their children's problems and the intensity of care they require raise new dilemmas and questions about the commitment and responsibilities of families and communities.[10] The relative benefits and burdens to the many involved parties are more analogous to the problems faced by parents and families of developmentally disabled children than they are to the problems faced by families of children with time-limited illnesses.

INTEREST IN HOME CARE

The recent movement to home care for children with complex care needs in the United States is a result of many factors. Among these are the increasing numbers of children surviving with long-standing technologic needs; the recognition of the inadequacy of hospitals in meeting the developmental and social needs of children over time; the many movements toward empowerment of families and individuals in the face of what is seen as an increasing-

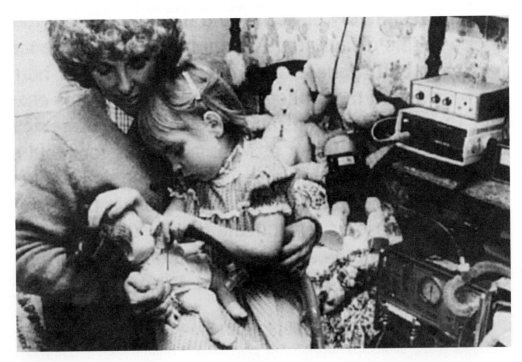

From Wong D: *Whaley & Wong's Nursing Care of Infants and Children*, ed 5, St Louis, 1995, Mosby–Year Book.

ly impersonal and paternalistic medical care system; and the push for cost containment and reduction in length of hospital stays.[8] The increasing portability and dependability of technologic devices such as ventilators and intravenous pumps make it possible to introduce into the home care that formerly was given only in hospitals or their intensive care units.

BENEFITS TO THE CHILD AND FAMILY

It is unarguable that children and caregivers can benefit enormously from home care. Impersonal and inflexible hospital routines are replaced by the comforts of the home and the spontaneity and casual intimacy of the family; the familiar comings and goings and mealtime banter have curative powers in themselves. In the home setting almost all children gain an enhanced sense of autonomy as families gain control over their care. The dominant perspective changes from one of sickness to one of recovery. Many children who have spent months or years in the hospital make great developmental and psychologic progress after coming home.[1]

Family members can experience the emotional and psychologic benefits as well. Despite the anxiety and difficulty attendant on first bringing a technology-assisted child into the home, the family may quickly grow to appreciate the presence and interdependence of all of its members. With its energies no longer divided between the hospital and the home, the family is better able to focus on both the sick child and on each other.

BENEFITS TO SOCIETY

A hospital intensive care unit is not an appropriate nor a cost-efficient locus for providing long-term care for children. Many studies[1-4,6] have demonstrated that home care for technology dependent children is less costly than hospital care. Recognizing the cost-effectiveness, public sector funding (Medicaid Title XIX) has expanded its eligibility criteria with the so-called Katie Beckett waiver program to allow for home care payments in lieu of hospitalization for this population of children. A retrospective study[7] of reimbursable services from Maryland Medicaid for 10 ventilator dependent children over a 2-year period suggests cost savings of $79,074 plus or minus $26,558 per child per year. Savings were calculated only on costs related to medical care and were broken down to include paid nursing care (69% of total cost), rehospitalization costs (18%), case management (3%), pharmacy and other outpatient costs (1%), speech and physical therapies (1%), and durable equipment and disposable supplies (8%). The study also indicated that the amount and cost of nursing care decreased after the first year at home, resulting in even more cost savings and greater cost containment.

In addition to the established cost savings, the benefits of pediatric home care to society can clearly be demonstrated by the full inclusion of these children into their families and communities. With the attention and support received in the home, children have the opportunity to live the least restricted lives possible and to develop fully as contributing members of their family and community. There are fewer and fewer children who, given proper support, are too sick or fragile to be with their own families or foster families in their community.

BARRIERS AND PROBLEMS

Despite the multiple benefits of home care, there are direct costs inherent to the process. The accepted cost savings, as dramatic as they are, only reflect the cost of medical care. Societal costs of higher taxes for expanded public funding are not considered; costs to families in terms of lost income because of work time missed are not part of the calculation, nor are costs associated with home modifications, increased electricity, transportation, or other out-of-pocket expenses. Cost savings estimates do not include the value of nursing care provided by unpaid family members (usually mothers). Also not considered is the psychologic effect on family members, added stress as a result of increased out-of-pocket expenditures, or the loss of leisure time.

The longevity of more children with long-term dependence on technology presents many new and difficult ethical and medical decisions and problems. The transition to home care from the hospital setting may be challenging and burdensome to parents. The very act of asking parents to take home children with complex medical needs and requirements for high and constant vigilance is in itself problematic. Families may be fearful as they contemplate the consequences of an equipment or technical breakdown; exhaustion may ensue. The losses of personal freedom and employment opportunity for the primary caretaker are very real and life changing. Problems of insurability for the primary family wage-earner are frequent, and job mobility and advancement may be lost. The effects on siblings because of the constant attention and concern paid to the affected child can be very significant and are often overlooked. All members must tolerate the loss of privacy that accompanies the permanent entry of health care professionals into the home. Parents often find themselves torn between traditional relationships to their children and the demands of being a case manager and at times a direct service provider, with the obligation to perform procedures on their child that cause pain or discomfort. Forced into these strange new roles, parents and children require extensive preparation and support in their transition to home care.

A COORDINATED PLAN

Experience has shown that the most successful home care outcomes result from a comprehensive, coordinated discharge process[12] (see Fig. 39-1). A well-organized multidisciplinary team, including the family, conducts the discharge planning process by considering medical, social, environmental, financial, and community factors. Each member is assigned a specific role with an established time line for completion; one person should be designated as the care coordinator or case manager. The case manager, usually a nurse, may be a hospital staff member, a representative from the insurance company/payer, a home health nurse or an independent case management agency. The responsibilities of the case manager are to oversee the coordination of all aspects of the discharge process and to provide follow-up and monitoring once the child has left the hospital. The individual assigned the role of case manager should possess solid technical, clinical, and communications skills and a comprehensive understanding of the resources available in the community. The case manager is also responsible for cost management and is often asked to provide cost comparisons to the agencies or organizations paying for the child's care. Cost analyses are an important part of the home care package, and a case manager who is familiar with community standards of practice will help guarantee that families receive the highest quality of care in the most cost-efficient manner.

The establishment of a child-specific multitiered coordinated home care plan must begin early in the child's hospital stay. Early identification of appropriate medical and allied health resources in the hospital and the community is essential if the home care experience is to be successful. All of the professionals (physicians, nurses, therapists, and others) participating in the home care plan must be willing to assume nontraditional roles and share with families the control over caregiving decisions. Personnel within the hospital must be willing to be cooperative partners with those outside of the institution, to share strategies and responsibilities for home care planning and continuing care, and to demonstrate their commitment to the philosophic concept that medical services are only part of the child's and family's needs. Community providers complement those necessary medical services; they provide a myriad of social, educational, and organizational supports and act as advocates for children and families with the various funding agencies. The discharging medical institution must, in turn, ensure that children will be able to return to the hospital if the need arises.

Coordinating Center for Home and Community Care
Process Flowchart

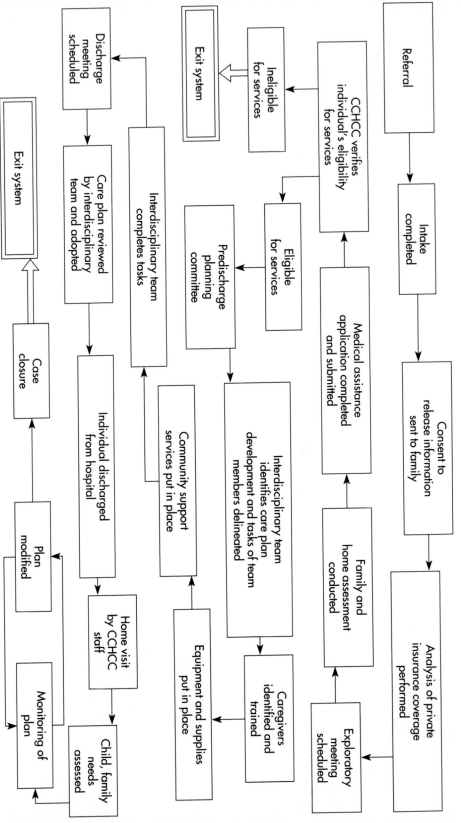

FIG. 39-1. Coordinating Center for Home and Community Care Process Flowchart.
Copyright CCHCC, 1989.

Planning

The first predischarge planning team meeting should focus on determining the medical care needs of the child at home. Will the child require in-home care by a skilled or licensed provider? What level of care is needed (i.e., are these skills that only a registered nurse can perform, or will a less-credentialed but well-instructed individual be appropriate for the medical care tasks)? How many hours of care does the family believe it can realistically provide? How often will the family require respite from this care? The answers to these questions require evaluation by and input from all members of the discharge planning team. The responsible physician should be prepared to write a prescription for home care that specifies the level and amount of in-home care by professionals or aides required per day, all treatments, medications, necessary durable medical equipment, disposable supplies, emergency protocols, therapeutic interventions, and any other special requirements. The physician should also discuss with the team the ongoing medical follow-up required by the child, such as any elective surgical procedures, clinic appointments, laboratory studies, and future adaptive equipment needs. Special considerations for transportation to and from appointments must also be anticipated. The physician must also discuss the home care plan, expected outcomes, and any other agreed upon protocols (resuscitation, emergency care, school placement) with the child's own pediatrician. Open and ongoing communication between the specialty physician and the community doctor will help ensure the continuity of care once the child leaves the hospital.

The case manager is accountable for coordinating and evaluating the effectiveness of the remaining items of the treatment plan and is also responsible for coordinating (but not necessarily providing) the family's training. The inpatient staff, serving as educators for the family, should use a comprehensive teaching assessment plan in preparation for discharge of a technologically assisted child to the home.[12] The care coordinator should help the family select the equipment vendors, home health agencies, and other providers by supplying families with lists of previously approved providers, qualities to look for in home care providers, and questions to ask of them. The case manager should also ascertain if there are any funding restrictions or providers, such as particular health maintenance organizations or preferred provider organizations, mandated by the insurance policy.

Discharge and Follow-Up

The child is ready to go home only after the child's condition is stable enough for discharge, the family is committed to and capable of carrying out a home care plan, the family has interviewed and chosen the home care providers and vendors and has successfully completed training, the equipment is in place at the home, the hospital and community physicians have discussed the treatment plan, and the payment mechanism is secure. A final discharge meeting should verify that all of the assigned tasks have been accomplished, that no new or unresolved issues remain, and that all team members are satisfied with discharge readiness. Once the child is at home, the family and care coordinator should then work together continually to monitor the home care plan and the child's health progress, and to review the appropriateness and quality of services. An in-home nursing care plan, developed by the primary home care nurse and the family, should be updated frequently to meet the changing needs of the child.

Through monthly visits in the home, the care coordinator should teach families the intricacies of the medical care and financing systems. The case manager should adhere to a strict protocol for transferring to parents the responsibility of becoming their child's care coordinator. Emphasis should be placed on safety measures, ordering necessary equipment and supplies, scheduling in-home nurses, communicating with insurers, and orchestrating the use of all essential services—in short, learning all the myriad details essential to a successful home care program for a technology-assisted child.

FUTURE NEEDS

It has been demonstrated that children who are dependent on technology can safely live at home, become active members of their community, attend school, and live full and productive lives.[1,6] However, many barriers to such successes still exist and threaten even well-designed home care efforts. The lack of comprehensive standardized arrangements for funding pediatric home care services continues to be a major impediment to successful transition from hospital to home for many children; wide variations in available funding continue to exist across states and regions. School systems vary widely in their ability to include all children into the least restrictive classroom settings. Standardization of transportation to and from school and curricula to train students and teachers to integrate technology-assisted children into classrooms would help decrease the fear and uncertainty that school systems presently experience.

There is a great need for standardization of cost and supply channels for equipment and medical supplies. Standards of practice for home care service and equipment vendors must be generated to ensure the best care and to contain costs to families and insurers.

Before- and after-school day care centers, drop-in day care centers, and trained community day care providers are an increasing necessity for children with these special health care needs. Affordable respite care services in the local community would allow families to replenish themselves for the endless task of caring for their technology-assisted children; availability of adequate educational and respite services may make the difference between successful and unsuccessful home care programs. Special programs for this population that enhance acceptance of technology-assisted children into the community and result in positive developmental benefits for the child become investments for society as a whole.

Reform of the American health care financing system must take into consideration the special needs of the families and caretakers of the technology-assisted child.[5,9] The loss of insurability and job mobility should be eliminated by guaranteeing portability of insurance and the elimination of prior condition clauses. A means for compensation for family members who devote themselves to the care of such children must be found or the apparent cost reductions obtained in transferring the locus of care from the hospital to the home will remain illusory. The personal sacrifices and opportunity losses of willing caretakers are a significant burden and inequity as the price paid for participating in what would seem to be a laudatory commitment.

The care of a technology-assisted or dependent child at home is a complex enterprise fraught with many problems and dilemmas and requiring great commitment from both professionals and caretakers. However, it has the potential of enormous rewards and benefits for the children and all who are involved in their care. It is a relatively new enterprise and its evolution will continue as the numbers of candidate children grow. Some of the technical, financial and organizational problems which face families who care for such children have clear, if politically problematic, solutions. The ethical and societal dilemmas posed by these children's care will require continuing discussion and thought. The challenge is to find ways to assist these very vulnerable children and their families and caretakers to achieve the remarkable benefits that home care can provide and, at the same time, permit all who provide that care, as well as the recipient children themselves, to share in those benefits.

ACKNOWLEDGMENT

We gratefully acknowledge the assistance of Beth Plunkett.

REFERENCES

1. Aday LA, Aitken MJ, and Wegener DH: *Pediatric home care*, Chicago, 1988, Pluribus Press.

2. Burr BH et al: Home care for children on respirators, *N Eng J Med 309*:1319-1323, 1983.

3. Fields AI et al: Outcome of home care for technology-dependent children: success of an independent, community-based case management model, *Pediatr Pulmonol 11*:310, 1991.

4. Frates RC, Splaingard ML, and Harrison GM: Outcome of home mechanical ventilation for children, *J Pediatr 106*:850-85, 1985.

5. Freedman SA and Clarke LL: Financing care for medically complex children. In Hochstadt NJ and Yost DM, editors: *The medically complex child: the transition to home care*, Chur (Switzerland), 1991, Harwood Academic Publishers.

6. Goldberg AI et al: Home care for life-supported persons: an approach to program development, *J Pediatr 104*:785-795, 1984.

7. Kaufman J: Case management services for children with special health care needs, *J Case Management 1*:53, 1992.

8. Kohrman A: Pediatric home care: a ten-point agenda for the future: In *Home care for children with serious handicapping conditions*, Washington, DC, 1984, The Association for the Care of Children's Health and the Division of Maternal and Child Health, U.S. Public Health Service, U.S. Department of Health and Human Services.

9. Kohrman AF: Facing the financing of care. In Stein REK, editor: *Caring for children with chronic illness: issues and strategies*, New York, 1989, Springer Publishing Co.

10. Kohrman AF: Psychological issues. In Mehlman M and Younger S, editors: *Delivering high technology home care*, New York, 1991, Springer Publishing Company.

11. Lantos J and Kohrman AF: Ethical aspects of pediatric home care, *Pediatrics 89*:920, 1992.

12. Sullivan-Bolyai S: All better: preparing parents to take their medically complex children home, *Continuing Care 9*:24, 1990.

CHAPTER **40**

Transportation of
Severely Disabled Children

LAWRENCE W. SCHNEIDER

Twenty-one years ago, the Education for All Handicapped Children Act*
became law and required that all handicapped children be provided the
opportunity for a public education, regardless of disability. One important
implication of this law was that thousands of severely disabled children
would be transported to and from school each day in various types of
wheelchairs and mobile seating devices. There was, however, no follow-up
with federally funded programs to establish criteria and procedures for
safe transportation of these students. As a result, most severely disabled
children in wheelchairs travel to and from school and in family vehicles.
Inadequate procedures and restraint equipment are used, which, in most
cases, do not adhere to basic crashworthiness design principles, and which
would not withstand the forces generated in a vehicle collision of even
mild or moderate severity.

For many years, Federal Motor Vehicle Safety Standard 222 (FMVSS
222)[2] has provided a measure of crashworthiness protection for able–bodied
students by requiring forward–facing, high–backed padded seats or com-
partments in large buses, and the use of seat belts in smaller buses (under
10,000 lb), but has exempted wheelchair–seated students. FMVSS 222 has
done this by defining disabled, wheelchair–seated students "as evidenced

*Public Law 94-142, Education for all Handicapped Children Act of 1975 (89 STAT.773)

421

by orientation of the seat in a direction that is more than 45 degrees to the left or right of the longitudinal centerline of the vehicle." In other words, the regulation has excluded severely disabled students from the crash protection standard by defining them to be oriented in a direction known to be least safe in a frontal vehicle crash.

It is well documented that school bus transportation is one of the safest modes of travel, with an accident rate only one fourth that of passenger automobiles. The provision of public education for disabled students however, often involves travel over longer distances, at higher vehicle speeds, and in smaller buses and van-sized vehicles, than is necessary for able–bodies students, thereby increasing exposure and risk to vehicle accidents. Yet, it is common for wheelchair–bound students to be transported with wheelchairs backed up to the side of the bus, facing the aisle, as shown in Fig. 40-1. Various types of inadequate and untested tiedown hardware are used to secure wheelchair wheels; lap belts and torso belts are placed over soft body regions; and rigid wheelchair structures and components, such as unpadded trays and armrests, are in close proximity to the students.

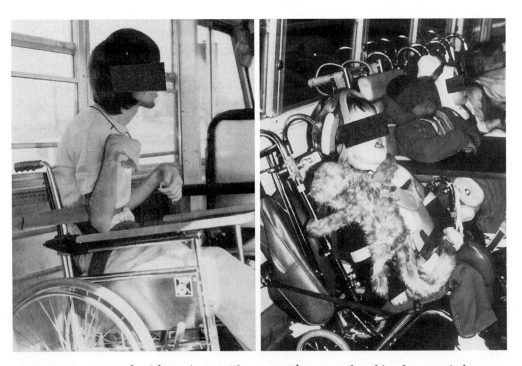

FIG. 40-1. Securing wheelchairs facing sideways with untested and inadequate tiedown hardware is the most common practice but is probably the least safe for occupant protection in frontal collisions.

Such examples of unsafe occupant packaging need not be the case if the people responsible for transporting these students will make safety a priority. The level of crash protection offered to disabled students can be greatly improved if general principles of occupant protection are followed, if equipment used to secure and restrain the wheelchairs and occupants are designed to withstand the forces generated in a crash, and if restraint devices, wheelchairs, and securement procedures are evaluated using standard dynamic test procedures. This chapter discusses the basic issues and principles involved in providing improved crashworthiness protection for children who must use wheelchairs as vehicle seats, and describes the progress made toward this goal.

INJURY CAUSATION AND OCCUPANT PROTECTION

The fact has been well established from accident investigations that the primary cause of serious injury to motor vehicle occupants in a crash is the human collision or second impact, where the occupant's body strikes components of the vehicle's interior after the vehicle has come to a stop as a result of the first collision.[1] Therefore, the goal of a well-designed occupant protection system is, first of all, to prevent the traveler from being thrown out of the vehicle and, secondly, to prevent or minimize the human collision within the vehicle by allowing the occupant to ride down the vehicle crash in the space available.

TRANSFER WHEN FEASIBLE

Vehicle safety engineers have long recognized the importance of seat design in providing effective occupant restraint and protection. Most wheelchairs on the market have not been designed for use as seats in motor vehicles. Effective occupant protection is usually best accomplished by transferring the wheelchair user to the vehicle seat so that the OEM's (original equipment manufacturer's) restraint systems, or other restraint system meeting federal safety standards, can be used. The wheelchair can then be stored and secured with effective tiedown hardware and procedures. For example, wheelchair–bound students may be transferred to a bus or van seat where a properly installed, four–point harness, such as the E–Z–On vest[4,5] can be used. For smaller children, child safety seats that comply with FMVSS 213[2] requirements can be secured on bus seats and modified, if necessary, to accommodate the needs of disabled children, as long as the basic structural integrity of the seats is not compromised.[3] Also, for children up to 60 inches tall who are too large for a standard child safety seat (i.e., over 40 lbs), there are a few larger safety seats, such as the Special Seat, the Orthopedic Positioning Seat, and Preston's Carrie Car Seat (Fig. 40-2), to which children can be transferred while in a motor vehicle.[3,5,6]

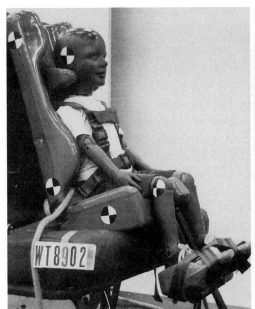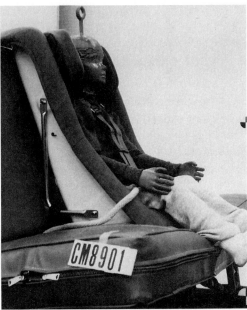

FIG. 40-2. Carrie Car Seat and the Special Seat for transferring children over 40 lb.

There are, of course, many children for whom transfer is not practical or acceptable because of their size and/or disabilities. In these cases, an effective occupant protection system must provide both wheelchair securement and occupant restraint designed to deal with crash–level forces and with adherence to basic crashworthiness principles.

A SYSTEMS PROBLEM

Providing safe transportation for children with severe disabilities is a systems problem that involves the wheelchair, the student with his or her unique disabilities, the wheelchair securement devices and occupant restraints, and the vehicle—its structural design and the strength of components to which restraint systems are attached. Effective occupant protection requires that each of these parts of the total system be taken into account and dealt with appropriately. Failure to consider any one part of the total system can result in ineffective occupant protection. For example, if an otherwise effective wheelchair tiedown system is attached to weak points of a vehicle, or with weak fasteners, the installation points may fail during impact loading, releasing the wheelchair and occupant to become free projectiles in the vehicle during a crash. Similarly, providing wheelchair securement without occupant restraint, or occupant restraint without effective and independent wheelchair securement, will compromise the level of occupant protection offered.

BASIC CRASHWORTHINESS DESIGN PRINCIPLES

While children with disabilities may have lower tolerance to injury from impact loads and body motions, several basic principles of occupant protection are still applicable to providing effective protection. The following design principles should be followed to the extent possible in transporting disabled students.

Restrain the Wheelchair Independent from the Occupant

A basic principle of crashworthiness safety is to not allow the mass of the vehicle seat to add to the forces applied to the occupant during a crash. Adhering to this principle is particularly important for people in wheelchairs or other special seating devices, as the chair mass can be 200 lb or more, and the occupant's tolerance to impact loading is likely to be less than that of an able–bodied person. This safety principle implies that the wheelchair must be secured to allow minimal movement during a crash, and to prevent the wheelchair from tipping over, collapsing, or breaking apart in a manner that could injure the user or other vehicle occupants. The wheelchair tiedown system should secure the wheelchair independent of the occupant. The same belts should not be used to restrain both the wheelchair and the occupant so the forces used to restrain the wheelchair are not imposed on and through the occupant's body.

Independent vs. Parallel Occupant Restraints

Securing the wheelchair independent of the occupant does not mean that the occupant should be secured independent of the wheelchair. In fact, the opposite situation is preferred, where occupant restraints (i.e., the lap belts and the lower anchorage of the shoulder belt) are anchored to the wheelchair or to the tiedown components as near to the hip of the occupant as possible. This integrated or serial configuration for the occupant restraint system and wheelchair securement system is illustrated in Fig. 40-3. Although this configuration will produce higher restraint loads on the vehicle attachment points and tiedown hardware, dynamic testing has demonstrated that such forces can be effectively managed using reasonable and acceptable hardware. More importantly, this approach offers improved occupant protection by increasing the opportunity to achieve a good fit of the occupant restraints and by eliminating the possibility of the wheelchair mass adding to the forces applied to the occupant.

The parallel or independent configuration shown in Fig. 40-4 can be effective if appropriate hardware testing is conducted to ensure that the wheelchair does not impose additional forces on the occupant. However, the system should be considered less desirable from an occupant protection standpoint for the same reasons that the integrated configuration is consid-

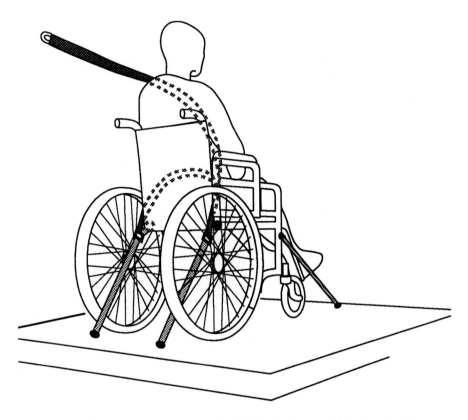

FIG. 40-3. A four-point, strap-type wheelchair tiedown with integrated (in series) three-point occupant restraint system.

ered to offer a better approach. In general, it is more difficult, and perhaps even impossible in some situations, to achieve a good fit of the restraint belts on the wheelchair occupant when the lap and shoulder belts are anchored to the vehicle floor. It is also difficult to determine in dynamic testing if some wheelchair securement is provided by the parallel occupant restraint system. If, for example, there is more stretch or give in the tiedown belts or wheelchair components than in the occupant restraints, the wheelchair may be partially restrained through forces acting on the occupant.

Provide Both Upper and Lower Torso Restraints

The purpose of an occupant protection system is to prevent or minimize contact of the occupant's body with vehicle structures. Both upper and lower torso restraints are needed to minimize knee, chest, and head excursions. While a properly positioned lap belt alone will prevent an occupant from being ejected from or thrown about inside the vehicle, the torso can still jack-knife forward, and the chest and head can impact with nearby vehicle structures and components, or with nearby occupants and wheelchairs. In addition, the spinal flexion or jackknifing of the torso that occurs without upper torso restraint may be sufficient to produce central nervous system trauma for severely disabled people. Finally, the use of upper torso restraint will reduce the tendency for the occupant to submarine under the lap belt, an undesirable kinematic which results in lap belt forces being applied to the more vulnerable organs of the soft abdomen rather than the pelvic bone.

The ideal restraint system, especially for small children, is a four– or five–point harness that is integrated into, and securely attached to, the seat frame of the wheelchair, as is done in child safety seats. In many cases, however, this method of restraint cannot be used due to the size of the child or limitations in the strength of the seat and wheelchair frame. In these cases, an integrated three–point restraint system offers the next–best level of protection.

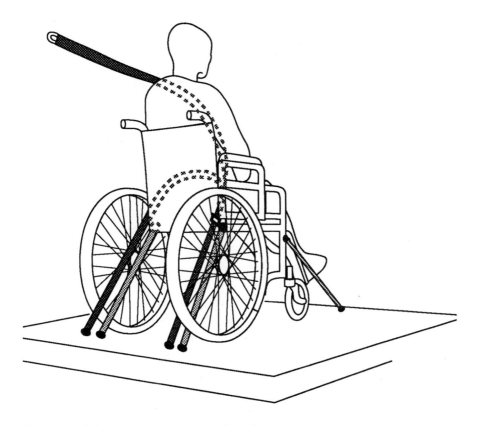

FIG. 40-4. A four-point, strap-type wheelchair tiedown with independent (in parallel) three-point occupant restraint system.

Apply Forces to Skeletal Structures

An important principle that has often been ignored in the case of wheelchair–seated motor-vehicle occupants is to apply restraint forces to the bony regions of the body and not to the soft tissues regions such as the abdomen. This means keeping the angle of the lap belt at 45 degrees or greater to the vertical so that it stays on the pelvic bone. The shoulder belt should be positioned so that the forces are applied to the clavicle or collar bone as well as the chest, and attached to the lap belt near the hip of the occupant, rather than over the lap so it doesn't pull the lap belt up onto the soft abdomen during impact loading.

Seat belts are frequently used to provide postural support and seating stability for people in wheelchairs. Seat belts are often wrapped around the back of the wheelchair at the level of the abdomen or chest. Belts should not be used as crash restraint systems and should be designed to break away before imposing high injury-producing forces.

Face Wheelchairs and Occupants Forward

The issue of occupant orientation is one that involves the statistics of vehicle crash directions. Analysis of thousands of accidents has established that more than 50% of motor vehicle accidents involving serious and fatal injuries have frontal impact as the primary component. These statistics have been taken into account in FMVSS 222 that requires all school buses to be manufactured with forward–facing, high–backed, padded seats to provide impact protection during frontal crashes. However, as indicated previously, wheelchair–seated students and passengers have customarily been transported facing sideways and backed up to the side wall of the bus, often with several wheelchairs, travel chairs, or stroller-type chairs next to each other. From an occupant protection standpoint, this is probably the least safe way for anyone to travel.

The safest direction for an occupant to face is rearward, if a properly designed and energy-absorbing structure is provided to absorb and distribute impact loads over the occupant's back and head during a frontal crash. This may, however, prove to be a costly, impractical, and unacceptable approach.

Occupant protection for disabled students can be improved, however, by facing the wheelchair forward and by providing adequate spacing between chairs. Comments from transportation professionals who have implemented the change to forward–facing wheelchairs indicate that students may also experience less travel fatigue, apparently from not having to brace against the lateral jerking movement as the vehicle starts, stops, and changes speeds, or from not having to watch the passing scenery through the opposite-side windows.

Pad Vehicle Interior Surfaces

In the previous section, the importance of providing adequate space around each occupant to prevent second impact with other occupants, other wheelchairs, or vehicle structures is mentioned. In addition to the precaution of added space, vehicle structures near wheelchair–seated travelers should be covered with energy–absorbing padding of sufficient thickness and density to prevent injury during impact loading. Plastic and steel trays or other equipment attached to the wheelchair should be removed and secured during transportation so that the rigid edges do not injure the wheelchair occupant and so the attached equipment does not break loose and injure other occupants in a collision.

Use Dynamically Tested Equipment

Wheelchair securement and occupant restraint equipment should be evaluated using dynamic testing. These tests are typically conducted on an impact sled such as that shown in Fig. 40-5. The forces developed in the tiedown and restraint equipment depend primarily on the sled impact velocity and deceleration, the size and weight of the anthropomorphic crash dummy, and the mass of the wheelchair.

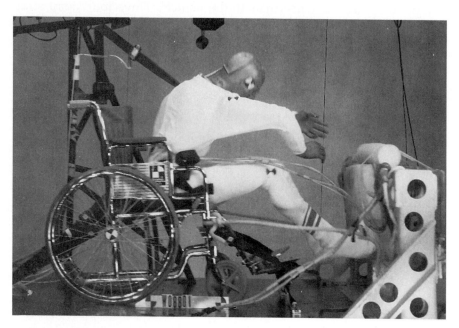

FIG. 40-5. Dynamic testing of wheelchair tiedown and occupant restraint system on the University of Michigan Transportation Research Institute's impact sled.

The level of crash severity for which a wheelchair tiedown and occupant restraint system should be tested (i.e., the impact velocities, decelerations, resulting restraint forces) depends on the vehicle size and the travel modes in which the equipment will be used. For systems intended only for use in large school buses that travel only on city streets, testing with a crash pulse of 10 to 20 mph and 10 to 15–G deceleration (1 G = acceleration of gravity = 32.2 ft/sec^2) is reasonable. However, for vans or van-sized school buses that travel on expressways, a 30–mph crash velocity is appropriate. Because most tiedowns and restraints are manufactured for general use, 30–mph, 20–G crash conditions similar to those required in FMVSS 213 for child safety seat testing, are usually used in conjunction with an average male crash dummy (170 lb) and a conventional electric wheelchair with simulated battery mass (160 lb) to evaluate crashworthiness performance.

EFFECTIVE TIEDOWN/RESTRAINT SYSTEMS

Several manufacturers now offer vehicle wheelchair tiedown and occupant restraint systems that comply with the general principles presented, and that have been dynamically tested using 30–mph, 20–G crash conditions. For school bus transportation, the most widely used type of wheelchair tiedown adaptable to different sizes and styles of wheelchairs utilizes four belts or straps to secure the wheelchair to the vehicle. Three four–point strap–type tiedown systems that have been dynamically tested for 30–mph, 20–G frontal crash conditions are Q'Straint, the Protector, and FE500. The Q'Straint and Protector systems include an integrated three–point occupant restraint system, while the Kinedyne FE500 system uses an independent three–point occupant restraint system.

The Strap-Lok tiedown/restraint system and the Transit–Lok and Secure–Lok systems use other types of securement hardware rather than straps, and use four wheelchair attachment points, but only two vehicle anchor points. These systems use separate and independent lap and shoulder-belt systems and have successfully restrained both a power wheelchair and 50th–percentile–male test dummy for 30–mph, 20–G frontal crash conditions.

Table 40-1 lists and describes wheelchair tiedown and occupant restraint systems that have been successfully sled tested in recent years. Because production systems may have been modified since the tests, consumers should contact the manufacturer for assurance that a particular system is still available and that it has been tested as currently designed and manufactured. Also, because there is not yet a national standard that defines the performance of a successful system, copies of test films and test reports should be requested to verify and compare performance.

Table 40-1. Tiedown/Restraint Systems Successfully Tested for
30-mph, 20-G Impact Conditions

Name of Tiedown/ Restraint	Manufacturer*	Type of Tiedown	Type of Restraint
Q'Straint	Q'Straint	4 straps to 4 points on chair and floor	Integrated 3-point
Protector	Ortho Safe Systems, Inc.	4 straps to 4 points on chair and floor	Integrated 3-point
FE500	Kinedyne, Inc.	4 straps to 4 points on chair and floor	Independent 3-point
Strap-Lok	Creative Controls, Inc.	2 rear straps to chair axles, 1 front strap to bar across chair frame, 2 floor anchor points	Independent 2-point lap belt plus independent 2-point shoulder belt
Transit-Lok Secure-Lok	Gresham Driving Aids, Inc.	2 steel hooks to chair axles, bar with strap or 2 straps to front of chair frame, 2 floor anchor points	Independent 2-point lap belt plus independent 2-point shoulder belt

*See listing at end of chapter for manufacturer address and phone number.

WHEELCHAIRS AND WHEELCHAIR TESTING

As indicated previously, the problem of providing safe transportation for the wheelchair–seated passenger is a systems problem. An extension of this systems concept is the fact that a tiedown/restraint system that is effective for one type or size of wheelchair may not be equally effective for a different wheelchair. To date, all the tiedown/restraint systems listed in Table 40-1 have been successfully tested using conventional manual and 3P–type power wheelchairs constructed with welded tubular steel frames. Wheelchairs that differ in structural design and materials should be dynamically tested to compare their crashworthiness potential with successfully tested tiedown systems, and to determine the optimal wheelchair attachment points.

For example, the Q'Straint and Ortho Safe systems have been tested and shown to be effective for securing travel chairs, such as those made by Orthokinetics, Inc. and Sunrise Medical, Inc., or the stroller-type chairs, such as those shown in Fig. 40-6. It is important to note that a wheelchair does not have to be heavy to be strong enough to sustain a crash with the occupant in the wheelchair. In fact, the heavier the wheelchair, the higher the forces that its structure must withstand. The important thing is for the wheelchair frame to be structurally designed to handle the loading paths imposed by the occupant and wheelchair, and that four designated and tested attachment points, or other wheelchair tiedown interface hardware, be available on the wheelchair frame to enable effective wheelchair securement.

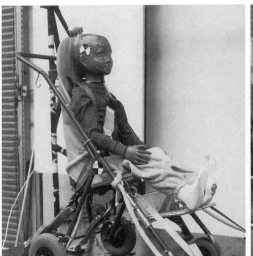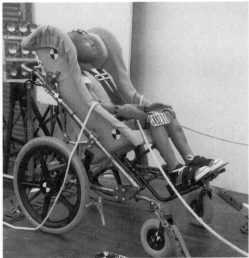

FIG. 40-6. Alvema Series 10 Push Chair by Physio E.R.P. and Snug Seat Postural Seating System in strollers that have been dynamically tested at 30 mph, 20–G frontal crash conditions.

Table 40-2 lists examples of different types of wheelchairs that have been successfully tested on the UMTRI (University of Michigan Transportation Research Institute) sled for 30–mph, 20–G frontal crash conditions. As with wheelchair tiedown and occupant restraint equipment, consumers should request copies of reports and films of dynamic tests from the manufacturer, and should make sure that the structural design of the wheelchair of interest is the same as that used in the tests.

OTHER IMPACT DIRECTIONS

The primary concern in crashworthiness protection is frontal impact, and this has been the primary concern in sled impact testing to date. Consideration should also be given, however, to the fact that vehicles experience impacts from the side and rear, and that vehicle rollover may occur. In fact, in most accidents, the impact direction is angled to the front, side, or rear of the vehicle. Thus, while a frontal crash test is typically used to evaluate the general strength of tiedown/restraint hardware, designers of tiedown equipment and wheelchairs should consider the need for strength and stability in other loading directions. The occurrence of angled and nonfrontal impacts call for the placing of padding between the occupant and rigid wheelchair components, such as armrests, and the use of high-backed wheelchairs or head supports attached to the backs of the wheelchairs to reduce the likelihood of neck injuries during rear impacts.

Table 40-2. Examples of Wheelchairs Dynamically Tested for 30–mph, 20–G Frontal Impact Conditions

Wheelchair Type/Name*	Wheelchair Tiedown	Occupant Restraint	Test Dummy
E&J 3P Power	Various	Various	50th %ile Male (170 lb)
Convaid 4T Cruiser stroller	Q'Straint 4-point	Q'Straint 3-point	50th %ile Male (170 lb)
Snug Seat Postural Seating System in heavy-duty mobility base	Kinedyne 4-point	5-point harness	3-Year-Old (35 lb)
Orthokinetics Travel Chair	Q'Straint 4-point	Q'Straint 3-point	5th %ile Female (100 lb)
Quickie No. 900 Series Travel Chair (formerly STC Travel Chair)	Prototype 4-point with top tether	5-point harness to seat	6-Year-Old (60 lb)
Tumble Forms Carrie Seat in Carrie Rover	Q'Straint 4-point	Q'Straint 3-point	5th %ile Female (100 lb)
Amigo Three-Wheel Sentra Scooter	Q'Straint 5-point	Q'Straint 3-point	50th %ile Male (170 lb)
Tumble Forms Carrie Seat and Carrie Rover	Q'Straint 4-point	Q'Straint 3-point	3-Year-Old (35 lb)
Physio E.R.P. Alvema Series 10 Push Chair	Q'Straint 4-point	Q'Straint 3-point	6-Year-Old (60 lb)
Kid-E-Plus Bus Transportable Model	Q'Straint 4-point	5-point harness to stroller seat	6-Year-Old (50 lb)

*Customers should check with manufacturers for exact models of wheelchairs tested. See listing at end of chapter.

DISCUSSION

Much progress in providing safe transportation for children in wheelchairs can be made by understanding and applying the basic principles of occupant crash protection, and by using established test procedures and facilities to dynamically evaluate wheelchairs, wheelchair securement, and occupant restraint hardware. Over the past 10 years, significant improvements have been made in the wheelchair tiedowns and occupant restraint equipment available to the consumer, and many manufacturers of this safety equipment now routinely conduct dynamic sled tests to evaluate their products. Still, in the absence of any standards, there is much equipment on the market that has not been tested and for which the performance in a crash must be questioned. People responsible for the transportation of wheelchair–bound children must make educated and informed decisions about the equipment that is purchased and the procedures that are used.

While further improvements in wheelchair tiedowns and occupant restraints can be realized, the greatest remaining obstacle to providing safe transportation for handicapped children is the lack of consideration of motor-vehicle transportation in the design of wheelchairs. In recent years, many new wheelchair models that offer improved positioning and versatility to their occupants have become available. These new chairs present new problems in the provision of effective securement in motor vehicles and effective restraint of wheelchair occupants. In accordance with the increasing use of wheelchairs as seats in motor vehicles, wheelchair manufacturers must consider this important application of their products. Manufacturers must not only provide designated and dynamically tested attachments points for securement to the vehicle, but must also consider the potential interaction of the wheelchair occupant with the wheelchair components, which can result in injury under impact conditions.

In response to a lawsuit filed by a Michigan–based transportation company claiming that FMVSS 222 discriminated against handicapped children by not providing a comparable level of occupant protection to students in wheelchairs, The National Highway Traffic Safety Administration (NHTSA) has recently modified (January 1994) FMVSS 222 to require that all school bus OEM tiedown and restraint equipment be designed and installed for use with forward–facing wheelchairs. It further establishes static strength requirements for wheelchair tiedown and occupant restraint hardware.

While there is some question as to the ultimate effectiveness of this new regulation because it applies only to OEM school bus equipment and does nothing to improve the design of wheelchairs for use in motor vehicles, it does represent a long–overdue step by the federal government toward improving the level of occupant protection provided to disabled children in school buses.

There are several efforts underway to develop standards that will require dynamic testing to evaluate equipment, and that will specify forward–facing transportation of all wheelchairs and their occupants. The Canadian Standards Association (CSA), the Society of Automotive Engineers (SAE), and the International Standards Organization (ISO) are developing test procedures and performance criteria that will require 30–mph, 20–G sled testing of wheelchair tiedowns and restraints. The CSA, ISO, and a recently formed ANSI/RESNA Subcommittee on Wheelchairs and Transportation (SOWHAT) are also working on standards for transportable wheelchairs that offer safe and suitable seating for disabled occupants of motor vehicles. Completion of the implementation of these standards, and particularly those of SAE and SOWHAT, which include children in their scope, should significantly enhance the level of crashworthiness available to all handicapped children who must remain seated in their wheelchairs while traveling in motor vehicles.

REFERENCES

1. Mackay M: An historical perspective on impact biomechanics and some basic kinematics, Aldman B and Chapon A, editors: *The biomechanics of impact trauma*, BV/Amsterdam ICTS, 1984, Elsevier Sciences Publishers.
2. National Archives and Records Service, Office of the Federal Register: Child restraint systems, Code of Federal Regulations, Title 49, Transportation, Washington, DC, Oct 1992.
3. Richards DD: The challenge of transporting children with special needs, *Safe Ride News*, Spring 1989.
4. Shelness A: Transporting children with special needs, Part II: Protecting handicapped school children, *Safe Ride News* 6(3), 4.
5. Stoudt JD, Bull JJ, and Stroup KB: Safe transportation for children with disabilities; *American Journal of Occupational Therapy*, Jan 1988.
6. Stroup KB, Weber K, and Bull MJ: Safe transportation solutions for children with special needs, Proceedings of the thirty-first annual meeting of the American Association for Automotive Medicine, New Orleans, Sept 28-30, 1987.

BIBLIOGRAPHY

Benson J and Schneider LW: Improving the crashworthiness of restraints for handicapped children, Tech Rep 840528, Warrendale, Penn, 1984, Society of Automotive Engineers.

Brenner E and Giangrande RV: Wheelchair securement systems in transit vehicles: a summary report, Rep DOT-TSC-UMTA-81-43, Washington DC, 1981, U.S. Department of Transportation, Transportation Systems Center.

Bull MJ and Stroup KB: Premature infants in car seats, *Pediatrics* 75(2), Feb 1985.

Khadilkar AV and Will E: Crash protection systems for handicapped school and transit bus occupants, Rep DOT-HS-805-821, Washington DC, 1980, U.S. Department of Transportation, National Highway Traffic Safety Administration.

Linebaugh PE: Handicapped seating study committee report: Washtenaw intermediate school district transportation report, Ann Arbor, Mich, 1988, Washtenaw Intermediate School District.

Petty SPF: The safe transportation of wheelchair occupants in the United Kingdom, Proceedings from the eleventh International Technical Conference on Experimental Safety Vehicles, Washington DC, 1986, U.S. Department of Transportation, National Highway Traffic Safety Administration.

Schneider LW: Dynamic testing of restraint systems and tie-downs for use with vehicle occupants seated in powered wheelchairs, Rep UM-HSRI-81-18, Ann Arbor, Mich, 1981, University of Michigan Transportation Research Institute.

Schneider LW: Protection for the severely disabled: A new challenge in occupant restraint, Green RN and Petrucello E, editors: *The human collision: international symposium on occupant restraints*, Morton Grove, Ill, 1981, American Association for Automotive Medicine.

Schneider LW: Sled impact tests of wheelchair tie-down systems for handicapped drivers, Rep UMTRI-85-19, Ann Arbor, Mich, 1985, University of Michigan Transportation Research Institute.

Schneider LW, Melvin JW and Cooney CE: Impact sled test evaluation of restraint systems used in transportation of handicapped children, Tech Rep 7900074. Warrendale, Penn, 1979, Society of Automotive Engineers.

Seeger BR and Caudrey DJ: Crashworthiness of restraints for physically disabled children in buses, Kilkenny, Austral, 1983, The Crippled Children's Association of South Australia.

Standards Association of Australia: *Wheelchair occupant restraint assemblies for motor vehicles,* Australian Standard, AS 2942. North Sydney, NSW, 1987.

Stewart CF and Geinl HG: Wheelchair securement on bus and paratransit vehicles, Rep UMTA-CA-06-0098-81-1, Sacramento, Calif, 1981, California Department of Transportation.

Tiedown/Restraint Manufacturers of "Successfully" Tested Products

Creative Controls, Inc.
32450 Dequindre
Warren, MI 48092
Phone: 810-979-3500

E-Z-On Products, Inc.
500 Commerce Way
Suite 3
Jupiter, FL 33458
Phone: 800-323-6598

Gresham Driving Aids, Inc.
P.O. Box 405
Wixom, MI 48393
Phone: 800-521-8930

Kinedyne, Inc.
3701 Greenway Circle
Lawrence, KS 66044
Phone: 913-841-4000

Ortho Safe Systems, Inc.
P.O. Box 9435
Trenton, NJ 08650
Phone: 609-587-3859

Q'Straint
3085 Southwestern Blvd.
Orchard Park, NY 14127
Phone: 716-675-2222

Wheelchair Manufacturers Who Have Conducted Sled Impact Tests

Amigo Mobility International
6693 Dixie Highway
Bridgeport, MI 48722
Phone: 800-821-2710

Convaid Products, Inc.
P.O. Box 2409
Palos Verdes, CA 90274
Phone: 310-539-6814

Everest & Jennings, Inc.
1100 Corporate Square Drive
St. Louis, MO 63132
Phone: 800-235-4661

J.A. Preston, Inc.
(Tumble Forms Products)
P.O. Box 89
Jackson, MI 49204
Phone: 800-631-7277

Kid-Kart, Inc.
732 Cruiser Lane
Belgrade, MN 59714
Phone: 406-388-1080

Love Lift
1274 Industrial Avenue
Holland, MI 49423
Phone: 616-875-6054

Snug Seat, Inc.
10810 Independence Point Pkwy
Matthews, NC 28106-1739
Phone: 800-336-7684
(Also source of Special Seat)

Sunrise Medical/Quickie Designs, Inc.
2842 Business Park Avenue
Fresno, CA 93727
Phone: 800-456-8168

Taylor Made Healthcare
10 West 9th Avenue
P.O. Box 1190
Gloversville, NY 12078
Phone: 800-258-0942

PART FIVE

CONDITIONS

The following part on conditions is not intended as a definitive resource on the various medical problems considered under the topic of disability and chronic illness. Rather, the brief descriptions presented here may be helpful as a quick reference or overview when more extensive material is not immediately available or needed.

Further information about the conditions in this section may be obtained from textbooks devoted to health information regarding disabilities and chronic illness, review articles found through medical literature computerized databases, library resources, condition specific organizations such as the United Cerebral Palsy Associations, and the World Wide Web. The local library as well as the health sciences library at health professions training facilities will be able to assist in locating the most up-to-date material.

CHAPTER **41**

Conditions

LISA T. CRAFT
MARK L. WOLRAICH

PHYSICAL DISABILITIES

Cerebral Palsy

Definition. Cerebral palsy (CP), a nonprogressive disorder of movement and posture, results from injury to the brain during early development. Although the muscles, peripheral nerves, and spinal cord are normal, the brain is unable to control muscle movement.

Incidence. The incidence of cerebral palsy is 1.5 to 2 in a thousand live births and is higher in areas with poor prenatal care and increased incidence of prematurity. Although the incidence may be declining, the prevalence (number of cases in the community) may be increasing, as technologic advances increase the infant survival rate.

Etiology. Cerebral palsy may result from injury to the brain due to chromosomal abnormalities, maternal infections (toxoplasmosis, rubella, cytomegalovirus, or herpes), or insufficient oxygen or blood reaching the brain, as in toxemia and placenta previa. However, researchers have recently challenged the role of birth asphyxia as a major cause of CP.[31,32] Intracranial hemorrhage (more common in premature infants), high bilirubin levels (jaundice), or meningitis can also lead to brain damage.

Prevention of CP involves maternal immunization for infectious agents, improved prenatal care, and prevention of premature delivery.

Clinical description. Clinical manifestations of cerebral palsy may not be apparent during the first few months of life. Delayed achievement of motor milestones, abnormal movements, and abnormalities detected by physical examination will develop during the first year or two of life.

Children with spasticity will have reduced movement or stiffness due to hypertonia, usually resulting from injury to the corticospinal (pyramidal) tract or motor cortex. About 60% of all cases of CP will have spasticity, further described as diplegia (involvement of the trunk and all extremities, with legs more involved), hemiplegia (involvement of one side of the body), quadriplegia (equal involvement of both arms, both legs, head, and trunk), or paraplegia (involvement of only legs).

Children with dyskinesia, also known as extrapyramidal CP, have involuntary, nonpurposeful movements, including athetosis and dystonia. Tone may vary or be increased, especially with certain body positions or emotional states. Dyskinetic CP usually results from injury to the basal ganglia, is quadriplegic in distribution, and is found in 20% of cases of CP.

Children with ataxia have a broad-based, lurching gait and balance difficulties. Injury to the cerebellum is the usual cause and accounts for about 1% of cases of CP.

Children with mixed CP will show a combination of spasticity, dyskinesia, and ataxia. This occurs in about 30% of cases.

Most children with cerebral palsy have associated disabilities, including mental retardation (in 60% to 70%), learning disability, and seizures (in 30% to 40%). Other common problems are visual, hearing, and speech-language impairment, feeding and growth problems, constipation, dental disease, and behavior problems.

Management. Successful management of a child with cerebral palsy involves team provision of specialist services, including orthopedics, neurology, ophthalmology, dentistry, physical therapy, occupational therapy, speech pathology, and orthotics. Services are often coordinated with early intervention programs, special preschool programs, and regular school programs.

Needs. A child with cerebral palsy needs assistance to optimize all areas of functioning and to achieve as much independence as possible in daily life. Early intervention to provide appropriate medical, educational, social, and family support services is of great importance.

Muscular Dystrophy

Definition. Muscular dystrophy refers to a group of genetically determined muscle disorders, many of which are progressive and disabling. Muscle biopsy often shows characteristic changes.

Incidence. Duchenne muscular dystrophy, the most common dystrophy, occurs in approximately 30 in 100,000 live-born males, with a prevalence of 2 to 3 in a population of 100,000. The Becker type has an approximate incidence of 3 in a population of 100,000. Facioscapulohumeral dystrophy occurs with an approximate incidence of 5 in a population of 100,000 and prevalence of 0.2 in 100,000. The incidence of myotonic dystrophy is approximately 15 in a population of 100,000, with a prevalence of 5 in 100,000.

Etiology. The muscular dystrophies are inherited diseases. The Duchenne type and Becker type of muscular dystrophy are X–linked and thus usually affect boys. A gene defect in the Xp21 region of the X chromosome produces a reduced muscle content of the protein dystrophin which is less than 3% of normal in the Duchenne type and 3% to 20% of normal in the Becker type. The mode of inheritance is usually autosomal recessive for limb–girdle dystrophy and autosomal dominant for facioscapulohumeral dystrophy and myotonic dystrophy, with less known about the specific genetic defect for these types.

Clinical description. Duchenne muscular dystrophy almost always occurs in boys. Parents may notice problems when children first begin to walk, walk on tiptoe, have repeated falls, have a waddling gait, and have difficulty rising from the floor (Gower's sign). Diagnosis is often made after 4 years of age, as progressive weakness and calf enlargement are noted. Because of cerebral maturation children between the ages of 4 and 6 years often appear to improve. Thereafter increasing weakness and contractures lead to more difficulty with walking and climbing stairs. Children often require wheelchairs by ages 12 to 14. Pulmonary compromise develops, often leading to need for assisted ventilation and later to ventilator dependency. Most patients survive to age 20 but few survive past 30 years. Boys with Becker muscular dystrophy resemble those with the Duchenne type but have a later age of onset (6 to 10 years) and slower progression of the disease. Children with limb–girdle muscular dystrophy usually experience onset of the disease after age 10 with weakness of the proximal girdle muscles. Facioscapulohumeral dystrophy may begin in late childhood or early adulthood, with symptoms of weakness of the muscles of the face, shoulders, and arms.[34] After age 10 children with myotonic dystrophy usually begin to experience weakness or stiffness of the hands, weakness of the facial muscles (leading to a hatchet face appearance), and delayed muscle relaxation after a contraction. Newborns with the congenital form may exhibit poor sucking ability and respiratory distress.

Management. Management includes genetic counseling and rehabilitative efforts (physical therapy, occupational therapy, and respiratory therapy) to maintain optimal function and minimal deformity.[27] Children often require educational intervention because of learning disability or subnormal intelligence, which are especially common in Duchenne and Becker dystrophy. Psychosocial issues that must be dealt with include poor self-image, depression, anger, dependency, and family stress.

Needs. Continued search for a cure or method to slow the progression of muscular dystrophy is needed. Steroids (prednisone) may slow the progression of weakness and improve strength and function. Researchers are evaluating the effects of myoblast transfer (injection of normal muscle cells into a patient's muscle) and gene therapy that would allow the patient's own muscle cells to produce normal dystrophin.

Amputations

Definition. Amputation is the loss of part of a limb or of an entire limb.

Incidence. Congenital amputations are estimated to occur in 2 to 8 children in 10,000 births, with variation often noted among communities.

Etiology. Maternal infections (such as varicella), drug use (such as thalidomide), and undetermined genetic factors can produce congenital amputation or limb reduction. Amputation or reduction may also be associated with identifiable syndromes, or may be the result of amniotic constriction bands (Streeter's dysplasia). Acquired amputation results from trauma or from surgical treatment of diseases such as osteogenic sarcoma.

Clinical description. Amputations may be partial or complete and may be transverse or longitudinal. Congenital amputations may involve the terminal end of an extremity, or intermediate parts may be absent, with the terminal end present. Absence of the thumb (or presence of a rudimentary thumb) and below-elbow amputation are among the more common congenital upper extremity amputations.

Children with congenital amputation or limb defects may have other anomalies consistent with a syndrome. Holt-Oram Syndrome includes upper limb defects plus heart anomalies. Cornelia de Lange's Syndrome involves limb anomalies, plus small size, mental deficiency, and characteristic facial features.

Management. Surgical treatment must be individualized for the specific defect. Treatment of congenital amputations includes reconstructive surgery, when feasible, or amputation revision to produce a stump that is suitable for prosthesis fitting. A child with an absent thumb may have a remaining digit transferred to the thumb position. For children with traumatic amputations, technologic advances often allow successful replantation of digits or limbs, but return of normal function is not always obtained.

Early fitting of a prosthesis is usually preferred for children with congenital amputations, allowing them to reach developmental milestones at the usual time. However, early or later use of a prosthesis depends on the type and severity of defect and whether it is unilateral or bilateral. With less severe defects, children may function well until a later age.[4] For children with traumatic or surgical amputations, early fitting of prostheses provides positive psychologic benefit, reduces the sense of loss, and encourages rehabilitation.[24]

Needs. Children with amputations need psychologic support as they adjust to loss of a limb and to functioning with prostheses.

CHRONIC ILLNESS

AIDS

Definition. Acquired immunodeficiency syndrome (AIDS) in the pediatric age group involves immunodeficiency and subsequent opportunistic infections in patients who are infected with the human immunodeficiency virus (HIV). Other types of immunodeficiencies, congenital infections, malignancies, and malnutrition may mimic AIDS.

Incidence. Approximately 2000 children in the United States have AIDS, although many more may be asymptomatic or do not yet meet the criteria for diagnosis. Prevalence has been steadily increasing and is higher among minorities and the poor. However, the AIDS epidemic continues to spread and is not limited to poor urban communities.

Etiology. Children may develop AIDS following exposure to contaminated blood or blood products. This most often occurs during transfusions to infants during the newborn period or to children with coagulation disorders (such as hemophilia). Blood bank screening of donated blood for the detection of HIV (since 1985) has produced a dramatic decline in this risk. The majority of cases of pediatric AIDS are now caused by perinatal transmission from HIV-infected mothers who usually are drug users or sexual partners of drug users.

Clinical description. Infants who are infected by perinatal exposure usually show symptoms of AIDS within the first two years of life, while those infected by blood products typically have a later onset of symptoms. Most children with AIDS exhibit failure to thrive, hepatosplenomegaly, interstitial pneumonitis (lung disease), lymphadenopathy, persistent diarrhea, recurrent bacterial infections, and opportunistic infections. The term AIDS–related complex (ARC) describes children who are infected with HIV and have non-specific symptoms but have not yet had serious infection. Many children with AIDS also have neurologic abnormalities, such as seizures, ataxia, motor weakness, and loss of developmental milestones. They are at risk for delayed cognitive and motor development.[1,9]

Management. Management of children with AIDS involves careful routine physical examination, modified schedule of immunizations, nutritional assessment, testing of immune function, and treatment (along with prophylaxis) of infections. Ideally, these children should receive formal assessment of cognitive, speech–language, motor, and social-emotional function on an annual basis. While there is currently no specific cure for AIDS, the efficacy of intravenous gamma globulin therapy and antiviral therapy are being evaluated.

Needs. Children with AIDS need comprehensive care from medical, health care, and social services. Also important are efforts to provide coordinated care for both mothers and children who are infected with HIV. Efforts to slow the rise in the number of AIDS patients include education on family planning and reduction of risk behavior, continued investigation of antiviral treatment, and work toward the development of an effective vaccine.

Rheumatic Disease

Definition. Rheumatic diseases are clinical syndromes involving inflammation of connective tissues throughout the body. They are also known as collagen-vascular diseases, connective tissue diseases, and autoimmune diseases.

Incidence. Incidence and prevalence vary among the specific conditions. For example, approximately 0.6 in 100,000 children have a diagnosis of systemic lupus erythematosus (SLE). Frequency is higher in females and African-Americans. Several other types of rheumatic diseases also affect girls more frequently than boys.

Etiology. The etiology of rheumatic diseases is unknown, although production of autoantibodies against many tissue components is involved. Genetic susceptibility, hormonal factors, viral infections, and trauma play a role in determining disease occurence.[10]

Clinical description. Juvenile rheumatoid arthritis (JRA) may be systemic (with fever, rash, and anemia), pauciarticular (involving four or fewer joints), or polyarticular (involving five or more joints). About 75% of children with JRA experience permanent remission by adulthood. Systemic lupus erythematosus (SLE), the "great imitator," produces diverse clinical manifestations that may involve the skin, joints, kidneys, lungs, and central nervous system. Dermatomyositis involves skin lesions and inflammation of the muscle, leading to symmetrical weakness, mostly of proximal muscles. Scleroderma involves varying degrees of fibrosis and destruction of skin, soft tissue, muscle, and internal organs.[28]

Management. Management includes medical treatment, physical and occupational therapy, nutritional training, and family education and counseling. Treatment centers on the reduction of inflammation, which results in disuse and weakness, as well as damage to vital organs, such as the central nervous system, eyes, heart, and kidneys. Drug therapy may include nonsteroidal antiinflammatory drugs (NSAIDs), slower acting antirheumatic drugs (SAARDs), steroids, and cytotoxic drugs.[8]

Needs. Children with rheumatic diseases need extra attention paid to school performance, since physical disability and frequent absence may place them at risk for academic failure. Provision of special adaptive physical education and assistance with physical limitations also require attention. Counseling should address the stress of the disease and restriction of normal lifestyle.

Epilepsy

Definition. A seizure (or convulsion) results from a sudden paroxysmal electrical discharge in the brain and produces an abrupt change in consciousness, behavior, or motor activity. The location, type, and spread of the electrical discharge determine the type of seizure. Epilepsy refers to a chronic condition with recurrent seizures that are not provoked by any known acute event, such as trauma or fever.

Incidence. Epilepsy is present in 0.5% to 1% of the population and is more common in children with other central nervous system problems, such as cerebral palsy, hydrocephalus, and mental retardation. Epilepsy is more common in children than adults, and many children outgrow their disorder.

Etiology. Congenital defects, perinatal injury, infection (such as meningitis and congenital infections), brain tumors, and head trauma may damage the brain and result in epilepsy. In most cases, however, the cause of epilepsy is unknown (idiopathic).

Clinical description. Seizures are usually classified as partial or generalized, based on clinical and EEG findings. Partial seizures begin focally and are considered simple partial if consciousness is not affected, and complex partial if consciousness is impaired. Children with these seizures may display unusual, repetitive motor acts.

Generalized seizures begin in both hemispheres of the brain simultaneously. They include absence (petit mal) seizures, which involve staring spells lasting for a few seconds, and tonic-clonic (grand mal) seizures, which involve stiffening and jerking movements. Tonic-clonic seizures are usually accompanied by incontinence and followed by drowsiness.

Management. The decision to begin anticonvulsant medication is based on the age of the patient, the type and frequency of seizure, and psychologic consequences, as well as the etiology of the seizures. Recent data suggest that the majority of children with a first unprovoked seizure do not have recurrences and thus may not need treatment.[38] A patient who is treated with anticonvulsants requires monitoring of seizure control, side effects, psychosocial issues, and school performance. A child with intractable epilepsy may be a candidate for epilepsy surgery.[14]

Needs. Improved knowledge about appropriate use of anticonvulsant medication is required to avoid suboptimal treatment leading to continued seizures, as well as toxicity from inadequate monitoring. Family education and counseling are also necessary to insure optimal compliance and outcome.

Congenital Heart Defects

Definition. Congenital heart disease (CHD) includes structural or functional heart disease that is present at birth, although it may not be recognized until much later. CHD may be associated with cyanosis (resulting from poor oxygenation), as with transposition of the great arteries, tetralogy of Fallot, truncus arteriosus, and tricuspid atresia. Little or no cyanosis is associated with other defects, such as ventricular septal defect, atrial septal defect, patent ductus arteriosus, and coarctation of the aorta.

Incidence. The incidence of CHD is approximately 4 to 10 in 1000 live-born infants, but is much greater in aborted or stillborn infants. The risk of having another child with CHD is 2% to 6%. A child with CHD has a 1% to 10% chance of CHD in his future offspring. These risks may be much higher in some families.[19]

Etiology. Approximately 5% to 8% of children with CHD will have a chromosomal abnormality, such as Down syndrome (trisomy 21) or Turner's syndrome (45,X). Another 3% have classic mendelian single-gene defects, as with Marfan syndrome or Noonan's syndrome. Teratogens, such as viruses, drugs, and radiation, also damage the developing embryo and produce cardiovascular defects. For most children, however, the specific cause of congenital heart disease cannot be identified.

Clinical description. The type and severity of the heart defect determine what symptoms an infant or child displays. An infant with serious CHD, such as transposition of the great arteries and tetralogy of Fallot, may have cyanosis and difficulty breathing during the newborn period. Newborns or older infants and children may also have dyspnea, tachypnea, feeding problems, poor physical development, and recurrent pneumonia. Congestive heart failure may also develop. Children with small defects, such as atrial septal defect and ventricular septal defect, may have no symptoms but will have a murmur noted on physical examination.

Management. Careful physical examination and use of chest X-ray, electrocardiogram, and echocardiogram aid in early detection and management of CHD. Medication may be required for treatment of congestive heart failure or for stabilization prior to the corrective surgery required for some children. Attention must also be given to development and to nutrition, as some children are unable to take in an adequate diet.

Needs. Children who have serious CHD, are medically fragile, and frequently hospitalized need attention paid to their learning and developmental needs, requiring cooperation between medical and education professionals. Children who require corrective surgery deserve even closer scrutiny, because of the risk of permanent brain injury, resulting in seizures, motor disorders, mental retardation, and learning disabilities.[15]

Diabetes

Definition. Type 1 diabetes, also known as insulin–dependent diabetes mellitus or juvenile diabetes, is a common disorder of energy metabolism resulting from reduced or absent insulin production.

Incidence and prevalence. Type 1 diabetes is the most common endocrine disorder of childhood and adolescence, affecting approximately 2 in 1000 youngsters. The prevalence of type 1 diabetes appears to be increasing.

Etiology. An incompletely understood interaction of genetic, immunologic, and environmental factors (such as viral infections) determines the development of diabetes. The familial tendency for the development of diabetes has long been recognized, and linkage to certain histocompatability antigens (HLA) has been established. However, the immune system and viral agents play a role in determining which genetically susceptible children develop diabetes.[39]

Clinical description. Young people with diabetes usually have recognizable symptoms such as polydipsia, polyuria, nocturia, anorexia, weight loss or poor weight gain, vision changes, or changes in behavior or school performance. Glucose in the urine and a blood glucose level above 200 milligrams/deciliter support the diagnosis.

Management. Treatment of diabetes involves insulin injections, along with adjustment of dosage and blood glucose monitoring, which is often done with home glucose monitors. Measurement of hemoglobin A1 C levels reflects glucose control over the previous 6 to 8 weeks, so that accuracy of reported home glucose levels and patient compliance can be monitored. An appropriate dietary plan and exercise play an important role in management.[16] Attention must also be given to management of acute complications, such as infections; and chronic complications, such as growth failure, retinal changes, neuropathy, renal function, and skin problems. Satisfactory diabetic control in children and adolescents is difficult to achieve but must be emphasized in order to prevent or delay complications.

Needs. Current research may determine whether type 1 diabetes can be treated or prevented by use of immunosuppressive therapy or pancreatic transplantation. Use of a permanent indwelling glucose sensor connected to an insulin infusing device may also be useful in achieving close control of blood sugar. Meanwhile, optimal outcome for children with diabetes requires continued education and psychosocial support for patients and families.

BIRTH DEFECTS

Craniofacial Anomalies

Definition. Craniofacial anomalies refer to congenital deformities of the cranium and face, although tumors and trauma also produce a minority of these defects.

Incidence. The most common congenital defect is cleft lip and palate; hemifacial microsomia is the second most common. Cleft lip and palate occur in about 1 in 600 Caucasian births, affecting African-Americans less often, and Asians more often. Craniosynostosis occurs in about 1 in 1000 live births, with 10% also having associated facial skeletal deformities.

Etiology. Both genetic and environmental factors influence development of craniofacial anomalies, so that the cause appears to be multifactorial. For cleft lip and palate, families with an affected child have an increased risk of recurrence in future children. Hemifacial microsomia is usually sporadic, with little chance of recurrence. Apert syndrome and Crouzon syndrome, which include craniosynostosis, are usually inherited in an autosomal dominant pattern.

Clinical description. Clefts may involve the lip, palate, or both and be complete or incomplete, unilateral or bilateral. Affected children can have significant feeding difficulties, susceptibility to middle ear infection, hearing impairment, and abnormal speech development. Children with hemifacial microsomia usually have asymmetric, unilateral abnormalities of the ear (including hearing loss), eye, mandible, or other facial structures. Premature closure of the sutures of the skull produces craniosynostosis, resulting in abnormal skull shape, such as tall or long and narrow. Children with Apert syndrome have craniosynostosis and other anomalies, such as syndactyly (fusion) of fingers. Those with Crouzon syndrome also have shallow orbits and underdevelopment of the maxilla.[29]

Management. The rare and complex nature of these defects necessitates an organized craniofacial team that may include a plastic surgeon, neurosurgeon, otolaryngologist, ophthalmologist, psychologist, dental professional, and speech and hearing personnel. Early correction, when safe, will minimize secondary growth defects and maximize sensory and motor input. Treatment seeks restoration of function, improvement in appearance and self-image, and maximization of growth potential.[30]

Needs. The families of children with craniofacial anomalies need sensitive and compassionate guidance during their children's surgeries and treatments. The children's psychosocial development and needs must also be attended to.

Spina Bifida

Definition. Spina bifida, also known as meningomyelocele, is a malformation of the spinal cord, skin, and vertebrae. The malformed spinal tissue pushes out through an open (bifid) spine. Spinal cord or nerve root dysfunction occurs, since the nerves below the defect are not properly connected to the spinal cord and brain.

Incidence. Spina bifida occurs in about 1 in 1000 live births, although the overall rate has been gradually declining. The incidence is somewhat greater in females and in those of English and Irish descent. The chance of having an infant with spina bifida increases if there are other affected family members.

Etiology. Interaction of multiple environmental and genetic factors produces spina bifida. Recent research has identified elevated maternal body temperature and deficiency of folic acid as potential causes.[44] Attention to these factors may lead to prevention of some cases.

Clinical description. The extent and location of the defect determine the type of neurologic deficits. Voluntary muscle movement, sphincter control, and skin sensation are lost below the level of the lesion. Children can thus present with varying degrees of paralysis, loss of bowel and bladder control, and pressure sores. Associated problems include hydrocephalus (often caused by a brain defect called Arnold-Chiari malformation, found in 80% of children with spina bifida), scoliosis or kyphosis, and tethered cord. Children may also have mental retardation, learning disabilities, or poor fine motor coordination of the upper extremities, usually the result of hydrocephalus.[26] A small number of children may have brain stem abnormalities leading to problems with breathing and swallowing and even death.

Management. Children with spina bifida require care from a team of specialists. Neurosurgical care includes repair of the spinal cord defect and placement of a ventriculoperitoneal shunt if hydrocephalus is present. Urologic care involves treatment of urinary tract infection, intermittent catheterization, and possible surgery. Orthopedic care includes bracing and surgery to minimize contractures and deformities and enhance ambulation. Occupational therapy, physical therapy, nutritional counseling, special education, and patient/family counseling are also needed for optimal care.

Needs. Children with spina bifida have complex needs which require careful coordination. Patients with the physical and intellectual capacity for independence also need close attention to their psychologic needs in order to prepare for independent living.

SENSORY DISORDERS

Auditory Impairments

Definition. Reduction in the ear's responsiveness to loudness and pitch results in auditory impairment, which can range from mild to profound. Hearing loss may be classified as conductive (usually the result of problems of the outer or middle ear), sensorineural (the result of problems with the inner ear or auditory nerve), or mixed.

Incidence. Approximately 3 to 6 in 1000 children have some type of auditory impairment, either present at birth or acquired during childhood.

Etiology. Genetic causes probably account for the majority of auditory impairment and include Usher syndrome, Treacher Collins syndrome, and Alport's syndrome. Malformation syndromes include Goldenhar's syndrome and cleft lip or palate.[36] Acquired causes include infections (such as meningitis, mumps, congenital rubella and cytomegalovirus), hyperbilirubinemia, complications of prematurity, head trauma, and ototoxic drugs.

Clinical description. Parents are often the first to express concern about an infant's hearing. Appropriate evaluation should be accomplished before reassurance is offered. Failure to develop normal speech and language is usually the primary symptom of hearing loss. Even deaf infants may begin to coo and babble but then will show lack of attainment of normal speech and language milestones. Hearing impairment may be an isolated handicap in an otherwise normal child or may be associated with mental retardation, cerebral palsy, autism, or visual impairment.

Management. Early diagnosis and treatment of hearing impairment is critical for preventing serious developmental handicap.[11] Children who have delayed speech and language, or failure to respond normally to sound, or whose parents are concerned about hearing, should receive audiological evaluation. Children with congenital infections; meningitis; prematurity; family history of childhood hearing loss; malformations of the head, neck, and ear; or other high-risk features should also be assessed. Formal audiological evaluations can be performed on infants or children of any age. Auditory brainstem response (ABR) may be used in infants or uncooperative children. Behaviorally reinforced or play audiometry can be used in older, cooperative infants and children. Following diagnosis, children should receive evaluation of underlying diseases and genetic factors. Treatment of hearing impairment may involve medical or surgical treatment and/or amplification by use of a hearing aid. Speech and language therapy and special education school services may be necessary.

Needs. Researchers continue to search for better electronic devices for early detection of hearing loss. The usefulness of cochlear implants for profoundly deaf children also needs further investigation.

Visual Impairments

Definition. Visual impairment results from problems in any part of the visual apparatus, including the outer layers of the eye, the lens, the retina, the extraocular muscles, and the brain. Impairment may be complete (blindness) or be milder, but still result in significant disability.

Incidence. About 1 in 4000 children are blind, with 1 in 20 children having significant but less severe visual impairments. Approximately 30% of children with multiple handicaps have visual defects.

Etiology. Congenital visual impairments may result from inherited conditions (congenital cataracts), chromosomal abnormalities (Down syndrome), or congenital infections (rubella). Perinatal events, such as retinal damage in premature infants (retinopathy of prematurity), may also cause visual defects. Postnatal causes include trauma, infection (cellulitis, Toxocara canis), and connective tissue diseases (Marfan syndrome). Strabismus, or misalignment of the eyes, may result in amblyopia or progressive loss of vision in one eye.

Clinical description. Parents may report that children fail to focus on faces or objects, hold objects close to the face, have difficulty with eye-hand coordination, cross their eyes, or have other unusual eye movements (nystagmus). Examination should search for nystagmus, strabismus, an abnormal "white" pupillary reflex, or changes in the retina. Abnormalities of visual acuity can be most accurately detected in children who are at least age 3, although visual evoked response (VER) testing may be used to detect problems in younger or delayed children. Visually impaired children may also display unusual self-stimulatory behaviors, such as rocking, eye pressing, and light gazing. They may exhibit other handicaps, such as cerebral palsy, mental retardation, or hearing impairment.[40]

Management. Management includes referral to a pediatric ophthalmologist who may prescribe glasses, patching, medication, or surgery. Children with other severe impairments (such as mental retardation or cerebral palsy) should receive the same evaluation and treatment, since visual impairment affects the degree of their other disabilities. Since visual impairment can produce delays in motor development, spatial orientation, and language development, children should also receive appropriate educational intervention, including infant stimulation programs, referral to organizations that work with blind children, and school special education services.[33] Visual training techniques, such as visual tracking and eye muscle exercises, have not shown any proven benefit.

Needs. Early detection is needed to provide effective treatment and avoid further impairment and developmental delays. Children at high risk for visual problems, including those who were premature, have other disabilities, or have family histories of visual problems, deserve especially close attention.

COGNITIVE DISABILITIES

Learning Disabilities

Definition. The term learning disabilities (LD) refers to a heterogeneous group of children who have difficulty with processing information and with academic productivity. The definition often includes documentation of a discrepancy between children's potential achievement (based on intelligence testing) and actual achievement (based on achievement testing), or of a discrepancy between verbal measures and performance measures on cognitive testing.

Incidence. Confusion over the best definition of LD makes documentation of incidence and prevalence difficult. Most estimates indicate that 7% to 10% of students are learning disabled. Prevalence is higher in males but not as much different as previously thought. Social class may influence prognosis, but children with LD are present in every socioeconomic level.

Etiology. No specific cause of LD has been identified, although differences in brain organization and metabolism have been demonstrated in some children. The frequent occurrence of LD in particular families is well-known and suggests a genetic influence. Other predisposing factors include perinatal factors (prematurity and low birthweight), health problems (recurrent otitis media or meningitis), environmental toxins (lead), cultural deprivation, and educational mismanagement.

Clinical description. Some children with LD demonstrate problems in early childhood, such as delayed or disordered language acquisition, difficulty following directions, attentional problems, hyperactivity, behavior problems, or clumsiness. These characteristics may persist as additional problems for some children.[5] At school age, children with LD typically experience general academic failure or show weakness in specific areas, such as reading, math, or written language. They may also display poor social skills and low self-esteem.

Medical evaluation may reveal neurological "soft signs" or clumsiness, as well as minor dysmorphic features, but these children do not otherwise have specific abnormalities.

Management. Vision and hearing deficits should be ruled out. Psychoeducational evaluation is necessary to specifically identify and categorize learning disabilities. Language evaluation may also be indicated. Following evaluation, children need assistance from special education services, such as resource rooms or tutoring. In the regular classroom, teachers may make modifications for children by requiring less writing, offering oral test administration, repeating directions, and avoiding display of the children's problems to peers. Children with LD may also need speech and language therapy, occupational therapy, and psychologic services.[42] Visual tracking and eye muscle exercises (visual training techniques) have not proven useful in treatment of LD.

Needs. Further research is needed to better define causes of LD. Early identification and provision of appropriate services must be sought, in order to ensure educational success, peer acceptance, and positive self-esteem.

Mental Retardation

Definition. Mental retardation (MR) refers to impaired intellectual functioning, usually defined as an intelligence quotient (IQ) below 70, and ranging in severity from mild to profound. Adaptive behavior is also impaired, such that children's coping skills, social abilities, and personal independence are below age and cultural expectations.

Incidence. The incidence of MR may be as high as 150,000 births in a year, but the inability to detect all cases at birth limits accurate determination. Prevalence is thought to be 1% to 3% of children, with the majority (75% to 85%) in the mild range. Mild MR is more often found in the lower socioeconomic levels, while moderate to severe cases are more evenly distributed among all levels.

Etiology. While severe MR in children is more likely to have an identifiable cause, the etiology of the majority of cases is unknown. Identifiable causes include hereditary disorders (inborn errors of metabolism, fragile X syndrome, tuberous sclerosis), early alterations of embryonic development (congenital infections, chromosomal disorders), other perinatal problems (prematurity, hypoxia), acquired childhood diseases (meningitis, head trauma, lead exposure), and environmental problems and behavioral syndromes (parental psychosis, emotional disorders).[13]

Clinical description. Children with MR often exhibit delayed motor milestones or delayed language development within the first two years of life. Those with mild MR may not be detected until school age when academic failure occurs. Most children with MR will have a normal physical examination. However, some will have dysmorphic features, as with Down syndrome or fragile X syndrome. These syndromes can often be confirmed, as with chromosomal testing for Down syndrome and identification of a fragile site or even DNA analysis for fragile X syndrome. Large or small head size, poor growth, associated motor disorders (cerebral palsy), and vision or hearing problems may also be present.[18]

Management. Children suspected of having MR should receive formal psychologic testing to diagnose MR and determine the degree of retardation. Children at all levels of MR need early intervention and special education services, which benefit even profoundly handicapped children. Children may also require services from physical therapists, speech therapists, ophthalmologists, and psychiatrists. The current trend for coordination of care has enabled the vast majority of mentally retarded children to live at home.

Needs. Primary prevention of mental retardation, along with early identification and intervention, are needed to reduce the economic and psychologic burdens. Families need support for coordination of services, financial burdens, respite care, advocacy within the school system, and long-term provision of care for their children.

Communication Disorders

Definition. Communication disorders involve impairment in understanding and/or transmitting information, including disturbances in speech production, comprehension, spoken and written language, or language-based learning.

Incidence. Speech and language impairment is the most common disability in childhood, occurring in about 11% of preschool children and 3% to 10% of school-age children. Disagreement about terminology and classification makes exact determination of incidence and prevalence difficult.

Etiology. Communication impairment is often seen in association with mental retardation, autism, cerebral palsy, cleft palate, or hearing impairment, which in turn may or may not have identified etiologies, such as genetic disorders, congenital infection, or prematurity. Other biologic, psychologic, and social factors that are not always identifiable also play a role in communication disorders.[12]

Clinical description. Children with an articulation disorder (speech impairment) have inaccurate production of speech sounds and speech that is difficult to understand, because of imprecise use of lips, tongue, teeth, and/or palate. Children who speak too softly or too loudly, have a vocal pitch that is too high or too low, or have abnormal voice quality are said to have voice disorders, resulting from abnormal use or function of the vocal cords. Disorders of fluency lead to unusual pauses, repetitions, and sound interjections in a child's flow of speech, or may be manifested as stuttering. Abnormal speech sound production is also seen in dysarthria (result of damage to motor pathways, as in cerebral palsy) and dyspraxia (inability to initiate and sequence oral motor movements). Language disorders may involve language comprehension (receptive language) impairment, such that children have difficulty understanding spoken and/or written messages. These children may understand single words but not sentences and may appear inattentive or disobedient. Children with impairment in oral language production (expressive language impairment) may have limited expressive vocabulary, difficulty finding an exact word, and trouble building complex sentences and expressing ideas. This may also extend to problems in written language. Language-learning disability describes school-age children with a language disorder associated with learning disabilities.[3]

Management. Evaluation includes audiologic and speech and language assessment, and often involves assessment of cognitive ability and medical evalution to assess underlying causes. School-age children may also need psychoeducational testing to look for learning disabilities. Treatment typically includes speech and language therapy, possibly in the setting of an early stimulation program for infants and young children or a special education program, including resource room, for school-age children.

Needs. Improved methods of early identification are needed to allow early intervention and avoidance of more severe communication impairment. High–risk children, such as premature infants and those with congenital anomalies, deserve careful screening.

BEHAVIORAL DISORDERS

Attention Deficit Hyperactivity Disorder (ADHD)

Definition. Attention Deficit Hyperactivity Disorder (ADHD), previously known as Minimal Brain Dysfunction (MBD), refers to children who are inattentive, impulsive, and hyperactive. These symptoms must have been present for at least six months and have started before age 7. Attention Deficit Disorder without Hyperactivity (ADD-H) describes children who have attentional deficits but not hyperactivity.

Incidence, prevalence, trends, and demographics. Prevalence reports have ranged from 1% to 20%, depending on the criteria used to define ADHD. More boys than girls are reported to have this disorder, although girls may be less aggressive or hyperactive and therefore less likely to be identified.

Etiology. Although some children with brain damage resulting from head trauma or meningitis may have symptoms of ADHD, most cases do not have an identifiable cause. A family tendency for ADHD has been recognized, but no specific genetic cause has been established. Abnormalities of neurotransmitters and neuroanatomy may also play a role. Exposure to toxins such as lead and alcohol (fetal alchohol syndrome) has been associated with this disorder, as well. Research has not demonstrated a connection with sugar or food additives.

Clinical description. Children with ADHD have levels of sustained attention, impulse control, and motor activity that are not appropriate for age and that affect school performance and/or home behavior management. There is no definite test or marker for ADHD, so diagnosis depends on close attention to history from parents and teachers. Standardized questionnaires or rating scales are useful to determine if children's behaviors are of sufficient degree and frequency to warrant a diagnosis of ADHD. Children may also have clumsiness (poor handwriting or sports abilities), poor social skills, and poor self–esteem. Physical exam may reveal minor dysmorphic features or neurological soft signs but does not otherwise necessarily aid in diagnosis.[37]

Management. Appropriate management first requires ruling out other disorders that may masquerade as or co-exist with ADHD. These include absence (petit mal) seizures, hearing or vision impairment, mood disorders, conduct disorder, oppositional defiant disorder, or learning disabilities. The basic components of management are training parents and teachers in behavior modification techniques, and possible use of medication. Children may also receive special education services based on a diagnosis of ADHD or associated learning disabilities. They may also require speech and language therapy, occupational therapy, social skills training, and counseling.[2]

Needs. Children with ADHD need early identification and intervention to avoid academic failure, disrupted home lives, poor peer relations, and low self-esteem. They also deserve close attention to other problems that may be associated with and compound the difficulties of ADHD.

Autism

Definition. Autism is a pervasive developmental disorder characterized by deficient social interaction, impaired communication, and limited range of play activities and interests. It is usually detected within the first 30 months of life.

Incidence. Estimates of the prevalence of autism range from 4 to 15 in a population of 10,000, with more frequent occurrence in boys. Distribution appears to be similar for all socioeconomic levels.

Etiology. In most cases of autism the cause is not known, although it may sometimes be associated with other diagnoses such as fragile X syndrome, tuberous sclerosis, or congenital rubella. A genetic basis is suggested in some families, since autism is more common in siblings of affected children. Earlier theories that poor parenting caused autism have been proven incorrect.

Autistic children often have a history of prenatal or perinatal difficulties, as well. Researchers have found that some children have neurophysiologic or neuroanatomic abnormalities, based on EEG, PET scan, MRI scan, or autopsy results. It may be that various etiologies affect a particular brain system, resulting in characteristic autistic behavior of varying degrees.

Clinical description. Impairment in social relationships may be apparent in infants who are not cuddly, seldom make eye contact, or show minimal social imitation. Toddlers and older children may show lack of interest in peers and seem unaware of other people. Deficits in communication may present as failure to acquire language at the expected time. Some children reportedly were using words but then stopped. About 50% of autistic children are nonverbal. Others develop language but do not use it to communicate. Unusual language features include echolalia which is repetition of what another person has just said or what was heard in the past (such as TV commercials). Children's ability to understand language is almost always affected, as well. A limited range of activities and interests may be visible as repetitive (stereotypic) movements, such as rocking or spinning in circles, and unusual sensory responses. Repetitive play patterns include lining up toys or flipping a light switch. Autistic children may also resist change in routine.

Signs of autism range from mild to severe and change with age and developmental level, so that affected children have different levels of disability. Some children also have associated problems, including mental retardation (in 70% to 80%), seizures, and hyperactivity.[35]

Management. Evaluation should include hearing assessment, speech and language testing, and psychologic testing. Children with autism benefit from special education to address problems with social relations, communication, and behavior. Although there is no specific medical treatment for autism, some children need judicious use of medication to treat seizures, hyperactivity, or severe behavior problems.

Needs. Comprehensive services are needed to provide lifelong appropriate intervention and family support, such as respite care or group homes. Improved methods of early identification, early intervention, and better treatment approaches are also needed.[25]

Emotional Disorders

Definition. Children with emotional disorders may display inappropriate behaviors or feelings under normal circumstances, be unable to establish interpersonal relationships, or show general unhappiness.

Incidence. The incidence and prevalence vary with the particular type of disorder. School-age children with emotional disorders make up the fourth largest of ten categories of children receiving special education.

Etiology. Although brain damage is sometimes associated with emotional disorders, most children do not have a specific known cause for such problems. Because some families have an increased incidence of disorders, a genetic predisposition is suggested. The role of environmental factors is demonstrated by the higher incidence of parental alcoholism, marital discord, or other family stresses in emotionally disturbed children.

Clinical description. Common emotional disorders include conduct disorders, anxiety disorders, and depression. Children with these disorders typically will display problems with academic performance, peer relations, and social functioning both at home and at school. Children with conduct disorders demonstrate severe, repetitive antisocial behavior, such as lying, stealing, fire-setting, and destroying property.[17] Children with overanxious disorders show excessive worry and fear not related to a specific situation, and are often restless and perfectionistic. Separation anxiety, which is sometimes incorrectly referred to as school phobia, describes children whose excessive anxiety (even panic) is a result of separation from parents, other attachment figures, or home. Features of childhood depression include withdrawn behavior, passivity, difficulty concentrating, sleep problems, and aggression.

Management. Referral for psychologic evaluation is usually the first step to provide appropriate diagnosis of children's emotional disorders. Along with educational assessment, this will also allow diagnosis of learning disabilities which, if untreated, may lead to secondary emotional problems. Special education may also be necessary for some children with emotional disorders. Counseling for patients and families is a critical component of management.[21]

Needs. The role of biologic and environmental factors in the etiology of emotional disturbances requires further investigation. Assessment of which treatment approaches provide the best outcome is also needed.

ENVIRONMENTALLY-INDUCED IMPAIRMENTS

Drugs And Alcohol Effects

Definition. Drugs and alcohol effects refer to fetal malformations, organ damage, or alterations in behavioral and intellectual function secondary to exposure during pregnancy, at any time from conception through labor and delivery.

Incidence. Incidence and prevalence vary, depending on the particular substance to which a fetus is exposed. For example, approximately 10% of infants exposed to phenytoin (for maternal seizure control) may have anomalies, while the incidence may be 20% for carbamazepine exposure. Inaccurate maternal reporting of cocaine and alcohol use make determination of incidence more difficult for these exposures. Estimates for incidence of fetal alcohol syndrome range from 2 to 6 in 1000 live births.

Etiology. Effects on the fetus may be the result of teratogenesis, direct toxicity, or neurobehavioral abnormalities. Teratogenesis refers to the production of structural malformations or birth defects, such as spina bifida, heart defects, or limb anomalies. Direct toxicity describes damage to organ function (without malformation), such as renal failure or seizures. Neurobehavioral effects are long-term, sometimes permanent, changes in intellectual function and behavior, and are often associated with a withdrawal syndrome in newborns.[7]

Clinical description. Infants exposed to maternal anticonvulsants may have growth retardation, a characteristic anticonvulsant face, cleft lip, or spina bifida. Antihypertensive agents, which are angiotensin-converting enzyme inhibitors, can produce kidney damage, skull hypoplasia, and growth retardation. Infants exposed to anticoagulants (warfarin) may have brain malformation and abnormalities of the nose, ears, and fingers. Ethanol use can lead to fetal alcohol syndrome, with a characteristic face, microcephaly, growth retardation, mental deficiency, and hyperactivity. Infants exposed to cocaine may have poor feeding, irritability, and increased risk of sudden infant death syndrome. They also appear to be at risk for long-term emotional and behavioral difficulties and learning problems.[20,41]

Management. Management must be individualized, based on the drug of exposure. Infants with known maternal drug use must be examined carefully to determine possible effects of the drug in the newborn period. These children also need careful long-term observation because of risk for developmental delay, learning disabilities, and emotional and behavioral difficulties that require psychologic or educational evaluation.

Needs. Continued research is needed to address the safety of the medications required to treat maternal conditions. Counseling and treatment are needed for mothers who abused drugs and/or alcohol during pregnancy. The role of drug and alcohol use by fathers in causing fetal abnormalities also needs further investigation.

Trauma (Traumatic Brain Injury; Spinal Cord Injury)

Definition. Traumatic brain injury (TBI) can be caused by blunt trauma or penetrating objects and ranges from mild to severe. Primary injury results from the immediate impact, while secondary brain damage can result from hypoxemia, cerebral edema, hemorrhage, or herniation. Traumatic spinal cord injury may be complete or incomplete (with a better prognosis for recovery). Because of anatomical differences in the immature spine, young children are more likely to have upper cervical spinal cord injury.

Incidence. Differences in reporting criteria, type, and severity of injury lead to variation in reported rates of injury. TBI is the most common form of accidental childhood injury. According to recent estimates, 1 of every 30 newborns will sustain significant head trauma by late adolescence. Incidence is higher for boys, nonwhites, and those in poverty. The incidence of spinal cord injury is low, with only 5% of such injuries occurring in children below age 15.

Etiology. Falls (usually at home), pedestrian or bicycle accidents associated with motor vehicle accidents (MVA), child abuse, and sports activities typically cause injury in young children. Seat belt injury in an MVA may also lead to spinal cord damage. Use of helmets by children on bicycles, skateboards, and rollerblades would reduce the incidence of head injury, as would seat belt and car seat use in automobiles. Researchers are evaluating drugs that block further damage from biochemical events following injury.

Clinical description. Children generally have a better outcome from TBI than do adults. Contrary to popular belief, children younger than age 5 may be more vulnerable to damage. Severity of injury, defined by initial depth of coma, duration of coma, and duration of posttraumatic amnesia, also determines outcome. Children with mild TBI (80% of cases) do not usually suffer significant behavioral or intellectual impairment. Those with moderate to severe TBI are more likely to have neurologic deficits, cognitive impairment, and psychiatric disturbances.[23] Common problems include socially disinhibited behavior, memory deficits, difficulty with visual-motor skills and motor dexterity, language deficits, and difficulty with school-related functions that require concentration, organization, and abstract thinking. For a child with spinal cord injury, the level and completeness of injury determine the potential for functional independence.

Management. Rehabilitation following injury requires a team approach to address multiple needs, including neuropsychologic assessment, speech and language therapy, occupational therapy, physical therapy, special education, dietary management, and counseling.[22] Children with spinal cord trauma also need attention to bladder, bowel, and skin care, as well as management of spasms and spasticity.

Needs. Early intervention with proper rehabilitative care must be available to achieve optimal outcome in function, independence, and quality of life.

Environmental Toxins (Lead)

Definition. Although there are many potential environmental toxins, lead is considered the most important pediatric environmental toxin. Lead poisoning refers to elevated blood lead levels that produce toxic effects. Levels greater than 60 microgram/deciliter are associated with acute encephalopathy. Since lower levels have been found to produce serious and permanent neurobehavioral deficits, 10 microgram/deciliter is now considered to be the level at which to consider intervention.

Incidence, prevalence. An estimated 4 million (about 16%) American children age 5 or younger have blood lead levels that could impair their development. Children who are African-American, poor, and live in urban areas are at greatest risk for lead poisoning, although children of all socioeconomic levels may be affected.

Etiology. Children may inhale or ingest lead from sources such as leaded paint and contaminated water, soil, and food. Certain industries produce higher air and dust lead levels to which children living nearby may be exposed. Children of parents who work in lead smelters or battery manufacturing plants may be exposed through contact with contaminated skin and clothing. Exposure to elevated maternal lead levels can also cause neurobehavioral effects in the fetus.[43]

Clinical description. Mild lead toxicity may produce myalgia and mild fatigue or lethargy. Moderate toxicity may produce general fatigue, headache, abdominal pain, vomiting, and weight loss. Children with severe toxicity experience severe abdominal cramps, paresis, seizures, coma, and even death. Elevated lead levels may produce obvious neuropsychologic sequela, such as mental retardation and behavioral dysfunction, while even low lead levels can produce deficits in intelligence, school performance, and behavior in otherwise asymptomatic children.[6]

Management. Screening all children from ages 6 months to 6 years identifies those with notable lead exposure as early as possible. Once an elevated blood lead level (above 10 or 15mcg/dL) is identified, environmental intervention must eliminate further exposure to lead. Dietary intervention decreases lead absorption by providing a diet rich in iron, calcium, and zinc. Children with lead levels above 45 mcg/dL should receive chelation therapy. Chelation therapy for those with levels between 10 and 44 is controversial, since acute encephalopathy is not an immediate risk and such therapy has not been proven to reverse or prevent neurodevelopmental deficits. The usefulness of oral chelating agents for different levels of exposure must also be clarified. Children with identified elevated lead levels need close monitoring of development and school performance.

Needs. Social issues often preclude provision of safe, lead-free housing for many children. Treatment of lead poisoning must include assessment of these issues, as well as determination of the most beneficial treatment.

REFERENCES

1. Aylward EH et al: Cognitive and motor development in infants at risk for human immunodeficiency virus, *AJDC 146*: 218-222, 1992.

2. Barkley RA and Murphy JV: Treating attention-deficit hyperactivity disorder: medication and behavior management training, *Pediatr Annals 20(5)*:256-266, 1991.

3. Bashir AS, Wiig EH, and Abrams JC: Language disorders in childhood and adolescence: implications for learning and socialization, *Pediatric Annals 16(2)*:145-156, 1987.

4. Beasley RW and de Bese GM: Upper limb amputation and prostheses, *Orthop Clin North Am 17(3)*:395-405, 1986.

5. Beauchamp G: Visual correlates of dyslexia and related learning disabilities, *Pediatr Annals 19(5)*:334-341, 1990.

6. Bellinger DC, Stiles KM, and Needleman HL: Low-level lead exposure, intelligence, and academic achievement: a long term follow-up study, *Pediatrics 90(6)*:855-861, 1992.

7. Berlin CM: Effects of drugs on the fetus, *Pediatr Rev 12(9)*:282-287, 1991.

8. Brewer EJ: Collagen vascular disease. In Gellis SS and Kagan BM, editors: *Current pediatric therapy*, ed 12, Philadelphia, 1986, WB Saunders.

9. Cohen SE, Mundy T, and Karassik B et al: Neuropsychological functioning in human immunodeficiency virus type 1 seropositive children infected through neonatal blood transfusion, *Pediatrics 88*:58-68, 1991.

10. Condemi JJ: The autoimmune diseases, *JAMA 268(20)*:2882-2892, 1992.

11. Coplan J: Deafness: ever heard of it? Delayed recognition of permanent hearing loss, *Pediatrics 79(2)*:206-213, 1987.

12. Coplan J: Evaluation of the child with delayed speech or language, *Pediatric Annals 14(3)*:202-208, 1985.

13. Crocker AC: The causes of mental retardation, *Pediatric Annals 18(10)*: 623-636, 1989.

14. Duchowny M: Surgery for intractable epilepsy: issues and outcome, *Pediatrics 84*:886-894, 1989.

15. Ferry PC: Neurologic sequela of open-heart surgery in children, *AJDC 144*: 369-373, 1990.

16. Ginsberg-Fellner F: Insulin-dependent diabetes mellitus, *Pediatrics Review 11(8)*:239-247, 1990.

17. Gottlieb SE and Friedman SB: Conduct disorders in children and adolescents, *Pediatr Rev 12(7)*:218-223, 1991.

18. Healy A: Mental retardation, *Pediatr Rev 9(1)*:15-22, 1987.

19. Hoffman JIE: Congenital heart disease: incidence and inheritance, *Pediatric Clin North Am 37(1)*:25-43, 1990.

20. Holmes LB: Fetal environmental toxins, *Pediatr Rev 13(10)*:164-369, 1992.

21. Hunt RD and Cohen DJ: Pyschiatric aspects of learning difficulties, *Pediatr Clin North Am 31(2)*:471-497, 1984.

22. Jaffe KM and McDonald CM: Rehabilitation following childhood injury, *Pediatr Annals 21 (7)*:438-447, 1992.

23. Johnston MV and Gerring JP: Head trauma and its sequela, *Pediatr Annals 21 (6)*: 362-368, 1992.

24. Lamb DW and Scott H: Management of congenital and acquired amputation in children, *Orthop Clin North Am 12(4)*:977-994, 1981.

25. Levitas A: Developmental and family effects of autism, *Pediatric Annals 19(1)*:52-58, 1990.

26. Mapstore JB et al: Relationship of cerebrospinal fluid shunting and IQ in children with meningomyelocele: a retrospective analysis, *Childs Brain* 11:112-118, 1984.

27. Miller G: Myopathies of infancy and childhood, *Pediatr Annals 18(7)*:439-453, 1989.

28. Miller ML (ed): Pediatric rheumatology, *Pediatric Clin North Am 33(5)*, 1986.

29. Murray JE, Kaban LB, and Mulliken JB: Craniofacial abnormalities. In Ravitch et al, editors: *Pediatric surgery*, Chicago, 1979, Mosby.

30. Murray JE: Reconstructive surgery for multiple congenital, cranial, facial, and hand anomalies. In Rubin IL and Crocker AC, editors: *Developmental disabilities*, Philadelphia, 1989, Lea & Febiger.

31. Naeye RL et al: Origins of cerebral palsy, *AJDC* 143:1154-1161, 1989.

32. Nelson KN and Ellenberg JH: Antecedents of cerebral palsy, *N Engl J Med* 315:81-86, 1986.

33. Nelson LB: The visually handicapped child, *Pediatric ophthalmology*, Philadelphia, 1984, WB Saunders Co.

34. Patterson MC and Gomez MR: Muscle disease in children: a practical approach, *Pediatr Rev* 12:73-82, 1990.

35. Rapin I: Autistic children: diagnosis and clinical features, *Pediatrics (suppl) 87(5)*:751-760, 1991.

36. Rapin I: Hearing disorders, *Pediatr Rev 14(2)*:43-49, 1993.

37. Shaywitz SE and Shaywitz BA: Diagnosis and management of attention deficit disorder: a pediatric perspective, *Pediatr Clin North Am 31(2)*:429-457, 1984.

38. Shinnar S. Berg et al: Risk of seizure recurrence following a first unprovoked seizure in childhood, *Pediatrics* 85:1076-1085, 1990.

39. Skyler JS and Rabinovitch A: Etiology and pathogenesis of insulin dependent diabetes mellitus, *Pediatric Annals 16(9)*:682-692, 1987

40. Smith V and Keen J (editors): Clinics in developmental medicine no. 73, *Visual Handicap in Children*, London, 1979, Spastics International Medical Publications.

41. Volpe JJ: Effect of cocaine use on the fetus, *NEJM 327(6)*:399-407, 1992.

42. Warren SA and Taylor RL: Education of children with learning problems, *Pediatr Clin North Am 31(2)*:331-343, 1984.

43. Weitzman M and Glotzer D: Lead poisoning, *Pediatr Review 13(12)*:461-468, 1992.

44. Werler MM, Shapiro S, and Mitchell AA: Periconceptual folic acid exposure and risk of occurrent neural tube defects, *JAMA 269(10)*:1257-1261, 1993.

BIBLIOGRAPHY

Blackman JA, editor: *Medical aspects of developmental disabilities in children birth to three*, revised ed 1, Rockville, Md, 1984, Aspen Systems.

Wolraich ML, editor: *The practical assessment and management of children with disorders of development and learning*, St Louis, 1987, Mosby.

PART SIX

PROVIDERS

One of the most positive developments in the care of children with disabilities and chronic illness has been the evolution of the service delivery team. While the concept of the team has many variations and themes, the relative contributions of a wide-variety of professionals have received appropriate emphasis. In some cases, traditional disciplines have adjusted to changing needs by incorporating new skills into existing training and practice. For example, physical and occupational therapists now provide opportunities for specialization in pediatrics, and within pediatrics, infancy. In other cases, new disciplines have evolved, such as the parent-infant educator. Some skills are shared, as in service coordination; other skills remain the exclusive domain of a particular professional group, although these barriers are of necessity breaking down quickly. Formerly, only a nurse would be permitted to suction a tracheostomy or catheterize the bladder of a child with meningomyelocele. Now, teachers are asked to perform these tasks when nurses are unavailable.

Despite the cross training and transdisciplinary models of practice, it is useful to define and describe the core training and primary professional expertise of the many disciplines involved in care of children with disabilities and chronic illness. Understanding what skills each person on the team can be expected to contribute will help in the assignment and sharing of tasks.

Many of the disciplines continue to define and refine their roles. Some professionals seek to expand roles, others, concerned about overextension and liability, are intent on restricting responsibilities. The following descriptions of service providers were based on consultations with spokespersons from the various disciplines and, hopefully, represent prevailing viewpoints.

CHAPTER **42**

Service Providers

JOHN C. MACQUEEN

The concept that community–based services for children with special health care needs (CSHCN) should be provided anticipates the availability of community–based teams of professional service providers that can deliver the needed services. The following section offers brief descriptions of some of the major professions that care for these children and their families. The section summarizes the training these professionals have received, where they work in the community, what services they provide, and how they function as members of community–based teams to ensure provision of the services described in this book.

AUDIOLOGIST

An audiologist is a person who can provide, on the basis of professional training, independent clinical services to persons with auditory, or hearing, disorders.

Audiologists must complete a college undergraduate education that provides a broad educational and preparatory professional experience. Upon graduation from such a program, audiologists receive a BA or BS degree and may be eligible to enroll in a master's degree program in audiology. Upon completion of professional and clinical practicum education, applicants must complete a Clinical Fellowship Year and pass the National Examination in Audiology to be certified audiologists. The professional education required for the Certificate of Clinical Competence in Audiology includes study of:

1. Auditory disorders, such as pathologies of the auditory system, as well as assessment of auditory disorders and their effects on communication

2. Habilitative/rehabilitative procedures, such as selection and use of appropriate amplification instrumentation for the hearing impaired, both wearable and group; evaluation of speech and language problems of the hearing impaired; and management procedures for speech and language habilitation and/or rehabilitation of the hearing impaired (may include manual communication)

3. Conservation of hearing, such as environmental noise control and identification audiometry

4. Instrumentation, such as electronics, calibration techniques, and characteristics of amplifying systems

Audiology services are provided in schools, hearing centers, clinics, hospitals, and in offices of private audiologists. The major activities of pediatric audiologists are assessing the severity and cause of hearing disorders, making recommendations about habilitative and rehabilitative procedures, and determining appropriate amplification instruments.

DENTIST

A dentist is a person who has received the professional training required to provide various types of dental services.

Dentists have satisfactorily completed at least two, but usually four years pre-baccalaureate study in an accredited college, have typically received a BS or BA degree, graduated from an accredited dental college, and been granted the degree of Doctor of Dental Surgery (DDS). Dentists must be licensed to practice dentistry in the state where they practice. Most dentists conduct their practices in some type of office setting which may be shared with other dentists.

During recent years dentistry has emphasized the practice of primary dental care, which includes dental education, preventive dentistry, regular routine dental care, and the correction of cavities. Children with mild to moderate chronic health problems may receive their dental care from a general dentist.

Some dentists pursue additional training in a dental specialty field for a period of one to six years, which results in certification, and then practice as one of the following recognized dental specialists:

1. Endodontists, who diagnose and heal diseases and injuries that affect the vitality of teeth

2. Oral and maxillo-facial surgeons, who provide diagnostic and surgical services for diseases, defects, and injuries in the head, neck, face, and oral cavity

3. Oral pathologists, who treat diseases of the mouth

4. Orthodontists, who treat problems related to misaligned teeth
5. Periodontists, who diagnose and treat diseases of the gums and bone supporting the teeth
6. Prosthodontists, who create oral appliances and replace missing natural teeth with dentures, bridges, and implants
7. Public health dentists, who specialize in preventing and controlling dental diseases in the population
8. Pediatric dentists, who specialize in providing dental services for children with major health problems and chronic disabling conditions

Many dentists serve as members of the community health team for CSHCN.

DENTAL HYGIENIST

A dental hygienist is a graduate of a two–year associate degree or a four–year baccalaureate degree program in dental hygiene. A dental hygienist must have a state license to practice.

The majority of dental hygienists are employed by private dental offices, where they function as members of the dental office team. Many dental hygienists are employed by clinics, public health programs, school systems, and other institutions. In these settings dental hygienists function more independently than do those employed by private dental offices.

The dental services provided by dental hygienists are determined by the dental hygienists' training and the type of dental care provided by their employers. These services may include, but are not limited to, functioning as skilled assistants to dentists, performing scaling (cleaning) of teeth, conducting dental examinations to identify needed dental care and oral examinations to identify oral pathology, providing preventive dental service, and educating patients in matters of dental self–care techniques.

DIETICIAN

A dietician is a person who has been trained in the science of nutrition and its application to disease prevention and treatment. Dieticians integrate and apply the principles of nutrition, biochemistry, physiology, food management, and behavior to help their patients achieve and maintain health.

Dieticians must meet specified education requirements, including course work in physiology, biochemistry, and nutrition, and hold bachelor's, master's, or doctoral degrees from accredited universities. After receiving their degrees, dieticians acquire supervised practical experience by completing either an approved Preprofessional Practice Program or an accredited Dietetic Internship. They are then eligible to take the Registration Examination for Dieticians and to be credentialed as registered dieticians (RD).

Many registered dieticians work in health care delivery settings such as hospitals, clinics, and long-term care facilities. Some registered dieticians are employed in other settings such as school food services.

With the rapid advance of the science of nutrition and its correlation with health maintenance and disease prevention and treatment, the dietician has become a community team member in effective health care delivery. Dieticians assess patients' blood chemistry, anthropometric measurements, and medical and diet history to determine nutrition status. Then in coordination with other team members, dieticians develop, administer, and evaluate patients' responses to nutrition therapies.

Dieticians are a vital component of the community team for conditions and diseases that have a special nutritional component, such as cerebral palsy, obesity, diabetes, PKU, and gastrointestinal disorders.

DIETETIC TECHNICIAN

A dietetic technician has completed an approved two–year, associate degree program that combines classroom learning and supervised practical experience. Graduates are eligible to take the Registration Examination for Dietetic Technicians (DTR). Most dietetic technicians work in some type of health institution and are supervised by a regular dietician.

EARLY INTERVENTION SERVICE PROVIDER

An early intervention service provider is a professional trained to provide special early intervention services to infants and small children who are developmentally delayed or disabled.

At this time there is no nationally recognized single curriculum, certification, or licensure that defines this group of professionals. New university programs designed to address the growing need for individuals skilled in early intervention have been established to provide formal training at the baccalaureate, master's, and, in some cases, doctoral and post-doctoral levels. The variety of training provided by these programs is reflected in the titles of their graduates, e.g., childhood specialist, infant–toddler developmentalist, early childhood special educator, infant–parent educator, developmental pediatrician, developmental therapist, etc. Policy-makers, particularly those at the state level, are also being called upon to make critical decisions about licensure and certification criteria for this group of practitioners.

Currently, the need for providers who can serve infants and young children and their families is being met in part through the utilization of professionals who are trained to serve older children with special needs and who have expanded their knowledge base and skills to address problems of younger children. This expansion has been achieved through participation in continuing education programs conducted by national professional organizations, medical centers, and state community service programs.

Early intervention service providers typically work in either center– or community–based early intervention programs as members of interdisciplinary teams which can include physical and occupational therapists, speech and language professionals, psychologists, physicians, nurses and others.

FAMILY MEDICINE PHYSICIAN

A family medicine physician is a medical specialist who is concerned with the total health care of the individual and the family. Family medicine physicians' practices integrate the biologic, clinical, and behavioral sciences. The field of family practice, unlike the fields of other specialists, is not limited by age or sex of the patient, or by a single organ system or disease entity.

Family medicine physicians are graduates of an accredited medical school and have been granted the degree of Doctor of Medicine (MD). These physicians must satisfactorily complete a three–year family practice residency program accredited by the Accreditation Council for Graduate Medical Education.

Many family medicine physicians practice in small groups or in some type of panel practice and are accorded the same basic considerations in regard to hospital privileges as are given to diplomates of other specialty boards. Family physicians are trained to provide first contact care, continuous care, comprehensive care, personal care, family care, and are trained in scientific general medicine.

Family medicine physicians have the information and skills needed to provide the primary medical care required by children who have complex medical problems. Examples of care provided by family physicians to CSHCN are the treatment of urinary tract infections in children with spina bifida, the treatment of upper respiratory tract infections in children with cleft palate, and the monitoring of the responses of children with seizure disorders to anticonvulsant drugs. Because family physicians are community–based physicians, they provide medical care as part of family care in the child's community. Family medicine physicians may participate in the provision of a continuum of care by providing, with the concurrence of the child's medical specialist, those parts of specialized care that are best provided in the community.

GENETIC COUNSELOR

A genetic counselor is a health professional who has received the training necessary to provide counseling related to genetic disorders. Genetic counselors obtain and interpret genetic histories; participate in assessment of individuals and families; conduct nondirective discussion of the risks of recurrence of genetic problems, as well as discussion of options for management of disorders and of reproductive alternatives; and assist patients with identification of additional resources.

Health professionals from a variety of disciplines may be certified as genetic counselors. Most hold degrees in human genetics, genetic counseling, or nursing. Currently the criteria for certification are undergoing reevaluation.

Genetic counseling can be provided by a team of health professionals. The composition of the team will vary according to the region of the country and the nature of the service provided, but the team usually includes a physician who has completed a fellowship in an area of clinical genetics and a master's-level genetic counselor. Master's-level genetic counselors have undergone specialized multidisciplinary training which prepares them for counseling related to a wide variety of genetic disorders and birth defects.

In some areas of the country, especially those in which genetic counseling is offered as part of an outreach program, genetic counselors are registered nurses who are genetic specialists. The majority of nurse genetic specialists are graduates of master's–level nursing programs; some have bachelor's degrees and advanced training in genetic health care and genetic counseling.

NURSE

A nurse is a health professional who can be involved with a broad range of health care provision, wellness, and health promotion. Nurses also coordinate health services that assist people to be healthy and achieve their optimal development.

The nursing profession is in a period of transition related to its training programs and levels of practices. Many registered nurses (RNs) continue to be trained in hospital–based or associate degree nurse training programs. At the university level, there are three recognized levels of nursing degrees: the Bachelor of Science in Nursing (BSN), the Master of Arts or Science in Nursing (MA or MSN), and the Doctor of Philosophy in Nursing (PhD).

Nurses with a BSN are primary health care providers who have received undergraduate training emphasizing the nursing process, nursing knowledge, nursing skills, communication, and leadership. On the basis of this training, nurses with a BSN can function in the following ways:

1. In hospitals as primary health providers
2. In clinics as members of teams that provide ambulatory care
3. In health programs as members of teams that provide community–based health care for children with special health care needs
4. In programs that provide home care, where nurses often provide primary care and organize and facilitate the delivery of coordinated services.

The current trend in health care delivery is toward emphasizing nursing as a service provided both inside and outside hospitals.

Nurses with master's degrees can specialize in child health nursing, adult health nursing, gerontological nursing, or community/family health nursing. In addition to providing primary health services, these nurses coordinate health care by organizing and facilitating the delivery of comprehensive, efficient, and appropriate services to individuals, families, groups, and communities. MA nurses also analyze, synthesize, and apply knowledge from the humanities, the physical and social sciences, and nursing theory. In coordinating health care, MA nurses assess patient needs, formulate nursing diagnoses, plan and implement therapeutic actions, evaluate the effectiveness of those actions, and conceptualize the total health needs of the patient, including legal and ethical aspects of care.

Nurses may also obtain additional training to become nurse practitioners. Pediatric Nurse Practitioners (PNPs) are child health nurse specialists. PNPs are a major health service provider in many child health clinics and programs. PNPs are often active participants in the community-based health team that is designed to provide contemporary services for CSHCN. These services may include, but are not limited to, performing physical assessments, developing nursing diagnoses and making recommendations for care, providing follow-up health services, monitoring the status and care provided to technology–dependent children who are receiving their care at home, and serving as community–based case managers for children with special health care needs.

PhD nurses are involved primarily with nursing administration and with nursing education.

A great deal of hospital nursing care continues to be provided by licensed practical nurses (LPNs) and licensed vocational nurses (LVNs), who receive their training in programs located in a number of sites including community colleges, as well as by nurses aides, who most often receive their instruction in a hospital–based program.

OCCUPATIONAL THERAPIST

An occupational therapist is a health and rehabilitation professional who provides services to patients of all ages who need, because of physical, developmental, emotional, or social deficits, specialized assistance in learning skills to enable them to lead independent, productive, and satisfying lives.

Registered occupational therapists (OTR) or certified occupational therapy assistants (COTA) must be graduates of an educational program that includes the study of human growth and development, with specific emphasis on the physiologic, emotional and social implications of illness and injury. The program must be accredited jointly by the American Medical Association and the American Occupational Therapy Association. In addition, OTRs or COTAs must have completed supervised fieldwork and passed a national certification exam. Registered occupational therapists hold a master's degree. Certified occupational therapist assistants (COTA) hold an associate degree.

Occupational therapists are trained to provide services for children who exhibit problems such as developmental delay; muscular dystrophy; developmental disabilities, including mental retardation, spinal bifida, and cerebral palsy; sensory integrative dysfunction; juvenile rheumatoid arthritis and related disorders; learning disabilities, including dyslexia, delayed motor development and dyspraxia; and orthopedic disabilities, traumatic injuries, burns, and amputations.

The goal of occupational therapy for infants and children is to assist them to the degree possible to achieve age–appropriate self–help, as well as play and leisure skills. More specifically, occupational therapists provide the following services:

1. Positioning
2. Neuromotor facilitation
3. Strengthening activities
4. Sensory stimulation/desensitization
5. Handling techniques during feeding
6. Food selection—in consultation with a nutritionist or physician
7. Self–feeding guidance
8. Changes in environmental stimulation

Occupational therapy services may be provided in a variety of settings, including the home, hospitals, clinics, public schools, early intervention programs, Head Start centers, university-affiliated programs, home health agencies, developmental day care facilities, rehabilitation centers, and private practices.

OSTEOPATHIC PHYSICIAN

An osteopathic physician is a physician who practices osteopathic medicine, which emphasizes the interrelationship of the body's structure and systems. The osteopathic philosophy of treating the whole person is applied to the prevention, diagnosis, and treatment of illness, disease, and injury.

Osteopathic physicians have completed a four–year period of medical study and clinical training in an accredited college of osteopathy and have received the degree of Doctor of Osteopathy (DO). Graduates of osteopathic medical schools complete at least a one–year rotating hospital internship, and may complete an additional two to six years of residency training in a medical specialty such as cardiology, surgery, pediatrics, or orthopedic surgery as required to be a certified medical specialist. Osteopathic physicians are licensed to practice medicine by the state in which they practice.

The majority of osteopathic physicians are primary care physicians who provide comprehensive care for the individual and family. Many osteopathic physicians practice in small group or panel practices, and many practice in relatively small communities. In their practice, osteopathic physicians use all diagnostic and therapeutic techniques, including drugs and surgery, to prevent and treat illnesses.

PEDIATRICIAN

A pediatrician is a medical specialist primarily concerned with the physical, emotional, and social health of children from birth to young adulthood. Pediatric care encompasses a broad spectrum of health services, ranging from preventive health care to the diagnosis and treatment of acute and chronic diseases. A pediatrician participates at the community level in preventing or solving problems in child health care and publicly advocates the causes of children.

Pediatricians have received a degree of Doctor of Medicine (MD) or Doctor of Osteopathy (DO) from an accredited medical school. Pediatricians have completed three years of accredited post-graduate hospital training in an accredited residency training program and have taken the National Board examination to become board-certified pediatricians. They are licensed to practice as physicians in the state where they practice.

Pediatricians may take additional fellowship training after their residency training in one of many specialties including adolescent medicine, pediatric cardiology, pediatric critical care medicine, pediatric emergency medicine, pediatric endocrinology, pediatric gastroenterology, pediatric hematology–oncology, pediatric infectious disease, neonatal–perinatal medicine, pediatric nephrology, pediatric pulmonology, pediatric rheumatology, pediatric rehabilitation, pediatric neurology, and developmental medicine. After completing this additional training, pediatricians may take a Specialty Board examination to become certified subspecialists in the field.

Pediatricians often elect to have a special interest practice that does not involve certification. The community-based care of many children with special health needs is provided by pediatricians with a special interest in children with disabilities.

Pediatricians have the ability, as it pertains to infants, children, and adolescents, to:

1. Assess and formulate a management plan for any medical or health maintenance problem.
2. Execute the management plan with patients and families, without further medical consultation, for all common problems of disease and health maintenance and for all medically life–threatening situations.
3. Consult, when appropriate, with physicians and other professionals regarding common problems and life–threatening situations .
4. Arrange for patients to receive additional consultation, know what to anticipate from the consultant, and personally guide further management with assistance, when appropriate, for unusual problems requiring subspecialty, surgical, or other specialized skills.

Most primary care pediatricians practice in group practices or in some type of panel practice. Many pediatric subspecialists practice in medical centers, where they provide tertiary level care and/or conduct biomedical research. An increasing number of primary care pediatricians who provide care for children with complex chronic health problems participate as members of a community health care team that coordinates services for their patients and their patients' families. Many are also involved with cooperative arrangements with medical center-based pediatric subspecialists to assure that their patients have access to a continuum of medical care. Some pediatricians serve as public health physicians in public health programs that provide health services for children with new morbidity problems.

PHYSICAL THERAPIST

A physical therapist is a professional member of the health team who is concerned with prevention, evaluation, and treatment of physical disabilities resulting from injury, illness, developmental processes, or the aging process.

Until recently, many physical therapists were trained in baccalaureate–degree or post baccalaureate–degree programs. Many of these programs, however, are now changing to master's degree programs. All programs include requirements in basic health sciences and clinical sciences, as well as opportunities to apply theory in supervised clinical practice. Upon graduation, a licensing examination is given. All physical therapists must comply with the licensing requirements of the state in which they practice.

Physical therapists practice in a variety of settings, including hospitals, clinics, schools, nursing homes, community health centers, home health agencies, rehabilitation centers, sports medicine centers, government agencies, and industries, and some physical therapists are in private practice. In most settings physical therapists function as an important member of the community care team of a child with special health needs.

Physical therapists use a variety of techniques to evaluate patients for evidence of disabilities, to correct disabilities, or to help patients adapt to them. Evaluation techniques include muscle testing, gait and postural evaluations, and functional activities assessments. Physical therapists use both manual techniques and physical agents to relieve pain; the latter include heat, cold, ultraviolet and infrared rays, functional electrical stimulation, and water (whirlpools and therapeutic swimming pools). Physical therapists also prescribe assistive devices and offer psychologic support to patients and their families during the process of overcoming or coping with a disability and regaining mobility.

Examples of patients treated by physical therapists include newborn babies with birth defects; children with muscular dystrophy or cerebral palsy; stroke and heart attack victims; the injured; amputees; paraplegics; people with impaired lung or heart capacity; and those in pain from arthritis, nerve injuries, bone fractures, and burns.

The American Board of Physical Therapy Specialties recognizes seven specialty areas: cardiopulmonary, clinical electrophysiologic, neurologic, pediatric, sports, orthopedics, and geriatrics. Those physical therapists who specialize in pediatric physical therapy (for CSHCN) are commonly involved with conducting developmental evaluations to identify normal and abnormal reflexes and to verify normal and abnormal development.

PHYSICAL THERAPIST ASSISTANT

Physical therapist assistants work under the supervision of a physical therapist. Their duties include assisting the physical therapist in implementing treatment programs according to the plan of care, training patients in exercises and activities of daily living, conducting treatments using special equipment, administering modalities and other treatment procedures, and reporting to the physical therapist on the patient's response.

Physical therapist assistants must complete a two–year education program, usually offered in a community or junior college. Graduates receive an associate degree. Licensure, registration, or certification is not required in all states for the physical therapist assistant to practice. States that require licensure stipulate specific educational and examination criteria.

PSYCHOLOGIST

A psychologist is a professional who, based on his or her training, is licensed or certified to provide psychologic services. These services are generally divided into three types: psychologic counseling services, school psychologic services, and industrial/organizational psychologic services.

A psychologist holds a BA or an MA degree from an approved department of psychology from an accredited college or university. Some psychologists complete an additional period of study in a clinical psychologic program accredited by the American Psychological Association and receive a doctoral degree in clinical psychology.

Professional psychology in general and school psychology in particular have had a long and difficult history of attempting to establish criteria for guidelines for the delivery of services. In the field of school psychology, there are wide variations in requirements among the many states.

A list of different psychologic services include the following:

1. Counseling psychologic services, including assessment and intervention, are provided by clinical psychologists for the purpose of understanding, predicting, and alleviating intellectual, emotional, psychologic, and behavior disability and discomfort
2. Assessment services are directed toward diagnosing the nature and causes, and predicting the effects of personal, social, and work dysfunction; and of the psychologic and emotional factors involved in, and consequent to, physical disease and disability
3. Intervention services are directed at identifying and correcting the emotional conflicts, personality disturbances, and skill deficits underlying a person's distress and/or dysfunction. These services are intended to help people acquire or alter personal and social skills, improve their adaptability to changing life demands, enhance their environmental coping skills, and develop a variety of problem-solving and decision-making capabilities
4. School psychologic services are provided by psychologists with a master's degree, as well as psychologists with a doctorate degree; at the present time, however, the great majority of psychologists employed by public school systems have master's degrees

The evaluation and assessment services for children and youth conducted by psychologists with an MA include screening, psychologic and educational testing of intellectual functioning, cognitive development, and behavior evaluation. In addition, clinical psychologists evaluate and assess affective behavior and neurophysiologic status.

The interventions for children and youth used by MA psychologists include procedures to facilitate their functioning in school. Intervention may include recommending, planning and evaluating special educational services. Clinical psychologists also may provide psychoeducational therapy and counseling affective educational programs.

Consultation and collaboration with school personnel and parents concerning specific school–related problems of students and the professional problems of staff may include activities to provide assistance in planning educational programs from a psychologic perspective, as well as consultation with teachers and other school personnel to enhance their understanding of the needs of particular pupils.

Psychologists are important members of the community team of professionals that provides services for children with special health care needs. As members of early intervention programs, psychologists may evaluate infants and small children for evidence of intellectual and developmental delay. As employees of or consultants to the public school system, psychologists may test preschool and school-age children to determine their ability to learn, identify the type and cause of children's behavior disorders and counsel teachers and parents on how to appropriately respond. As members of community teams, psychologists may evaluate children's skills and behavior as they relate to illness or disability and recommend or provide needed psychologic services.

RECREATION THERAPIST

A recreation therapist provides therapeutic recreation services to facilitate the development, maintenance, and expression of an appropriate leisure style for individuals with limitations.

Therapeutic recreation specialists have a baccalaureate degree or higher from an accredited college or university, with a major in therapeutic recreation or a major in recreation and an option in therapeutic recreation. Therapeutic recreation assistants have an associate of arts degree from an accredited educational institution, with either a major in therapeutic recreation or a major in recreation and an option in therapeutic recreation.

The therapeutic effect of recreation therapy is accomplished through providing programs and services that assist patients in eliminating barriers to leisure; developing leisure skills and attitudes; and optimizing leisure involvement.

There are three specific areas of therapeutic recreation services: therapy, leisure education, and recreation participation. These three service areas represent a continuum of care. Decisions about where and when each of the three service areas is provided are based on an assessment of patient needs and the service mandate of the sponsoring agency.

Therapeutic recreation services are provided in a variety of settings. The majority of patients in residential, treatment, and community settings need leisure education services in order to initiate and engage in leisure experiences. In settings where a comprehensive treatment approach is used, however, therapy focuses on team-identified treatment goals, as well as on addressing unique aspects of leisure-related functional behaviors.

SOCIAL WORKER

A social worker is a trained professional who promotes, restores, maintains, or enhances the functioning of individuals, families, households, social groups, organizations, and communities by helping them to prevent distress and to utilize resources. These resources may be found in people's intrapersonal or interpersonal capacities or abilities and in social services institutions.

Social work education takes place in four–year undergraduate and two–year graduate programs and leads to professional degrees at the baccalaureate and master's levels, respectively. The purpose of undergraduate social work education is to prepare students for beginning professional level of practice. Social workers with a BA degree usually work under the direction of a MSW.

Social work education at the master's level is directed toward preparing the students in one or more of the following fields of service: population groups, problem areas, professional roles, interventive modes, and advanced generalist practice. MSW–trained social workers may provide direct patient services, may supervise BA–trained social workers, and may be involved with administrative responsibilities.

Social work as an organized profession is practiced in a wide variety of settings, including major institutions of society such as public social service agencies, hospitals, school systems, and justice systems.

Social workers employed by public or private organizations that provide services for CSCN and their families may assist families by informing them about eligibility requirements, methods of applying for, and the locations of, available health services; they also may assist families in making appointments for these services. In addition, social workers provide families with information about public programs such as Early Periodic Screening Diagnosis Treatment (EPSDT) and Supplemental Security Income (SSI), which pay for medical care, as well as help families obtain services such as respite care and day care. Although social workers often provide families with appropriate counsel, their goal is to assist families to be independent.

SPECIAL EDUCATION TEACHER

A special education teacher is an educator who is primarily responsible for children who have been identified as disabled and in need of a specially designed educational program.

Special education teachers must, at a minimum, complete an undergraduate degree that provides training in the field of special education. A few states require a master's degree before a special education certificate or license will be issued. Each state's Department of Education sets certification or licensure requirements for special education teachers, and these requirements vary depending upon the type of special education certificate or license issued. Teacher training programs at colleges and universities must adhere to their respective state requirements so graduates can qualify for special education certificates or licenses.

Special education teachers are trained to provide the following services:

1. Assessing students placed to identify their strengths and weaknesses that may need to be addressed
2. Working with students, parents, and other professionals to develop Individual Education Programs (IEPs) that describe the students' specially designed educational programs
3. Working with regular classroom teachers to integrate special education students in programs and activities with non-disabled students
4. Monitoring student progress to determine the effectiveness of the special education programs as described in student IEPs

5. Keeping parents and other involved professionals informed concerning the progress of special education students
6. Participating in community–based inter-, multi- and trans-disciplinary service teams that may be composed of various service providers from the fields of health, welfare, mental health, to develop coordinated community plans of services for students who are experiencing difficulties while in school

SPEECH AND LANGUAGE PATHOLOGIST

A speech and language pathologist is a professional who has been trained to provide independent clinical services to people with communication (speech and language) disorders.

Speech and language clinicians must have completed a college undergraduate education that provides a broad educational foundation. Upon graduation, prospective speech and language clinicians receive a BA or BS degree and may then enroll in a master's degree program in speech and language pathology. Master's programs in speech and language pathology typically include the following content:

1. Understanding of speech and language disorders, including the various types of communication disorders, their manifestations, and their classifications and causes
2. Evaluation skills such as procedures, techniques, and instrumentation used to assess not only the speech and language status of children and adults but also the bases of disorders of speech and language
3. Management procedures, such as principles of remedial methods used in habilitation and rehabilitation for children and adults with various disorders of communication

Following completion of masters–level training, trainees must complete one year of clinical fellowship. (Those who have an interest in pediatric speech and language pathology take their clinical training in approved pediatric training centers.) After completing a clinical fellowship, professionals are eligible to take the National Examination to be certified as speech and language pathologists.

Some speech and language pathologists practice in speech and language and hearing centers, clinics, hospitals, or they have private practices. These speech and language pathologists function as important members of community–based teams for CSHCN. Most speech and language pathologists, however, are employed by public special education programs, where they serve as designated members of the required special education team which creates Individual Education Plans, and where they evaluate the speech and language skills of, and provide speech and language therapy for, children referred by classroom teachers.

SPEECH AND LANGUAGE AIDE

Speech and language aides are not required to have professional training in the field. These aides work under the supervision of speech and language pathologists to carry out a program of speech instruction designed by a speech and language pathologist. Most speech and language aides work in special education classrooms for the language impaired.

Index